Potential Carcinogenic Hazards from Drugs

UICC Monograph Series · Volume 7

Potential Carcinogenic Hazards from Drugs

Evaluation of Risks

Edited by

René Truhaut

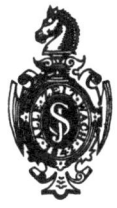

Springer-Verlag Berlin Heidelberg New York 1967

René Truhaut, Professeur, Chaire de Toxicologie,
Université de Paris, Faculté de Pharmacie, Paris, France. Chef de l'Unité de
Chimiotherapie expérimentale à l'Institut Gustave Roussy, Villejuif, Seine, France

ISBN-13: 978-3-642-87900-5   e-ISBN-13: 978-3-642-87898-5
DOI: 10.1007/ 978-3-642-87898-5

Title-No. 7518

Contents

Contents

Participants

Dr. S. B. DE C. BAKER, Biological Research Department, Imperial Chemical Industries Ltd., Alderley-Park, Macclesfield, Cheshire, Great Britain

Professor I. BERENBLUM, Chairman, U.I.C.C. Expert Panel on Carcinogenicity, The Weizmann Institute of Science, Department of Experimental Biology, Rehovoth, Israel

Professor E. BOYLAND, Chester Beatty Research Institute, Fulham Road, London S.W. 3, Great Britain

Professeur P. CHASSAGNE, Faculté de Médecine de Paris; adresse privée: 135, avenue Emile Zola, Paris 15ème, France

Professeur J. CHEYMOL, Chaire de Pharmacologie, Faculté de Médecine, 21, rue de l'Ecole de Médecine, Paris VIème, France

Dr. D. G. DAVEY, Chairman of The European Society for the Study of Drug Toxicity, Imperial Chemical Industries Ltd., Alderley Park, Macclesfield, Cheshire, Great Britain

Dr. G. DELLA PORTA, Istituto Nazionale per lo Studio e la Cura dei Tumori, Piazzale Gorini, 22, Milano, Italia

Dr. L. DE SOUZA, Crescent House, Ballard Estate, Bombay I, India

Professor F. DICKENS, Courtauld Institute of Biochemistry, The Middlesex Hospital Medical School, London W. I, Great Britain

Professor R. DOLL, Director, Medical Research Council's Statistical Research Unit, University College Hospital, Medical School, 115, Gower Street, London W. C. I, Great Britain

Professor H. DRUCKREY, Leiter der Forschergruppe Präventivmedizin, Stefan-Meier-Straße 8, (78) Freiburg i. Br., Bundesrepublik Deutschland

Professor A. C. FRAZER, Head, Department of Medical Biochemistry and Pharmacology, The High Medical School, University of Birmingham, Birmingham, Great Britain

Dr. J. HIGGINSON, Chairman, U.I.C.C. Committee on Geographical Pathology, University of Kansas Medical Center, Rainbow Boulevard at 39th Street, Kansas City, Kansas, 66103 U.S.A.

Doctor W. HUEPER, Chief, Environmental Cancer Section, National Cancer Institute, Bethesda 14, Maryland, U.S.A.

Dr. J. JUHÁSZ, Department of Pathological Anatomy, Experimental Cancer Research, Medical University, Ulloi-ut 26, Budapest VIII, Hungary

Professor L. KREYBERG, Institutt for Generell og Eksperimentell Patologi, Universitetet i Oslo, Rikshospitalet, Oslo, Norway

Professeur A. LACASSAGNE, Membre de l'Académie des Sciences, Laboratoire de Recherches de l'Institut du Radium de l'Université de Paris, 26, rue d'Ulm, Paris 5ème, France

Dr. A. LEHMAN, President, Research Division, Bureau of Biological and Physical Sciences, Department of Health, Education, and Welfare, Food and Drug Administration, Washington 25 D.C., U.S.A.

Professor P. MARQUARDT, Universität Freiburg i. Br., Hugstetter Straße 55, (78) Freiburg i. Br., Bundesrepublik Deutschland

Professor J. A. MILLER, Mc. Ardle Memorial Laboratory for Cancer Research, Medical School, University of Wisconsin, Madison, Wisconsin, U.S.A.

Dr. N. P. NAPALKOV, Vice-Director for Research, N.N. Petrov's Research Institute of Oncology, 68, Leningradskaya St., Pos. Pesochny-2, Leningrad, U.R.S.S

Madame le Docteur N. C. PARMENTIER, Département de la Protection Sanitaire, Commissariat à l'Energie Atomique, Fontenay-aux-Roses, Seine, France

Professor W. E. POEL, Director, Laboratory for Experimental Carcinogenesis, University of Pittsburgh, Graduate School of Public Health, Department of Occupational Health, Pittsburgh, Pennsylvania 15213, U.S.A.

Dr. F. J. C. ROE, Department of Experimental Pathology, Chester Beatty Research Institute, Institute of Cancer Research, Fulham Road, London S.W. 3, Great Britain

Dr. G. RUDALI, Chef du Laboratoire de Génétique, Institut du Radium, 26, rue d'Ulm, Paris Vème, France

Professor U. SAFFIOTTI, The Chicago Medical School, Institute for Medical Research, Division of Oncology, 2020, West Ogden Avenue, Chicago 12, Illinois, U.S.A.

Miss R. SCHOENTAL, Medical Research Council Laboratories, Toxicology Research Unit, Woodmansterne road, Carshalton, Surrey, Great Britain

Professeur L. M. SHABAD, Président du Comité de Prévention du Cancer de l'U.I.C.C., Institut d'Oncologie Expérimentale et Clinique, Académie des Sciences Médicales, Kashirskoye chaussee, 6, Moscou B-409, U.R.S.S

Professor P. SHUBIK, The Chicago Medical School, Institute for Medical Research, Division of Oncology, 2020, West Ogden Avenue, Chicago 60612, Illinois, U.S.A.

Dr. R. M. TAYLOR, Chairman of U.I.C.C. Cancer Control Commission, National Cancer Institute of Canada, 790, Bay Street, Toronto 2, Ontario, Canada

Professeur R. TRUHAUT, Directeur du Centre de Recherches Toxicologiques de la Faculté de Pharmacie de l'Université de Paris, 4, avenue de l'Observatoire, Paris, VIème, France. Chef de Service à l'Institut Gustave Roussy, 16 bis, Avenue Paul Vaillant Couturier, Villejuif, Seine, France.

Professeur M. TUBIANA, Chef du Laboratoire des Isotopes, Institut Gustave Roussy, 16 bis, Avenue Paul-Vaillant Couturier, Villejuif, Seine, France

Professeur G. VALETTE, Doyen de la Faculté de Pharmacie de l'Université de Paris, 4, avenue de l'Observatoire, Paris, VIème, France

Dr. G. J. VAN ESCH, Head, Laboratory of Toxicology, Ryles Institut von de volles Gezondheid, Sterrebos I, Utrecht, Holland

Monsieur C. AGTHE, Scientist Food Additives, Nutrition Division, O.M.S., Avenue Appia, 1211, Genève, Suisse

Dr. H. HALBACH, Chief, Division of Pharmacology and Toxicology, O.M.S., Avenue Appia, 1211, Genève, Suisse

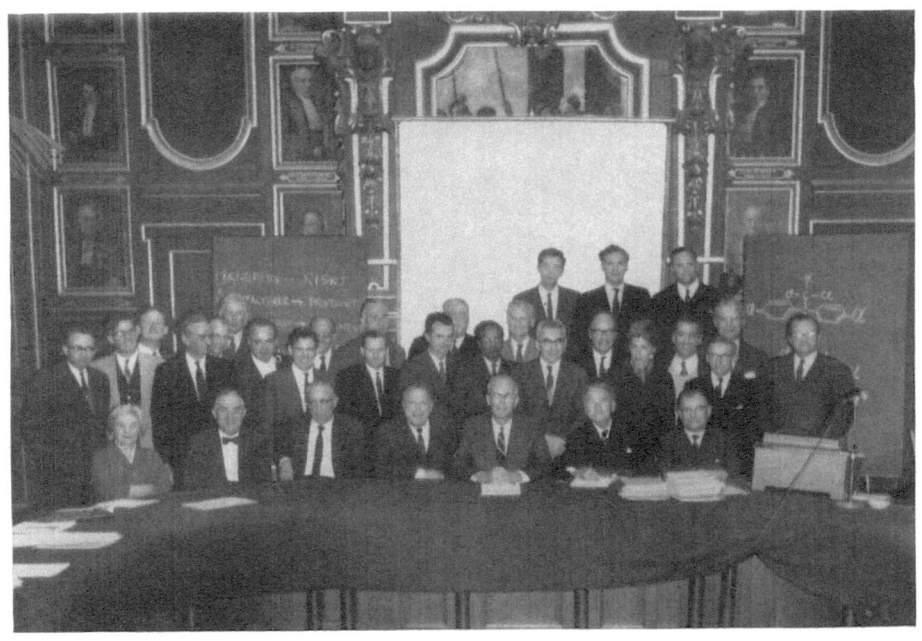

Les participants au Symposium dans la Salle des Actes de la Faculté de Pharmacie
de l'Université de Paris

Opening remarks

R. M. TAYLOR, M.D.

National Cancer Institute of Canada, Toronto 2, Ontario, Canada
Chairman of the UICC Cancer Control Commission

On behalf of the Commission on Cancer Control. I would like to welcome the distinguished scientists who have gathered here to discuss a most important subject. Since I am charged with responsibility for promoting the Union's activities in the field of cancer control, it will not be surprising to you if I say I believe that there is more to be gained from the application of current knowledge and techniques to the prevention of cancer than from any new method of treatment on the horizon or under development in the research laboratory.

We are surrounded by a bewildering array of new chemical compounds and exposed to a host of new drugs whose potential for causing cancer is largely unknown. Your deliberations will contribute to the lifting of this veil of ignorance and it will be a privilige for me to attend your sessions.

I would like to congratulate Professors L. SHABAD, R. TRUHAUT and N. P. NAPALKOV for their efforts in organizing the Symposium and to express the hope that your discussions will be useful and stimulating.

Opening remarks

Professeur L. M. SHABAD

Institut d'Oncologie expérimentale et clinique, Académie des Sciences Médicales, Moscou, U.R.S.S.

Président du Comité de Prévention de la Commission de Lutte Contre le Cancer de l'Union Internationale Contre le Cancer

Mesdames, messieurs, au nom du Comité de Prévention du Cancer, j'ai le plaisir et l'honneur de vous souhaiter la bienvenue à notre Symposium. J'exprime le sentiment de notre profonde gratitude à l'organisateur, mon cher ami le Professur TRUHAUT, au Président de la Commission du Contrôle du Cancer sous l'égide duquel travaille notre Comité, au Professeur TAYLOR, au Directeur de notre Centre à Genève le Docteur DELAFRESNAYE, et à tous nos chers Collègues qui ont consenti à participer aux travaux de ce Symposium.

La notion des agents cancérigènes est née de nos premières connaissances sur les tumeurs professionnelles de l'homme et s'est développée dans l'expérimentation animale. L'étude des agents cancérigènes chimiques nous a apporté beaucoup de faits concernant leur répartition dans l'environnement de l'homme. Maintenant ce ne sont pas des faits uniques et isolés comme les cancers professionnels, mais l'influence sur toute la population de tels facteurs comme les pollutions de l'air, de l'eau, des produits alimentaires. Les produits chimiques envahissent pour ainsi dire chaque jour de nouveaux domaines de notre vie non seulement dans l'Industrie mais aussi dans l'Agriculture, dans l'Urbanisation, dans les produits cosmétiques, dans la médicamentation.

Ce dernier problème attire aujourd'hui notre attention spéciale. On peut dire qu'il est encore plus délicat que celui des produits alimentaires. Ce problème est beaucoup moins étudié. Les médicaments, maintes fois et chez certains malades, sont utilisés pendant un temps prolongé, c'est une vraie application chronique, et il faut faire attention à la possibilité d'une cumulation. Dans certains cas les médicaments suspects (dans le sens de la possibilité d'une action cancérigène) sont administrés à des malades ayant déjà des lésions précancéreuses et on pourrait obtenir une accélération de leur développement. C'est surtout dans le traitement des femmes gravides et des enfants qu'il faut se méfier des médicaments qui pourraient avoir une influence cancérigène sur l'organisme du foetus, du nouveau né et de l'enfant qui est particulièrement susceptible aux agents cancérigènes, comme on l'a démontré récemment.

Dans notre Laboratoire nous avons observé par exemple des adénomes pulmonaires déjà après 4, 6 et 8 jours dans les cultures de poumons explantés du foetus de la souris qui a été traitée pendant la gravidité par l'uréthane.

Enfin un tout autre problème, c'est le traitement des malades cancéreux par des médicaments cancérigènes, comme par les rayons X.

Tous ces nouveaux problèmes doivent être étudiés sérieusement pour obtenir de nouveaux faits, élucider et coordonner les idées modernes et ouvrir de nouvelles voies pour le traitement et surtout la prévention des cancers humains, ce qui est notre tâche directe.

C'est au développement de la prévention qu'est consacré notre Symposium et nous commençons par donner la parole à Monsieur le Professeur R. Truhaut que je propose comme Président de notre Symposium.

Presentation de l'Ordre du Jour Avec Commentaires

Professeur RENÉ TRUHAUT

Président du Symposium

Mesdames, Messieurs, mes chers Collègues,

Je voudrais tout d'abord exprimer, au nom de Monsieur le Ministre de la Santé Publique et de la Population et de Monsieur le Directeur Général des Relations culturelles du Ministère des Affaires étrangères, au nom de mes collègues français et en mon nom personnel, de chaleureux souhaits de bienvenue à nos hôtes étrangers et leur dire quel honneur représente pour nous le choix de Paris pour la tenue de ce Symposium. En tant que membre du corps enseignant de la Faculté de Pharmacie de Paris, permettez moi d'ajouter que mes collègues et moi éprouvons une très grande fierté à accueillir les experts éminents que vous êtes. Il m'est agréable, à cet instant, d'exprimer à notre Doyen, mon ami le Professeur GUILLAUME VALETTE, mes sentiments de profonde gratitude pour avoir mis à la disposition de l'Union Internationale contre le Cancer notre Salle des Actes dont les murs sont ornés des portraits des pharmaciens les plus célèbres du passé, dont la contribution aux progrès des sciences, et notamment de la Chimie et de la Thérapeutique, fut si précieuse.

Je me dois aussi de saluer, de façon particulière, les représentants de l'Organisation Mondiale de la Santé, Le Docteur HALBACH, Chef de la Division de Pharmacologie et de Toxicologie, et le Docteur AGTHE, de la Division de Nutrition, que Monsieur le Directeur Général de cette organisation a bien voulu délégué pour le représenter à ce Symposium. J'y vois une nouvelle matérialisation de la liaison étroite et cordiale qui n'a cessé d'exister entre l'OMS et l'UICC.

Je tiens à saluer aussi Monsieur le Docteur DAVEY, Président de l'Association Européenne pour l'étude de la Toxicité des Médicaments.

Enfin, je voudrais vous transmettre les voeux de plein succès que je viens de recevoir

de Monsieur le Professeur A. HADDOW, Président de l'Union Internationale Contre le Cancer (U.I.C.C),

de Monsieur le Professeur O. MUHLBOCK, Président de la Commission de recherche de l'UICC,

de Monsieur le Docteur MURRAY SHEAR, Secrétaire Général de l'UICC,

de Monsieur le Docteur P. LOUSTALOT, Trésorier de l'UICC,

et de Monsieur le Docteur J. F. DELAFRESNAYE, Directeur de l'Office de Genève,

qui, par suite de l'obligation qui s'impose à eux de participer à une réunion du bureau de l'UICC à Genève, n'ont pas la possibilité, à leur grand regret et au nôtre, de participer à nos travaux.

Il en est de même, pour d'autres raisons, du Professeur LOWELL T. COG-

GESHALL, Vice-Président de l'Université de Chicago, Président de la Commission «on Drug Safety» de la "Society of Toxicology", qui, jusqu'au dernier moment, espérait pouvoir être des nôtres.

Je voudrais vous dire ma confusion devant le grand honneur que vous venez de me faire en suivant la proposition de mon très cher ami LÉON SHABAD de me confier la présidence de ce Symposium. Connaissant mes faibles mérites, j'y vois surtout, de votre part, une manifestation de courtoisie, à laquelle je suis très sensible; j'essaierai, de toutes mes forces, de ne pas vous décevoir.

Je me dois de rappeler les étapes successives de l'organisation de ce Symposium. Aussitôt après son élection à la présidence du Comité de prévention, lors du 8ème Congrès international du cancer tenu à Moscou en Juillet 1962, le Professeur LÉON SHABAD, avec son habituel dynamisme, se mit à la besogne et décida d'organiser à Genève, à la fin de Novembre 1963, une réunion de ce Comité consacrée principalement à l'étude des risques de cancérisation liés à la consommation des drogues. Les rapports présentés et les discussions auxquelles ils donnèrent lieu amenèrent les participants à émettre unanimement le voeu que soit organisé, sous l'égide de l'Union Internationale contre le cancer, un Symposium spécifiquement consacré à l'étude plus approfondie du même problème, dont l'importance avait été soulignée dans le rapport du premier Comité d'experts de l'Organisation Mondiale de la Santé pour la prévention du cancer (Genève 19—25 Novembre 1963 — Série des Rapports Techniques de l'OMS n°276). Ce vœu, transmis au Comité Exécutif de l'UICC, reçut l'approbation de ce dernier à Mexico en Février 1964, grâce au soutien du Docteur TAYLOR, Président de la Commission de lutte contre le cancer, et le choix de Paris,

suggéré par les membres du Comité de prévention comme lieu de réunion, fut confirmé.

Avec mes collègues, le Professeur SHABAD et le Docteur NAPALKOV, nous nous sommes mis alors à l'oeuvre pour élaborer le programme.

Il nous a semblé qu'il convenait d'inviter, à côté d'experts dans le domaine spécifique de la cancérogénèse, des spécialistes de la pharmacologie et de la thérapeutique, de manière à élargir nos débats et, en bénéficiant de l'exposé de leurs points de vue, à éviter des prises de position trop rigides.

C'est dans cet esprit que nous avons conçu le programme que nous vous avons soumis pour recueillir vos suggestions et que vous avez bien voulu approuver. La version définitive vous a été remise au début de cette première session. Comme vous pouvez le constater, nous avons prévu la présentation de rapports concernant les problèmes généraux relatifs aux méthodes d'essais et d'évaluation, qualitative et quantitative, de la potentialité cancérogène, ainsi qu'aux aspects biochimiques de la cancérogénèse.

Il s'imposait, également, de prévoir des rapports consacrés à l'étude de groupes particuliers de drogues, au sein desquels avaient été signalées des potentialités cancérogènes. Il nous a semblé qu'il convenait d'examiner, non seulement des drogues proprement dites, mais encore les traceurs utilisés dans un but de diagnostic et les matériaux plastiques utilisés en chirurgie. Nous entendrons, également, exposés respectivement par le Professeur FRAZER et par le Professeur CHASSAGNE, les points de vue du pharmacologue et du clinicien devant la révélation de la potentialité cancérogène de ces divers composés ou matériaux.

Nous aurons finalement une discussion générale qui sera ouverte par le

Professeur Lacassagne qui a bien voulu nous faire bénéficier de sa grande expérience en présentant ses commentaires.

J'espère qu'il nous sera possible, à la lumière des exposés présentés et des discussions qui leur feront suite, d'arriver à des résolutions susceptibles de contribuer à la prévention du cancer.

Dans le but de permettre de larges échanges de vues sur les faits présentés par les rapporteurs et de l'interprétation à leur donner, nous avons prévu de consacrer une partie importante du programme aux discussions qui sont souvent plus fécondes que la présentation d'exposés toujours quelque peu académiques. C'est la raison pour laquelle nous vous avons imposé d'envoyer suffisamment à l'avance vos rapports. J'ai pu ainsi, personnellement, les faire reproduire et les adresser à chacun d'entre vous. Vous avez donc pu vous préparer à intervenir dans les discussions. Je demande aux différents rapporteurs de se borner, en conséquence, à une présentation synthétique des informations contenues dans leur rapport.

Avant de conclure cette brève introduction à nos travaux, permettez-moi d'exprimer à mes collaborateurs, parmi lesquels, ne pouvant les mentionner tous, je tiens à citer les noms du Docteur Jouany et de Madame Pringuet, mes sentiments de gratitude pour l'aide qu'ils m'ont apportée pour l'organisation du Symposium.

Considerations Générales sur les Risques de Cancérisation Pouvant Resulter de l'Emploi de Certains Agents Chimiques en Thérapeutique

R. Truhaut

Professeur de Toxicologie à la Faculté de Pharmacie de Paris, Chef de l'Unité de Chimiothérapie Expérimentale à l'Institut Gustave Roussy, Villejuif, France

Le caractère subtil de la distinction entre médicaments et poisons est une notion classique, bien soulignée, entre autres, à la suite de Paracelse, par Claude Bernard dans ses leçons au Collège de France sur les substances médicamenteuses et toxiques. Si, à doses convenables, les substances médicamenteuses peuvent exercer des effets salutaires en soulageant et, éventuellement, en guérissant les malades, elles peuvent, en sens inverse, provoquer des effets nocifs, lorsque les doses administrées sont trop fortes ou, même à des doses strictement limitées à celles nécessaires à l'obtention de l'effet thérapeutique visé, lorsque des actions secondaires indésirables accompagnent cet effet, pouvant même alors être à l'origine de véritables «maladies médicamenteuses».

Mais, du fait que, contrairement à ce qui a lieu pour d'autres agents chimiques pouvant être absorbés par l'homme, tels que les agents chimiques de pollution de l'air, les additifs aux aliments ou les pesticides, l'absorption des médicaments est le plus souvent *passagère*, l'attention est en général plus particulièrement concentrée sur les effets de toxicité immédiate ou à court terme et l'étude des risques de toxicité à très long terme, pouvant résulter, dans certains cas, de l'administration d'une seule dose ou, le plus souvent, de l'absorption répétée pendant de longues périodes de petites doses ne provoquant isolément aucun effet nocif, est trop souvent négligée.

Les exemples classiques de la digitale et de ses hétérosides ainsi que des drogues génératrices d'assuétude et de toxicomanies, auxquels sont venus s'ajouter de nombreux autres, devraient cependant inciter à une plus grande prudence, surtout à une époque où l'extraordinaire accroissement des corps chimiques mis à la disposition des thérapeutes et la pratique, malheureusement de plus en plus répandue, des auto-médications inconsidérées n'ont fait que multiplier les risques.

Parmi ceux-ci, figurent les risques cancérogènes, dont l'importance, déjà discutée lors de la réunion du Comité de prévention du Cancer de l'U.I.C.C., tenue à Geneve en Novembre 1963, justifie l'organisation du présent Symposium.

Nous reprendrons, dans cet exposé introductif, le plan que nous avions suivi lors de la présentation de notre rapport à la réunion de Geneve.

Dans une première partie, nous présenterons, en les classant d'après le groupe chimique auquel ils se rattachent, les principaux produits, proposés ou utilisés comme médicaments, ayant manifesté, dans certaines conditions, des effets cancérogènes, soit chez l'homme, soit, beaucoup plus fréquemment, dans l'expérimentation sur des animaux de laboratoire, et dits alors corps «potentiellement cancérogènes».

Dans une deuxième partie, nous discuterons, sur un plan très général, de l'attitude à adopter en face de la révélation, épidémiologique ou expérimentale, de tels risques cancérogènes ou de l'absence d'information à leur égard.

Pour stimuler la discussion, nous poserons un certain nombre de questions auxquelles nous donnerons nos réponses personnelles qui seront ainsi soumises à votre examen critique et notamment à celui des Professeurs Frazer et Chassagne qui exposeront, à la dernière session de ce Symposium, les points de vue respectifs du pharmacologue et du clinicien.

La première partie de notre rapport sera beaucoup plus brève qu'elle ne l'à été à la réunion de Geneve, car, en établissant le programme du Symposium, nous avons prévu, en dehors de rapports généraux sur la méthodologie et les relations doses-effets, une série de rapports spécifiquement consacrés à l'étude de groupes particuliers de produits examinés dans notre rapport de Geneve et dans celui présenté lors de la 3ème réunion de l'Association Européenne pour l'Etude de la Toxicité des Drogues tenue à Lausanne en Janvier 1964 (Truhaut, 1964). Aussi, concentrerons nous plus spécialement notre attention, parmi les corps reconnus cancérogènes ou potentiellement cancérogènes dans certaines conditions, sur ceux pour lesquels aucun rapport n'a été inscrit à l'ordre du jour.

C'est pourquoi nous laisserons de côté l'examen: des *dérivés de l'arsenic* et de divers autres éléments, tels que le *chrome* le *nickel* le *cobalt* et le *sélénium*, dont parlera le Dr. Hueper. ainsi que des *radio-éléments*, utilisés, soit dans un but thérapeutique, soit comme traceurs à des fins de diagnostic, dont parleront le Professeur Tubiana et Madame le Docteur Parmentier.

Nous laisserons également au Docteur Roe le soin d'étudier les *complexes du fer avec des macromolécules du type dextrane*.

En ce qui concerne les produits médicamenteux pouvant contenir des hydrocarbures polycycliques cancérogènes, nous laisserons à nos éminents collègues Lijinsky, Saffiotti et Shubik le soin de vous entretenir des produits dérivés des *pétroles (paraffines huiles des paraffine, vaselines, cires de pétrole)*, à propos desquels se pose impérativement le problème de l'établissement des normes de pureté et de leur contrôle par des méthodes analytiques adéquates.

Nous dirons en revanche quelques mots des *goudrons*, qui entrent encore fréquemment dans la composition de pommades ou de lotions (émulsions aqueuses ou solutions alcooliques) utilisées pour des traitements, souvent très prolongés, d'affections cutanées chroniques, en particulier des diverses formes d'eczéma et du psoriasis.

Le *goudron de houille*, ou coaltar, est inscrit d'ailleurs à de nombreuses pharmacopées. Il est superflu de rappeler les effects cancérogènes cutanés provoqués, soit chez l'homme, soit chez les animaux de laboratoire, par des contacts répétés avec des goudrons obtenus à partir de la houille. Aussi n'est-il pas tellement étonnant que quelques observations, rares à vrai dire, de cancers cutanés paraissant s'être développés chez l'homme, à la suite d'applications répétées de préparations à base de goudrons en thérapeutique dermatologique, aient été publiées. On trouvera des références à cet égard en particulier celles relatives aux observations de VEIEL (1924), de DE JONG, MEYER et MARTINEAU (1924), de KOVTOUNOVITSCH (1927), de HODGSON (1948) et de ALEXANDER et MACROSSON (1954), dans un article de ROOK, GRESHAM et DAVIS (1956), article dans lequel ces auteurs rapportent eux-mêmes un cas d'épithélioma spinocellulaire localisé à la partie supérieure de la cuisse gauche, dans l'étiologie duquel l'application répétée, pendant 34 années, de pommade à base de goudron de houille parait pouvoir être incriminée. Nous rapellerons, à ce sujet, que STERNBERG (1923) a pu obtenir des épithéliomas cutanés chez la Souris par badigeonnages répétés avec trois types de préparations à base de goudrons (solutions dans divers solvants) utilisées dans une clinique de Francfort. Des constations dans le même sens ont été faites sur le même animal avec la préparation «liquor picis carbonis BP » par BERENBLUM (1948), qui, parallèllement, a caractérisé, par spectrographie de fluorescence, la présence de benzopyrène à la concentration de 0,02% dans cette préparation, en soulignant que cette concentration ne pouvait, à elle seule, permettre d'expliquer la haute activité cancérogène du produit. BERENBLUM, dans sa publication, attirait l'attention sur les risques pouvant résulter de l'application répétée d'une telle formulation. Nous ajouterons, à cet égard, aux observations mentionnées plus haut, celles de TRUFFI (1925) et de ROSMANITH (1953).

Les *goudrons de bois* sont beaucoup moins actifs que les goudrons de houille, d'après divers auteurs et en particulier d'après SCHMÄHL et REITER (1953), bien que SHUSTEROV (1926) ait pu, chez une femme, observer un cancer de la règion vulvaire, avec métastases dans les ganglions lymphatiques, à la suite d'applications répétées d'une préparation à base de goudron de bois de bouleau.

En revanche, *l'huile de cade,* obtenue par distillation pyrogénée du bois de *Juniperus oxycedrus* n'a pas manifesté de potentialité cancérogène dans les expériences de FAIVICHEVSKI et ALEXANDRE SHABAD (1956).

En ce qui concerne les *hydrocarbures chlorés* de la série grasse (chloroforme, tétrachlorure de carbone…), nous renvoyons au rapport de G. RUDALI. Nous croyons toutefois utile de souligner que le chloroforme, s'il n'est pratiquement plus utilisé comme anesthésique, est employé sur une échelle assez large dans certains pays comme conservateur et aromatisant des potions et, à ce titre, peut être absorbé, per os. à petites doses répétées pendant de longues périodes.

Par ailleurs, il nous paraît intéressant de signaler que la potentialité cancérogène du tétrachlorure de carbone paraît bien s'être manifestée chez l'homme dans une observation récente de SIMLER, MAURER et MANDARD (1964) d'un cancer du foie développé sur cirrhose chez un sujet soumis à des expositions répétées à l'hydrocarbure chloré utilisé comme extincteur. Il convient d'ajouter que, au moins dans certains pays, ceux d'afrique par exemple, où se rencontrent à l'état endémique des helminthiases intestinales, le tétrachlorure de carbone peut être utilisé, à doses répétées pendant de longues périodes, sur des groupes importants de populations. Il serait, à notre avis, préférable de recommander l'emploi d'anthelmintiques moins toxiques.

Dans la série des glycols, où se rencontrent des produits souvent utilisés comme solvants de produits médicamenteux, le *diéthylèneglycol,*

$$CH_2OH—CH_2—O—CH_2—CH_2OH,$$

administré de façon prolongée au rat à la concentration de 2 à 4% dans le régime, a provoqué des cancers de la vessie dans les expériences de FITZHUGH et NELSON

(1946). En revanche, le *triéthylène-glycol*:

$$CH_2OH-CH_2-O-CH_2-CH_2-O-CH_2-CH_2-OH$$

a fourni, dans les mêmes conditions, des résultats négatifs confirmés par Robertson et coll. (1947) sur le Rat et sur le Singe. Il en a été de même du *propylèneglycol*,

$$CH_3-CHOH-CH_2OH$$

par ailleurs beaucoup moins toxique en raison de sa transformation métabolique en acide lactique, dans les expériences de ces derniers auteurs et dans celles de van Winkle et Newman (1941) et de Ambrose (1942) chez le Chien et le Rat et de Morris et coll. (1942) chez le Rat.

En ce qui concerne les corps possédant une ou plusieurs fonctions *lactone*, nous renvoyons au rapport de F. Dickens, en soulignant toutefois l'exemple spectaculaire de la *β.propiolactone*, dont l'emploi comme antiseptique pour la stérilisation des greffes artérielles et des sérums pour transfusion, ainsi que comme agent de désinfection de l'air des salles d'hôpitaux, avait été préconisé.

Dans le groupe des produits médicamenteux possédant dans leur molécules une ou plusieurs fonctions *phénoliques,* la potentialité cancérogène du *phénol ordinaire* et de divers composés phénoliques a été étudié par Bouthwell et coll. (1955, 1956, 1959) et Rusch et coll. (1955). Expérimental sur la Souris, ces auteurs ont montré que l'application répétée sur la peau de phénol ordinaire et de divers phénols substitués se traduisait par une action promotrice vis-à-vis de la cancérisation cutanée sous l'influence d'une seule dose de diméthyl 9.10 benzo 1.2 anthracène (DMBA). Le phénol seul s'est, par ailleurs, révélé capable de provoquer des tumeurs cutanées (papillomes et cancers). Ces résultats ont été confirmés par Salaman et Glendenning (1958). Il est précisé dans la publication de Bouthwell et Bosch (1959) que cet effet can-

cérogène du phénol peut être obtenu avec un composé rigoureusement pur. Plus de cinquante composés phénoliques dérivés du phénol ont été soumis aux investigations. Les résultats obtenus ont mis en évidence l'influence de la nature et de la position des substituants dans la molécule initiale. Le *β.naphtol* a été trouvé légèrement actif, cependant que le tetrahydro *β*.naphtol (tetralol) a manifesté une activité promotrice comparable à celle du phénol ordinaire.

En considérant ce groupe des composés phénoliques, il convient de rappeler les observations relatives aux effets cancérogènes de la *créosote*. Cette dénomination s'applique malheureusement à des produits de composition fort variable, obtenus par distillation entre 200° et 400° de goudrons de houille ou de bois ou de certaines fractions pétrolières. On y trouve en tout cas toujours des composés phénoliques en proportion plus ou moins importante, notamment, dans le cas de la créosote officinale de la Pharmacopée française (8ème édition 1965, p. 336), du créosol ou éther monométhylique de l'homopyrocatéchine, accompagné de

Créosol

gaïacol, crésylols, o.éthylphénol (phlorol) etc. Les créosotes de houille sont moins riches en composés phénoliques et plus riches en hydrocarbures aromatiques polycycliques que les créosotes de bois.

Cookson (1924) a publié une observation d'épithélioma cutané avec métastases multiples chez un ouvrier d'une fabrique de créosote ayant été exposé pendant 33 ans à ce produit. Ce n'est que beaucoup plus tard que la potentialité cancérogène de la créosote pour la peau de la Souris a été mise en évidence par les expérimentations de Woodhouse et Irwin (1950), Poel et Kammer (1957), Lijinsky, Saffiotti et Shubik (1957) et Bouthwell et Bosch (1958). Roe, Bosch et Bouthwell (1958) ont noté en outre, chez le même animal, la production d'adénomes pulmonaires après badigeonnages répétés de la peau avec une créosote commerciale employée pour la conservation des bois. Il faut bien Souligner, avec Lijinsky, Saffiotti et Shubik (1957), que les composés responsables de la potentialité cancérogéne de certains échantillons de créosote restent, pour la plupart, à identifier.

Se rattachent également à la série des composés phénoliques les *tanins,* dits souvent acides tanniques. Sont désignés sous cette dénomination des produits divers qui se rencontrent dans un très grand nombre de végétaux, particulièrement dans les feuilles et les écorces, et qui ont la propriété de se combiner à la peau fraîche en la rendant imputrescible et peu perméable. Ils possèdent un certain nombre de propriétés chimiques communes dues en grande partie à la présence dans leur molécule de fonctions phénoliques (cf entre autres, Perrot et Goris, 1909; Freudenberg, 1921). Leur constitution est complexe; ils renferment toujours, à côté de molécules phénoliques, du glucose engagé dans des liaisons osidiques. On les classe en général en deux groupes principaux:

1. Les tanins pyrogalliques hydrolysables, donnant, par distillation sèche, du pyrogallol ou trihydroxy 1.2.3 benzène.

Le type en est le tanin de la noix de galle d'Alep, ou acide gallotannique, inscrit à divers Pharmacopées, qui est composé d'un certain nombre de glucosides plus ou moins complexes de l'acide gallique, ou acide pyrogallolcarbonique,

Acide gallique

et de l'acide ellagique, ce dernier résultant de la combinaison de deux molécules d'acide gallique, avec estérification de la fonction carboxyle de chacune d'elle par un oxhydryle phénolique empruntée à l'autre molécule. Il convient de citer parmi ces glucosides le pentagalloylglucose.

2. Les tanins condensés ou catéchiques, dans lesquels les noyaux phénoliques sont liés dans les molécules, par les valences du carbone et non plus par l'intermédiaire des atomes d'oxygène. Le type de ces tanins, peu solubles dans l'eau et ayant une tendance marquée à l'oxydation et à la polymérisation en donnant des produits insolubles fortement colorés, est le tanin de cachou.

Un certain nombre de tanins ont été expérimentés sur l'animal, à la suite de l'observation d'accidents hépatiques chez des brûlés traités par ces produits. Administrés par injection sous-cutanée au Rat, ils provoquent la formation d'hépatomes, ainsi que l'ont montré, entre autres, Korpassy, Kovacs et Mosonyi (1949, 1950, 1959, 1961) et Kirby (1960), expérimentant, soit l'acide gallotannique ou divers tanins hydrolysables, soit des tanins condensés.

Cette potentialité cancérogène ne se manifeste pas per os, mais il faut noter, avec Boyd Bereczky et Godi (1965), qu'à doses suffisantes l'acide tannique, administré au Rat per os, est susceptible de provoquer la mort ($DL_{50} = 2,26\,g/Kg$), avec, entre autres symptômes, en cas d'issue fatale retardée, l'apparition d'une nécrose du foie traduisant bien un tropisme hépatique.

Ces observations imposent, selon nous, une certaine prudence dans l'emploi des tanins en thérapeutique, en particulier lorsqu'ils sont injectés, par exemple dans certaines formes-retard d'administration de la vitamine B_{12}.

Dans le groupe des *composés quinoniques*, d'après TAKIZAWA (1940) dont les résultats n'ont toutefois pas été confirmés par BUTENANDT (1950), la *p. benzoquinone* et l'*α naphtoquinone*

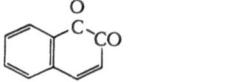

Parabenzoquinone

β-Naphtoquinone   α-Naphtoquinone

provoquent, chez la Souris, après badigeonnages cutanés, la formation d'épithéliomas. Dans les même conditions, la β naphtoquinone n'a pas manifesté d'activité.

Par ailleurs, dans les expériences de BOUTHWELL et BOSCH (1959) sur la Souris, la *naphtoquinone 1.4* (ou α naphtoquinone) et son *dérivé méthylé en 2* ont manifesté une légère activité promotrice vis-à-vis de la cancérisation cutanée par le diméthyl 9.10 benzo 1.2 anthracène. Rappelons que la *lutéoskyrine*, l'un des principes toxiques du *Penicillium islandicum*, moisissure susceptible de contaminer le riz en lui communiquant des propriétés cancérogénes vis à vis du foie, au moins chez le Rat, est une bis dihydro-anthraquinone.

Le caractère carcinophore bien connu du *groupe aminé NH_2* présent comme substituant sur des noyaux aromatiques conduit à suspecter a priori la potentialité cancérogène des médicaments porteurs d'un tel groupe sur leurs molécules. Cette notion fondamentale a souvent été oubliée.

C'est ainsi que, en 1953, avait été commercialisé, comme analgésique une formulation renfermant comme principe actif de l'*acétylamino 2. carbazole*

Acétylamino 2. carbazole

dont la structure est très voisine de l'acétylamino 2 fluorène

Acétylamino 2 fluorène

dont la haute activité cancérogène, chez toute une série d'espèces animales et par diverses voies d'administration, est bien connue.

A vrai dire, d'après les recherches expérimentales de MILLER et coll. (1955) sur le Rat, le remplacement dans l'acétylamino 2 fluorène du groupe CH_2 médian reliant les 2 noyaux benzéniques par un groupe NH fait disparaître la potentialité cancérogène vis-à-vis du foie, du conduit auditif et de l'intestin grêle, et diminue considérablement celle vis-a-vis de la glande mammaire. Il n'en demeure pas moins que deux femelles, sur les 13 d'un lot de 25 rats soumis à l'administration d'acétylamino 2 carbazole dans le régime pendant 8 mois, ont présenté des adénocarcinomes mammaires apparus au 10ème mois, alors qu'aucune tumeur n'était observée chez les témoins.

Dans la série des *sulfamides,* même si l'on met à part les résultats positifs obtenus par HAEREM (1948), par injection sous-cutanée de sulfanilamide chez la Souris (sarcomes spinocellulaires au point d'injection) et par BJERRE HANSEN et BICHEL (1952) chez la Souris et le Rat par administration par la même voie de divers sulfamides, il convient de mentionner l'obtention par BONSER et CLAYson (1964, 1965) de cancers de la vessie, par administration prolongée (65 semaines) à la Souris (souche Ab×I F) d'un régime renfermant 0,01% d'*éthylsulfonyl 4. naphthalène sulfonamide*, composé qui, d'après les observations de PAGET (1958) et de SEN GUPTA (1962), provoque une hyperlasie de l'épithélium vésical chez la Souris et chez le Rat. Les auteurs, dont les résultats positifs s'ajoutent à ceux de HUEPER (1962) avec un autre sulfamide, indiquent avoir obtenu des proliférations malignes par implantation directe du produit soumis à l'investigation dans l'épithélium vésical. Ils soulignent la sensibilité plus élevée des animaux femelles comparativement aux animaux mâles et indiquent que l'administration préalable d'acétylamino-2-fluorène ou de diméthyl 9.10 benzo 1.2 anthracène n'augmente pas le pourcentage des tumeurs obtenues. Ils estiment souhaitable d'étendre les expérimentations à d'autres souches de souris et à d'autres espèces animales.

BLACK et STEVENSON (1962) ont effectué l'étude pharmacodynamique d'une drogue dénommée *Alderlin* ou *Pronethalol* répondant à la formule suivante:

Alderlin (Pronethalol)

qui s'est révélée être un puissant inhibiteur des récepteurs cardiaques adrénergiques, aussi bien chez l'animal que chez l'homme, et dont l'emploi dans le traitement de certaines arythmies cardiaques avait pour cette raison été envisagé. Les essais de toxicité effectués sur diverses espèces animales paraissaient exclure tout risque pouvant résulter d'un tel usage. Mais, dans une expérimentation effectuée sur la Souris, ALCOCK et BOND (1964) ont vu apparaître, sous l'influence d'une administration répétée per os de ce composé, à des doses allant de 10 à 200 mg/kg, des lymphosarcomes, principalement d'origine thymique, après deux mois et demi de traitement et des réticulosarcomes de l'intestin et, moins fréquemment, du foie, après 7 mois et demi de traitement. Les autres espèces animales expérimentées (rat, cobaye, chien, singe) ne paraissent pas posséder la réceptivité de la souris à l'action cancerogène de ce composé.

La formation d'un groupe éthylène-imine ou éthylène-oxyde à l'extrémité de la chaine latérale lors des transformations métaboliques a été suggérée pour expliquer cette action. Des recherches sont actuellement en cours pour évaluer la validité de cette hypothèse.

Certains dérivés de la *quinoléine* ou benzopyridine ont manifesté dans certaines conditions une potentialité cancérogène.

Le premier composé de cette série ayant donné lieu à des constatations dans ce sens est le *Styryl 430* ou dérivé acétylé de l'hydroxyde du (p. aminostyryl) 2 (p. acétylaminobenzoyl) amino.6.méthylquinoléinium.

Ce composé hydrosoluble avait été préconisé pour la chimiothérapie des trypanosomiases. En procédant à son expérimentation, BROWNING et ses coll. (1936) constatèrent qu'il provoquait chez la Souris, après injection par voie souscutanée, l'apparition de sarcomes au point d'injection. Il faut noter que la

Styryl 430

présence d'un reste de p. aminophényl-éthylène le rapproche dans une certaine mesure des dérivés de l'amino 4 stilbène dont la potentialité cancérogène est bien connue.

Comme autres dérivés de la quinoléine ayant reçu des applications en thérapeutique et reconnus potentiellement cancérogènes dans certaines conditions, il faut encore mentioner:

l'hydroxy 8 quinoléine, ou orthoxy-quinoléine, composé ayant des propriétés chélatantes analogues à celle des ortho.amino phénols,

Hydroxy 8. quinoléine

dont le sulfate est utilisé comme anti-septique et désinfectant.

Boyland, Watson et coll. (1956, Allen, 1957) ont obtenu chez la Souris, des cancers de la vessie en 40 semaines environ, à la suite de l'implantation de «pellets» renfermant ce composé associé à du cholestérol. Par ailleurs, Hoch-Ligeti (1956, 1957), avec une préparation anticonceptionnelle à activité spermicide, à base d'hydroxyquinoléine, d'acide borique et d'acétate de phénylmercure, administré à des rats, soit par voie intra-vaginale, soit per os, a obtenu des cancers de diverses localisations, particulièrement au niveau de la glande mammaire, du foie, de l'utérus, du thymus et du cerveau. L'auteur souligne toutefois, à juste titre, qu'on ne saurait incriminer avec certitude l'hydroxy 8 quinoléine.

Nous avons personnellement soumis deux espèces animales, le Rat et la Souris, à l'administration pendant toute leur vie d'un régime renfermant une concentration aussi élevée que 5.000 ppm de sulfate d'hydroxy 8. quinoléine. Nous n'avons observé aucun effet nocif significa-

tif et particulièrement aucune augmentation significative du nombre des tumeurs comparativement aux témoins (Truhaut, 1960, 1963). Il nous semble que les différences entre les résultats observés par les divers investigateurs en fonction de la voie d'administration sont importantes à considérer en ce qui concerne les applications en thérapeutique. S'il nous paraît prudent de déconseiller l'emploi de l'hydroxy 8. quinoléine comme contraceptif spermicide, la plupart des autres emplois thérapeutiques actuels ne nous semblent pas comporter de risques cancérogènes.

Le *N. oxyde de la nitro ¦4. quinoléine*,

N oxyde de nitro
4. quinoléine

dont la haute potentialité cancérogène a été mise en évidence par les expérimentations de Nakahara et coll. (1957 bis 1958) sur la Souris, par badigeonnages et par injection.

Les résultats de ces auteurs ont été confirmés par Lacassagne et coll. (1960 bis 1961), qui ont précisé qu'il existait des différences très importantes de réceptivité à la cancérisation cutanée par badigeonnages selon les lignées de souris et mis en évidence la potentialité cancérogène du *N. oxyde de nitro-4 quinaldine*, homologue du N.oxyde de nitro 4 quinoléine. D'après Takayama, le Rat est également réceptif à l'action cancérogène cutanée du N.oxyde de nitro 4 quinoléine (Takayama, 1962).

Par ailleurs, Mori (1959—1962) a obtenu chez la Souris des adénocarcinomes pulmonaires avec métastases, par injections sous-cutanées répétées de ce composé qui possède, en outre, une haute activité mutagène comme l'ont montré les expérimentations de OKABAYASHI (1955).

On touvera la discussion de ces mécanismes possibles d'action, parmi lesquels figure la combinaison avec les groupements sulfhydrylés (thiols) biologiques, dans un article de NAKAHARA (1964).

Il convient de noter que son produit de réduction, le *N-oxyde d'hydroxylamino 4 quinoléine* est également potentiellement cancérogène, ainsi que l'ont montré SHIRASU et OHTA (1963) dans leurs expériences sur la Souris par injections souscutanées.

Tous ces faits, sur lesquels nous ne pouvons nous étendre davantage, nous font souhaiter que les dérivés nitrés de la quinoléine, préconisés pour des applications thérapeutiques, tels que la *nitro 4. hydroxy 8 quinoléine,* utilisée pour le traitement des infections intestinales avec des posologies relativement élevées et prolongées, soient, bien qu'ils ne possèdent pas les deux centres chimiques réactifs NO_2 et $N = O$ dont la présence simultanée a certainement une importance considérable, soumis à une évaluation de la potentialité cancérogène.

Les dérivés de l'*acridine,* ou diphénopyridine, dont certains, telle l'Euflavine,

Acridine

sont utilisés sur une très large échelle comme antiseptiques de la gorge chez les enfants sous forme de dragées à sucer, ont été considérés comme suspects par certains auteurs pour deux raisons principales :

1. Leur affinité pour les acides nucleiques, que nous avons nous-même étudiée dans le cas de la *quinacrine* ou atébrine (1962).

Quinacrine (Atébrine)

2. Leur caractère mutagène, mis en évidence, au moins dans le cas des amino-acridines (Jaune d'acridine, orangé d'acridine), sur certains bactériophages et certains végétaux (D'AMATO (1950), FREESE (1959)). TRAININ *et coll.* (1964) ont essayé de provoquer des tumeurs cutanées avec le jaune d'acridine et l'orangé d'acridine, en les appliquant après un traitement promoteur à l'huile de croton. Leurs résultats dans cette direction ont été négatifs et, par ailleurs, ils n'ont observé aucune augmentation significative de fréquence des adénomes pulmonaires chez les souris traitées comparativement aux témoins. Dans la littérature scientifique, nous n'avons trouvé qu'un résumé d'une publication concernant la production de tumeurs chez l'animal sous l'influence d'un dérivé aminoacridinique, en l'espèce la trypaflavine, dite aussi acriflavine ou euflavine, publication de SUSANA EZCYZA (1952) d'après laquelle l'injection répétée au rat, par voie sous-cutanée, de ce composé, aurait permis d'obtenir des sarcomes au point d'injection.

Aucune preuve valable n'a donc pu être apportée jusqu'ici à l'appui de la suspicion mentionnée plus haut. Mais, à notre avis, la mise en évidence de propriétés mutagènes chez les aminoacridines, quelles que soient les réserves légitimement exprimées, entre autres, par BURDETTE (1955), par RONS (1959) et par TRAININ (1964) en ce qui concerne l'existence d'une relation étroite entre l'activité mutagène et la potentialité cancérogène, devrait déjà inciter à ne pas les utiliser inconsidérément chez les enfants.

Dans le groupe des *colorants,* un grand nombre de composés se rattachant à des séries diverses ont été reconnus potentiellement cancérogènes. Or, un certain nombre de ces colorants ont été et sont parfois encore utilisés à des fins thérapeutiques. Nous nous bornerons à les citer en renvoyant, pour les données expérimentales concernant leur potentialité cancérogène, à une revue générale que nous avons publiée sur ce sujet (TRUHAUT, 1958).

1. Le *Soudan III* (Tolylazotolylazo β-naphtol) ou *Rouge organol IV*, dit encore *Ecarlate de Biebrich*,

Rouge Organol IV

très longtemps et parfois encore employé comme agent favorisant la formation épithéliale, en particulier sous forme de tulle gras dans le pansement des plaies, brûlures, ulcères et dermatoses.

2. Le *dérivé diacétylé de l'o.aminoazotoluène,* employé jusqu'à une date récente, sous le nom de *Pellidol,*

o. aminoazotoluène

comme agent antiseptique et kératoplastique, sous forme de pommades dans le traitement des plaies et de diverses dermatoses.

3. La *chrysoïdine,*

Chrysoïdine

colorant azoïque utilisé dans certains pays, jusqu'à une époque toute récente, comme désinfectant de la gorge, dans les angines en particulier, alors, que, comme

l'a bien démontré ALBERT (1954, 1956—1960), il provoque, après administration prolongée per os dans le régime, un très haut pourcentage d'hépatomes chez le Rat.

4. Le *Bleu trypan,*

Blue trypan

colorant azoïque utilisé en usage externe, sous forme de pommade ou de solution, comme désensibilisant, anesthésique et désinfectant dans le traitement des lésions cutanéo-muqueuses à virus neurotropes (zona, herpès, varicelle, etc.) et aussi par voie parentérale (injection intra-veineuse), entre autres, dans le traitement de la sclérose en plaques.

En dehors de sa potentialité cancérogène se manifestant électivement au

Pellidol

niveau du système réticulo endothélial, ce colorant manifeste des effets tératogènes chez différentes espèces de mammifères.

En présence des différences d'activité parfois très marquées des divers échantillons de Bleu Trypan, soumis aux investigations, certains ont pensé que les effets tératogènes pourraient être dus aux impuretés souvent présentes dans les produits commerciaux, en particulier une fraction colorée en violet pourpre, dite benzopurpurine, et une fraction colorée en rouge. D'après DIJKSTRA et GILL-

MAN (1961), la prolifération des cellules réticulo-endothéliales du foie serait due à cette impureté qu'ils ont séparée par chromatographie du colorant sur colonne d'alumine. Mais, en ce qui concerne l'activité tératogène, les travaux de TUCHMANN-DUPLESSIS et Mme MERCIER-PARO (1959), confirmés par ceux de LLOYD et BECK (1962), ont nettement démontré que la benzo-purpurine et les autres impuretés étaient dépourvues d'activité tératogène dont est responsable le Bleu trypan lui-même.

5. Le *Vert Lumière SF,* colorant de la série du triphénylméthane,

Vert Lumière SF (Vert Sulfo J.)

dénommé également *Vert Sulfo J* ou *Vert acide J,* préconisé comme antiseptique et antiallergique sous forme de collyres en ophthalmologie.

En ce qui concerne les colorants, nous mentionnerons, sans nous étendre, l'emploi d'un certain nombre d'entre eux pour colorer certaines formes médicamenteuses, notamment les comprimés et les pilules dragéifiées, formes sous lesquelles sont le plus souvent absorbés divers médicaments d'usage courant, parfois pendant de longues périodes. Nous nous bornerons à souligner qu'avant d'inscrire un colorant sur les listes de produits autorisés pour un tel emploi, il faut l'avoir soumis à une expérimentation toxicologique rigoureuse comportant l'évaluation de la potentialité cancérogène.

Il en est de même des composés fluorescents, dits *compensateurs* ou *azurants optiques* («brighteners» ou «optical blea-chers»), parfois employés pour donner une belle couleur blanche aux gazes et aux cotons médicamenteux et dont certains sont des dérivé du *p. diméthylaminostilbène,*

p. diméthylamino-stilbène

composé dont la potentialité cancérogène a été bien démontrée et ne disparait qu'après l'introduction de groupes sulfoniques dans les deux moitiés de la molécule:

Nous ne ferons que mentionner comme composés potentiellement cancérogènes utilisés ou pouvant être utilisés en thérapeutique:

— *l'hydrazide de l'acide isonicotinique*

— la *thiourée,* le *thiouracile,* le *thioacétamide* et les agents antithyroïdiens en général

— *l'uréthane ordinaire* (carbamate d'éthyle)

— les divers *agents alcoylants* cytotoxiques utilisés en chimiothérapie anticancéreuse

— les *alcaloïdes* à noyau de pyrrolizidine présents dans certains Seneçons parfois utilisés comme emménagogues

— le glucoside des noix de Cycas (*cycasine*)

— les *oestrogènes* et les *progestatifs,* puisque ces produits ont été spécifiquement étudiés dans les rapports respectifs de J. JUHASZ, N. P. NAPALKOV, E. BOYLAND, R. SCHOENTAL et de W. E. POËL.

Nous nous permettons toutefois d'attirer l'attention sur quelques points:

1. Parmi les substances ayant un certain degré de parenté avec les dérivés de l'hydrazine, la *métatolylsemicarbazide,*

Métatolylsemicarbazide

commercialisée sous le nom de Marétine comme analgésique et antipyrétique, succédané de la phénylsemicarbazide (cryogénine), provoque, d'après Jamai et Balo (1938), des leucoses chez la Poule.

2. L'utilisation encore répandue dans certains pays de l'*uréthane ordinaire,* ou carbamate d'éthyle, comme antialgique et son emploi, à des concentrations allant jusqu'à 40%, pour la préparation de solutés injectables de chlorhydrate de quinine ne nous paraissent pas souhaitables. Le Professeur Shubik, auquel on doit d'importantes recherches sur ce composé, a accepté de parler de sa potentialité cancérogène comme producteur, non seulement, comme on l'a cru longtemps, d'adénomes pulmonaires multiples chez la Souris ou de tumeurs cutanées, après badigeonnages de la peau ou administration par voie parentérale, suivis d'un badigeonnage avec un promoteur, en l'espèce l'huile de croton, chez la même espèce, mais encore de tumeurs de diverses localisations chez différentes espèces animales (souris, hamster). Nous ajouterons que Rivière et coll. (1964), soumettant des hamsters dorés à des applications cutanées répétées d'une solution d'uréthane à 50% dans l'acétone, ont obtenu, après plusieurs mois, un nombre important de tumeurs mélaniques.

3. Dans le groupe des alcaloïdes, les effets co-cancérogènes exercés par la *réserpine,* alcaloïde des Rauwolfia, actuellement très utilisé dans le traitement de l'hypertension artérielle et de divers troubles psychiques comme tranquillisant neuroleptique, vis-à-vis de la cancérisation hépatique par le Jaune de beurre, qui, en sa présence, se trouve considérablement accélérée, ainsi que l'ont montré Mme. Hurst, Lacassagne et Rosenberg (1958). Cet exemple de synergie devrait, à notre avis, attirer l'attention sur l'intérêt qui s'attache, en matière de prévention des risques cancérogènes, à ne pas étendre inconsidérément les emplois thérapeutiques d'une telle substance sensibilisant le foie à certains agents chimiques potentiellement cancérogènes, et de la réserver pour les maladies où son action comporte des conséquences bénéfiques indiscutables.

4. Parmi les drogues végétales, figure le bois de racine de Sassafras, *Sassafras officinale,* (Lauracées), entrant, sous forme de fines lamelles et à faible pourcentage (en général 0,50 gr à 1 gr pour 100 gr), dans la composition de formules pour la fabrication de tisanes dites dépuratives. Or l'essence de Sassafras contient 75 à 80% de *safrol* ou *allyl-4.methylène-dioxy-1.2-benzène,*

Safrol

dont l'action cancérogène hépatique a été reconnue chez le Rat, soumis à l'administration de régimes en renfermant des concentrations *relativement élevées,* par les experts de l'«U.S. Food and Drug Administration» (1960), dont les résultats ont été confirmés par Homberger et coll. (1961). Est-il prudent de continuer à tolérer la présence du sassafras dans les formulations servant à préparer des tisanes dépuratives? Ou bien, peut on considérer que les doses de safrol absorbées par les habitués de la consommation de telles tisanes sont suffisamment minimes pour justifier l'octroi d'une tolérance, comme cela a été fait aux Etats Unis, en ce qui concerne l'emploi, comme condiments alimentaires, de la cannelle, de la noix de muscade et d'autres produits naturels contenant de petites quantités de safrol?

5. En ce qui concerne l'interprétation des résultats des expérimentations effectuées avec des progestatifs sur des espèces de l'ordre des Rongeurs, il convient de souligner qu'elle est rendue très délicate par le fait que, contrairement aux Mammifères et à l'homme en particulier, les Rongeurs ne présentent pas un cycle sexuel à 2 phases et ne sont soumis à l'influence des hormones progestatives que pendant la gravidité.

6. Un certain nombre de drogues sont considérées comme suspectes en ce qui concerne la potentialité cancérogène. Il s'agit, entre autres:

— de la *Phénylbutazone*, ou dioxy-3.5.diphényl 1.2.n.butyl 4.pyrazolidine,

Phénylbutazone

qui, d'après un certain nombre d'observations rassemblées par ROE (1966), paraît pouvoir provoquer, chez des sujets soumis à l'absorption de cette drogue, des leucémies aiguës.

— de *l'oxolamine*, ou phényl 3.β.diéthylamine éthyl.5.oxadiazole.1.2.4, agent antitussif dont, d'après BARRON (1963), l'administration orale prolongée

au rat provoque des lésions précancéreuses au niveau de l'épithélium vésical, cependant que, chez le Chien, un tel traitement fait apparaitre une hyperplasie de cet épithélium.

Par ailleurs, certaines drogues manifestent, dans certaines conditions, des effets co-cancérogènes particulièrement marqués. Il en est ainsi par exemple, de *l'anthraline* (anthratriol)

OH OH OH

Anthraline
(Anthratriol)

drogue utilisée dans le traitement du psoriasis et de diverses affections cutanées, possédant 3 fonctions phénol dans la molécule. Dans les expérimentations de BOCK et BURNS (1963) sur la Souris, elle s'est révélée être, après applications répétées à très faibles concentrations (0,01 p. 100), un promoteur très actif de la cancérogénèse cutanée par le diméthylbenz(a)anthracène. Il faut cependant souligner qu'aucune production de cancer des téguments n'a été observée chez des sujets humains soumis à des applications cutanées d'anthraline consécutivement à des applications prolongées de pommade à base de goudron de houille (ROOK et coll, 1956).

Essai d'Etablissement d'une Doctrine de Prévention du Cancer en ce qui concerne l'emploi des Agents Chimiques en Thérapeutique

Le problème est beaucoup plus délicat que dans le cas des additifs aux aliments, car, ainsi que nous l'avons signalé dans notre introduction, toute substance médicamenteuse peut, dans certaines conditions, manifester des propriétés toxiques et c'est au médecin qu'il incombe de prendre une décision concernant son usage, en «pesant» les bénéfices et les risques à plus ou moins long

terme. Encore faut-il qu'il soit informé et ceci comporte comme corollaire un enseignement scolaire et post-scolaire adéquat et naturellement aussi la mise en œuvre d'expérimentations adéquates pour l'évaluation toxicologique et cancérologique des drogues.

Comme prévu, nous poserons un certain nombre de questions:

1. Quelle est l'attitude à adopter sur le plan de la prévention en ce qui concerne les drogues reconnues cancérogènes à la fois chez l'homme et dans l'expérimentation animale, le thorotrast (ThO$_2$) par exemple.

A notre avis, il s'impose, en principe, d'en recommander la prohibition.

Ce principe peut cependant ne pas être appliqué de façon trop rigide.

Si nous considérons, par exemple, le diéthylstilboestrol, il ne saurait être question d'en recommander la prohibition, car, d'une part, il est à doses fortes, le seul agent vraiment efficace pour soulager les malades atteints de cancers inopérables de la prostate, qui, de toute façon, dans l'état actuel de nos connaissances, sont condamnés à plus ou moins court terme, et, d'autre part, l'emploi à faibles doses de cet oestrogène contre les déséquilibres hormonaux et dans le traitement des cancers du sein de la femme âgée présente indiscutablement plus de bénéfices que de risques.

En revanche, il nous paraît très fortement recommandable d'éviter soigneusement toute administration qui ne s'impose pas et de limiter la posologie et la durée d'administration au strict minimum nécessaire pour l'effet thérapeutique à obtenir.

2. Quelle est l'attitude à adopter en ce qui concerne les drogues reconnues potentiellement cancérogènes chez certaines espèces animales sur la base de travaux valables?

La réponse à cette question nous apparaît plus délicate, car la méthodologie dont nous disposons est loin d'être parfaite et ceci limite singulièrement les possibilités d'interprétation en ce qui concerne les risques pour l'homme.

Cette réponse ne peut donc être univoque et doit, à notre avis, tenir compte d'un certain nombre de facteurs:

a) si la drogue ne manifeste des effets cancérogènes que dans des conditions très éloignées de celles réalisées lors de ses emplois en thérapeutique, son utilisation nous paraît pouvoir être continuée, en tenant compte, par exemple, du mode d'administration très différent et aussi du mécanisme d'action. Tel est le cas de l'utilisation per os de certains dérivés de la cellulose, tels que la carboxy-méthyl-cellulose, provoquant, par injections sous-cutanées répétées, des sarcomes locaux (Lusky et Nelson, 1957), mais fournissant des résultats négatifs par ingestion (Shelanski et Clark, 1948).

b) Si, au contraire, la drogue a manifesté ses effets cancérogènes dans des conditions comparables à celles réalisées lors de ses emplois en thérapeutique et si, par ailleurs, elle peut être aisément remplacée par un ou des produits fonctionellement équivalents, il nous semble pour le moins prudent de recommander son interdiction. Tel est, à notre avis, le cas de l'uréthane, du tétrachlorure de carbone et de l'acétylamino 2 carbazol.

c) Si la drogue est plus difficilement remplaçable et exerce des effets vraiment très bénéfiques, il convient de laisser au médecin la liberté et la responsabilité de la décision, en tenant compte du fait que les risques cancérogènes se manifestent le plus souvent à très long terme. L'exemple de la penicilline est à cet égard spectaculaire. Il serait, de toute évidence, outrancier d'en interdire l'emploi en raison de sa potentialité cancérogène à long terme. Il en est de même pour l'isoniazide, dont l'emploi a permis les progrès que l'on sait dans la lutte contre la tuberculose. Il en est de même encore de la griséofulvine, antibiotique à propriétés fongicides dont l'emploi a permis de juguler la teigne favique.

Mais, s'il est relativement facile au médecin d'apprécier le bénéfice de l'emploi d'une drogue, la situation est beaucoup moins favorable en ce qui concerne l'appréciation des risques, car, très souvent, les données qui les concernent sont publiées dans des revues très spécialisées qui ne sont lues par les praticiens que de façon très exceptionnelle. Combien de médecins, par exemple, sont au courant de la production d'hépatomes multiples chez la Souris soumise à l'administration orale prolongée de griséofulvine à la concentration de 0,5 à 1% dans les expériences de HURST et PAGET (1963)?

Il s'impose donc, à notre avis, d'établir un plan de diffusion auprès du corps médical des informations adéquates sur les risques, en relation avec la posologie, la voie et la durée d'administration, la répétition éventuelle du traitement et l'âge des sujets traités.

A cet égard, il convient d'être plus particulièrement prudent dans le cas des enfants, en considération de *l'importance du facteur temps* dans la révélation éventuelle d'effets cancérogènes. Une très grande prudence doit être également observée en ce qui concerne l'administration de substances suspectes à la femme enceinte, car il ne faut pas oublier que le passage de certains cancérogènes à travers la barrière placentaire a été démontrée, par exemple, dans le cas de l'uréthane, par GILLMAN (1951) et par KLEIN (1954) expérimentant sur la Souris, et que le foetus est en général particulièrement sensible à leur action[1]. Le passage dans le lait de nombreux cancérogènes impose des précautions analogues dans le cas des femmes qui allaitent.

Bien entendu, il s'impose également de recommander à l'industrie chimique

la recherche de produits de remplacement.

d) dans le cas très spécial des drogues cytotoxiques utilisées dans le traitement des affections cancéreuses, l'attitude à adopter nous paraît être, de toute évidence, celle que nous avons définie à propos de l'emploi du diéthylstilboestrol dans le traitement du cancer de la prostate, attitude basée sur la considération primordiale du bénéfice à obtenir, sans oublier que les risques ne peuvent en général se manifester qu'à une échéance si longue qu'elle dépasse de loin la probabilité de survie des malades. Une telle attitude vaut d'ailleurs pour l'emploi des rayonnements ionisants, doués également d'action cancérogène dans certaines conditions, dans le traitement des affections cancéreuses.

En revanche, l'emploi de tels agents pour d'autres affections que des cancers nous paraît devoir être prohibé. Il doit, à notre avis, en être ainsi par exemple de l'emploi de l'aminoptérine contre le psoriasis et des agents alcoylants recommandés par certains comme antiphlogistiques.

A notre avis, il est hautement désirable de dresser une liste

1. de drogues dont l'usage devrait être prohibé,

2. de drogues dont l'usage est à éviter chez les femmes enceintes et les enfants,

3. de drogues dont l'usage devrait être réservé exclusivement aux traitements de certaines maladies et exclu pour le traitement d'autres affections ou pour certains usages, ce qui comporte comme corollaire l'exigence d'une prescription médicale pour leur délivrance,

4. de drogues dont l'usage prolongé devrait être déconseillé, ce qui comporte le même corollaire,

5. de drogues pour lesquelles la prudence est à conseiller aux prescripteurs.

---

[1] Entre la rédaction de cet article et la correction des épreuves, nous avons eu connaissance des résultats de DRUCKREY *et coll.* (Nature, **210**, 1378—1379, 1966 et Naturwissenschaften **53**, 410, 1966) concernant la cancérogénèse diaplacentaire par diverses substances de la série des nitrosamines et composés apparentés, tels que la nitroso-méthylurée.

L'établissement et la diffusion de telles listes incombent, selon nous, à l'Union Internationale contre le Cancer.

3. Quelle est l'attitude à adopter en ce qui concerne les drogues qui n'ont fait l'objet d'aucune expérimentation ou d'une expérimentation inadéquate en ce qui concerne l'éventualité d'effets cancérogènes.

Avant de répondre à cette question, remarquons qu'elle concerne des drogues dont l'emploi en thérapeutique a été retenu et comporte par suite un certain bénéfice dont il faudra tenir compte.

A notre avis, parmi ces drogues, celles devant être administrées de façon prolongée et/ou employées chez les enfants et les femmes enceintes et aussi celles employées sur une large échelle pour des auto-médications sans prescription médicale, devraient faire l'objet d'une expérimentation spécialement orientée vers la révélation des risques cancérogènes, en adoptant un protocole expérimental tenant compte des conditions d'emploi et tout spécialement de la voie d'administration.

Cet impératif nous paraît s'imposer plus spécialement

a) pour les drogues dont la structure chimique ou celle des métabolites auxquels elles donnent naissance présentent des analogies avec des substances reconnues cancérogènes ou potentiellement cancérogènes. Tel est, en particulier, le cas des drogues dont les molécules sont porteuses de groupements leur conférant des propriétés alcoylantes. C'est, également, en appliquant un tel critère de suspicion par analogie de structure que Schmähl et Reiter (1954) ont été conduits à expérimenter la *phénacétine*

$$C_2H_5O-\langle\rangle-NH-CO-CH_3$$

Phénacétine

en raison de sa parenté avec la *dulcine* ou p. éthoxyphénylurée

$$C_2H_5O-\langle\rangle-NH-CO-NH_2$$

Dulcine

reconnue potentiellement cancérogène chez le Rat par Fitzhugh et Nelson (1950). Ils l'ont, en conséquence, administrée per os à des rats à doses relativement élevées et pendant 600 jours, avec observation des animaux jusqu'à leur mort. Leurs résultats ont été négatifs. Cela ne signifie pas d'ailleurs que des risques autres que les effets cancérogènes ne puissent résulter chez l'homme de la consommation répétée de cette drogue analgésique et légèrement tranquillisante pendant de trop longues périodes. Il est bien connu, en effet, que cette consommation a pu être à l'origine de néphrites.

C'est là un exemple à suivre. Les dérivés de l'hydrazine employés en thérapeutique (antituberculeux, modificateurs des réactions du système nerveux central) devraient ainsi, à la lumière des résultats obtenus et des observations concernant l'isoniazide et l'hydrazine elle même (cf rapport de J. Juhasz), être tous soumis à des investigations systématiques comportant des enquêtes épidémiologiques sur les sujets soumis à des traitements thérapeutiques par ces composés.

b) pour les drogues manifestant certains effets et notamment des effets cytotoxiques et surtout des effets mutagènes assez souvent associés à l'activité cancérogène. Tel est le cas, par exemple, des aminoacridines.

c) pour des drogues susceptibles de réagir avec les acides nucléiques, avec, comme conséquences éventuelles, l'altération de leur structure et la perturbation de leurs fonctions fondamentales dans la division et la croissance cellulaires.

4. Quelle est l'attitude à adopter vis-à-vis des drogues nouvelles?

La réponse à cette question est très délicate, en raison de la longueur et du coût élevé des expérimentations nécessaires pour révéler la potentialité cancérogène, avec, en plus, les difficultés fréquentes d'interprétation que nous avons soulignées.

Des exigences trop sévères risquent en effet de décourager la recherche thérapeutique dans l'industrie, d'autant que les drogues, dont la fabrication et la commercialisation est envisagée, sont loin de connaître toutes le succès et, pour la grande majorité d'entre elles, sont même destinées à être abandonnées.

Cependant, en tenant compte du fait que la potentialité cancérogène, bien qu'en relation certaine avec la structure chimique et notamment avec la présence de certains groupes actifs dont beaucoup d'ailleurs restent à fixer, a été révélée dans des molécules de configuration très diverse, il s'impose, à notre avis, de recommander, comme principe, qu'elles soient soumises à une expérimentation à long terme comportant l'étude des effets cancérogènes éventuels, cette recommandation devant devenir impérative avant toute autorisation définitive lorsque l'un des critères que nous avons précédemment mentionnés sous le point 3 est à prendre en considération: administration prolongée, emploi chez l'enfant et la femme enceinte, vente envisagée sans prescription médicale, structure chimique voisine de celle de produits reconnus potentiellement cancérogènes, propriétés physico-chimiques ou biologiques souvent associées avec la potentialité cancérogène. Même si l'interprétation des résultats d'une telle expérimentation est délicate, il est préférable de recueillir les données concernant l'éventualité d'effets cancérogènes plutôt que de laisser l'homme servir de cobaye pour la révélation de tels effets, comme ce fut le cas pour l'action tératogène du talidomide, considéré au moment de sa commercialisation comme l'un des hypnotiques les moins toxiques et même le moins toxique de tous ceux connus jusque là.

La prévention de ce mal du siècle qu'est le cancer nous paraît justifier l'exigence que nous formulons. Nous tenons à bien souligner qu'elle n'a pas pour objectif d'exclure automatiquement, sur la base d'une révélation de potentialité cancérogène, la possibilité d'emploi en thérapeutique de médicaments nouveaux représentant un progrès majeur dans la lutte contre les maladies.

Le but est de fournir aux médecins prescripteurs une catégorie d'informations indispensables pour leur permettre de peser, sur des bases objectives, non seulement les bénéfices, mais aussi les risques éventuels et notamment les risques cancérogènes pouvant résulter de l'emploi des drogues.

C'est la condition qui nous parait indispensable pour exclure, autant que faire se peut, l'éventualité d'apparition et d'emploi d'une drogue qui serait susceptible de provoquer le cancer chez l'homme.

La leçon tragique du talidomide ne doit, à cet égard, jamais être oubliée.

Bibliographie

ALBERT, Z., Induction of adenomas and carcinomas in the liver of mice by prolonged feeding with chrysoidine. *Pol. Tyg. lek.* 9 (48), 1565—1566 (1954).

— Wplyw przewleklego karmienia chryzoidyna na powstawanie gruczolaka i raka watroby u myszy. *Arch Immunol. Ter. dosw.* 4, 189—242 (1956). Cf. également ALBERT, Z., and

Orlowski, M., Some peculiar biological and biochemical properties of a mouse hepatoma induced by chrysoidin: I — Biological and biochemical characteristics of the hepatoma. *J. Nat. Cancer Inst.*, 25, 443—455 (1960) et Some peculiar biological and biochemical properties of a mouse hepatoma induced by chrysoidin: II — Activity of glucose-6-phosphatase. *J. Nat. Cancer Inst.* 25, 461—465 (1960).

Alcock, S. J., and Bond, P. A., Observations on the toxicity of alderlin (Pronethalol) in laboratory animals. *Proceedings of 4th meeting of the european Society for the stidy of drug toxicity; Cambridge. Excerpta med. — Internat. Congr. series*, No 81, 30 (1964).

Alexander, J. O'. D., and Macrosson, K. I., Squamous epithelioma probably due to tar ointment in a case with psoriasis. *Brit. med. J.* 1954 II, 1089.

Allen, M. J., Boyland, E., Dukes, C. E., Morning, E. S., and Watson, J. G., Cancer of the urinary bladder induced in mice with metabolites of aromatic amines and tryptophan. *Brit. J. Cancer* 2, 212—228 (1957).

Ambrose, A. M., Some toxicological and pharmacological studies on 3.5-dinitro-o-cresol. *J. Pharmacol. exp. Ther.* 76, 245—251 (1942).

Barron, C. N., Observations on the chronic toxicity of 3.Phenyl 5.β.diethylaminoethyl-1.2.4.oxadiazole in the rat and dog. *Exp. Molec. Path.* 2 (Suppl.), 1—27 (1963).

Berenblum, I., Liquor picis carbonis (B.P.) A carcinogenic agent. *Brit. med. J.* 1948 II, 601.

Bjerre Hansen, P., and Bichel, J., Carcinogenic effect of sulfonamides. *Acta radiol.* (Stockh.) 37, 258—265 (1952).

Black, J. W., and Stephenson, J. S., Pharmacology of a new adrenergic beta receptor-blocking compound (nethalide). *Lancet* 1962 II 311—314.

Bock, F. C., and Burns, R., Tumor promoting properties of anthralin (1.8.9. anthratriol). *J. Nat. Cancer Inst.* 30, 393—397 (1963).

Bonser, G. M., and Clayson, D. B., A sulphonamide derivative which induces urinary tract epithelial hyperplasia and carcinomas of the bladder epithelium in the mouse. *Brit. J. Urol.* 36, 26—34 (1964).

Boutwell, R. K., and Bosch, D., The carcinogenicity of creosote oil: Its role in the induction of skin tumors in mice. *Cancer Res.* 18, 1171—1175 (1958).

— — The tumor promoting action of phenol and related compounds for mouse skin. *Cancer Res.* 19, 413—424 (1959).

Boutwell, R. K., Rusch, H. P., and Bosch, D.: The action of phenol and related compounds in tumor formation. *Proc. Amer. Ass. Cancer Res.* 2, 6—7 (1955).

— —, and Booth, B., Tumor production by phenol and related compounds. *Proc. Amer. Ass. Cancer Res.* 2, 96 (1956).

Boyd, E. M., Bereczky, K., and Godi, I., The acute toxicity of tannic acid administred intragastrically. *Canad. med. Ass. J.* 92, 1292—1297 (1965).

Boyland, E., and Watson, G., Hydroxy-anthranilic acid, a carcinogen produced by endogenous metabolism. *Nature* (Lond.) 177, 837—838 (1956).

Browning, C. H., Gulbransen, R., and Niven, J. S. F., Sarcoma production in mice by single subcutaneous injection of a benzoyl-aminoquinoline styryl compound. *J. Path. Bact.* 42, 155—159 (1936).

Burdette, W. J., The significance of mutation in relation to the origin of tumors: A review. *Cander Res.* 15, 201—226 (1955).

Butenandt, A., cité par Druckrey, H., Beiträge zur Pharmakologie cancerogener Substanzen; Versuche mit Anilin. *Naunyn-Schmiedebergs Arch. exp. Path. Pharmak.* 210, 137—158 (1950).

Clayson, D. B., and Bonser, G. M., The induction of tumours of the mouse bladder epithelium by 4-ethylsulphonylnaphthalene 1-Sulphonamide. *Brit. J. Cancer* 19, 311—316 (1965).

Cookson, H. A., Epithelioma of the skin after prolonged exposure to creosote. *Brit. med. J.* 1924 I, 368.

D'Amato, F., cité par Trainin, N., Kaye, A. M., and Berenblum, I., Influence of mutagens on the initiation of skin carcinogenesis. *Biochem. Pharmacol.* 13, 263—267 (1964).

De Jong, S. I., Meyer, J. et Martineau, J., Cancer du goudron chez l'homme (Epithelioma spino-cellulaire développé au niveau d'un eczéma variqueux traité depuis 8 ans par des applications de goudroline). *Bull. Ass. franc. Cancer* 13, 326—329 (1924).

Dijkstra, J., and Gillmann, J.: Chromatographic separation of biologically active components from commercial trypan blue. *Nature* (Lond.) 191, 803—804 (1961).

Ezeyza, S., Neosalvarsan, Sulfato de Atropina y tripaflavina en Ratas Inyectadas Subcutaneamente: Carencia de Poder cancerigeno de los dos Primeros y produccion de un sarcoma en el Lugar de la Inyeccion de Tripaflavina. *Sem. méd. (B. Aires)* 1, 778—780 (1952).

FAIVICHEVSKY, V. A., et SHABAD, A. L., Etude du pouvoir blastomogéne possible de l'onguent Vishnevsky (traduction française du titre russe). *Exp. Chir.* No 6, 53—57 (1956).

FITZHUGH, O. G., and NELSON, A. A., Comparison of the chronic toxicity of triethylene glycol with that of diethylene glycol. *J. industr. Hyg.* **28**, 40—43 (1946).

— — Comparison of the chronic toxicities of synthetic sweetening agents. *Fed. Proc.* **9**, 272 (1950).

FREESE, E., The specific mutagenic effect of base analogues on phage T 4, *J. molec. Biol.* **1**, 87—105 (1959).

— The difference between spontaneous and base-analogue induced mutations of phage T 4; *Proc. nat. Acad. Sci.* (Wash.) **45**, 622—633 (1959).

FREUDENBERG, K., In: ABDERHALDEN, Nachweis, Isolierung, Abbau- und Aufbaustudien auf dem Gebiete der Gerbstoffe. *Handbuch der biologischen Arbeitsmethoden*, Abt. I, Teil 10, S. 439—544. (1923).

HAEREM, A. T., Tissue response to sulfanilamide in mice. *Proceedings of the Society for experimental biology and medicine*, **45**, 536—539 (1940); Carcinogenic effect of sulfonamide. *Proc. Soc. exp. Biol.* (N.Y.) **68**, 330—332 (1948).

HOCH-LIGETI, C., Effect of spermicidal contraceptives on the uterus of rats. *Proc. Amer. Ass. Cancer Res.* **2**, 118 (1956). Cf. également effect of prolonged administration of spermicidal contraceptives on rats kept on low. protein or on full diet. *J. nat. Cancer Inst.* **18**, 661—685 (1957).

HODGSON, G., Epithelioma following the local treatment of pruritus ani with liquor picis carbonis. *Brit. J. Derm.* **60**, 282 (1948).

HOMBURGER, F., FRIEDLER, G., KELLEY, T., and RUSSFIELD, A. B., 4 allyl-1,2-methylenedioxybenzene (safrole) as a new tool for the study of pathogenesis of toxic hepatic cirrhosis and adenomatosis. *Fed. Proc.* **20**, 288 (1961).

HUEPER, W. C., Environmental and occupational cancer hazards. *Clin. Pharmacol. Ther.* **3**, 776—813 (1962).

HURST, E. W., and PAGET, G. E., Protoporphyrin, cirrhosis and hepatomata in the livers of mice given griseofulvin. *Brit. J. Derm.* **75**, 105—112 (1963).

HURST, L., LACASSAGNE, A., et ROSENBERG, A. J., Action de la réserpine sur la cancérisation du foie chez le rat. *C. R. Soc. Biol.* (Paris) **152**, 441—443 (1958).

JAMAI, K., u. BALO, L., cited by DRUCKREY, H., Krebserzeugende Eigenschaften bei Arzneimitteln. *Münch. med. Wschr.* **9**, 295—297 (1956).

KIRBY, K. S., Induction of tumours by tannin extracts. *Brit. J. Cancer* **14**, 147—150 (1960).

KLEIN, M., Induction of lung adenomas following exposure of pregnant, newborn and immature male mice to urethan. *Cancer Res.* **14**, 438—440 (1954).

KORPASSY, B., Liver injury by tannic acid. *Schweiz. Zz. Path.* **12**, 13—22 (1949).

— The hepatocarcinogenicity of tannic acid. *Cancer Res.* **19**, 501—504 (1959).

— Tannins as hepatic carcinogens. *Progr. exp. Tumor Res.* (Basel) **2**, 245—290 (1961).

—, and KOVACS, K., Experimental liver cirrhosis in rats, produced by prolonged subcutaneous administration of solutions of tannic acid. *Brit. J. exp. Path.* **30**, 266—272 (1949).

—, et MOSONYI, M., Carcinogenic activity of tannic acid. Liver tumors induced in rats by prolonged subcutaneous administration of tannic acid solutions. *Brit. J. Cancer* **4**, 411—420 (1950).

KOVTOUNOVITCH, G. P., Cancerous ulcer of the skin of the abdomen after continuous application of tar ointment. *Wratchebnaya Gazeta* **4**, 272—273 (1927). Résumé in *Cancer Rev.* **2**, 450 (1927).

LACASSAGNE, A., BUU-HOI, N. et ZAJDELA, F.: Production de sarcomes, chez la Souris, par injections de 4-nitroquinoléine-N-oxyde et de 4-nitroquinaldine-N-oxyde. *C. R. Soc. Biol.* (Paris) **154**, 528—530 (1960).

— — — Inégale efficacité du 4-nitroquinoléine-N-oxyde dans la production d'épithéliomas de la peau chez deux lignées différentes de souris. *C. R. Soc. Biol.* (Paris) **155**, 444—446 (1961).

LE PECQ, J. B., LE TALAER, J. Y., FESTY, B., B., et TRUHAUT, R., Inhibition de la désoxyribonucléase (DNase) par complexation de l'acide désoxyribonucléique à l'aide de certains colorants. *C. R. Acad. Sci.* (Paris) **254**, 3918—3920 (1962).

LIJINSKY, W., SAFFIOTTI, V., and SHUBIK, P., A study of the chemical constitution and carcinogenic action of creosote oil. *J. Nat. Cancer Inst.* **18**, 687—692 (1957).

LLOYD, J. B., and BECK, F., The teratogenic activity of purified samples of trypan blue. *Biochem. J.* **83**, 30—31 (1962).

LUSKY, L. M., and NELSON, A. A., Fibrosarcomas induced by multiple subcutaneous injections of carboxymethylcellulose (CMC), polyvinylpyrrolidone (PVP) and polyoxy-éthylenesorbitan and monostéarate (Tween 60). *Fed. Proc.* **16**, 318 (1957).

MILLER, J. A., SANDIN, R. B., MILLER, E. C., and RUSCH, H. P., The carcinogenicity of compounds related to 2-acetylaminofluorene. II — Variations in the bridges and the 2-substituent. *Cancer Res.* **15**, 188—198 (1955).

MORI, K., and YASUNO, A., Preliminary note on the induction of pulmonary tumors in mice by isonicotinic acid hydrazide feeding. *Gann* **50**, 107—110 (1959). Cf. également MORI, K., Preliminary note on adeno-carcinoma of the lung in mice induced with 4-nitroquinoline N-oxide. *Gann* **52**, 265—270 (1961); Induction of pulmonary tumors in rats by subcutaneous injections of 4-nitroquinoline I-oxide. *Gann* **53**, 303—308 (1962).

MORRIS, H. J., NELSON, A. A., and CALVERY, H. O., Observations on the chronic toxicities of propylene glycol, ethylene glycol, diethylene glycol, ethylene glycol mono-ethyl-ether and diethylene glycol mono-ethylether. *J. Pharmacol.* **74**, 266—273 (1942).

NAKAHARA, W., Newer studies on the carcino-genic action of quinoline N-oxide derivatives. *Arzneimittel-Forsch.* **14**, 842—844 (1964).

— FUKUOKA, F., and SAKAI, S., The relation between carcinogenicity and chemical structure of certain quinoline derivatives. *Gann* **49**, 33—41 (1958).

— —, and SUGIMURA, T., Carcinogenic action of 4 nitroquinoline-N-oxide. *Gann* **48**, 129—137 (1957).

OKABAYASHI, T., Antifungal substances. VIII—The mutagenic activity of 4-nitroquinoleine N-oxide on fungi. *Hakkô Kôgakn Zasshi* **33**, 513—516 (1955).

PAGET, G. E., The morphological evaluation of toxic action. *A symposium on the evaluation of drug toxicity* (ed. A. L. WALPOLE and A. SPINKS). London: J & A. Churchill 1958.

PERROT, L., et GORIS, A., Essai d'une terminolo-gie des corps désignés généralement sous le nom de „tanins". *Bull. Sci. pharmacol.* **16**, 189—191 (1909).

POEL, W. E., and KAMMER, A. G., Experimen-tal carcinogenicity of coaltar fractions: the carcinogenicity of creosote oils. *J. Nat. Cancer Inst.* **18**, 41—50 (1957).

RIVIERE, M. R., OBERMAN, B., ARNOLD, J. et GUERIN, M., Tumeurs mélaniques déve-loppées chez les Hamsters dorés après appli-cation cutanée d'uréthane. *C. R. Soc. Biol.* **158**, 2254—2257 (1964).

ROBERTSON, O. H., LOOSLI, C. G., PUCK, T. T., WISE, H., LEMON, H. M., and LESTER, W., Tests for the chronic toxicity of propylene glycol and triethylene glycol on monkeys and rats by vapor inhalation and oral ad-ministration. *J. Pharmacol. exp. Ther.* **91**, 52—76 (1947).

ROE, F. J. C., The relevance of predinical as-sessment of carcinogenesis. *Clin. Pharmacol Therap.* **7**, 77—111 (1966).

—, BOSCH, D., and BOUTWELL, R. K., The carcinogenicity of creosote oil: The induc-tion of lung tumors in mice. *Cancer Res.* **18**, 1176—1178 (1958).

ROOK, A. J., GRESHAM, G. A., and DAVIS, R. A., Squamous epithelioma possibly induced by the therapeutic application of tar. *Brit. J. Cancer* **10**, 17—23 (1956).

ROSMANITH, J., Un cas de cancer du goudron sur lupus érythémateux. (traduction fran-çaise du titre) *Pracov. Lék.* **5**, 270 (1953).

RUSCH, H. P., BOSCH, D., and BOUTWELL, R. K., The influence of irritants on mitotic activity and tumor formation in mouse epidermis. *Acta Un. int. Cancr.* **2**, 699—703 (1955).

ROUS, P., Surmise and fact on the nature of cancer. *Nature* (Lond.) **183**, 2, 1357—1361 (1959).

SALAMAN, M. H., and GLENDENNING, O. M., Tumour promotion in mouse skin by sclero-sing agents. *Brit. J. Cancer*, 434—444 (1957).

SCHMÄHL, D., u. REITER, A., Prüfung von Räuchereiprodukten auf krebserregende Wir-kung. *Z. Krebsforsch.* **59**, 397—401 (1953).

— — Fehlen einer cancerogenen Wirkung beim Phenacetin. *Arzneimittel-Forsch.* **4**, 404—405 (1954).

SEN GUPTA, K. P., Hyperplasia of urinary tract epithelium induced by continuous ad-ministration of sulphonamide derivatives. *Brit. J. Cancer* **16**, 110—119 (1962).

SHELANSKI, H. A., and CLARK, A. M., Physio-logical action of sodium carboxymethyl-cellulose on laboratory animals and human subjects. *Food Res.* **13**, 29—35 (1948).

SHIRASU, Y., and OHTA, A., A preliminary note on the carcinogenicity of 4-hydroxy aminoquinoline N oxide. *Gann.* **54**, 221—223 (1963).

SHUSTEROV, G., Cité par SHABAD, L., Communi-cation personnelle 1926.

SIMLER, M., MAURER, M., et MANDARD, J. C., Cancer du foie sur cirrhose au tétrachlorure de carbone. *Strasbourg méd.* **15**, 910—918 (1964).

STERNBERG, A., Beiträge zur experimentellen Krebserzeugung durch Teer. *Z. Krebsforsch.* **20**, 420—431 (1923).

TAKAYAMA, S., Effect of 4-nitroquinoline N-oxide painting on azo dye hepatocarcinogenesis in rats, with note on induction of skin fibrosarcoma. *Gann* **52**, 165—171 (1961).

— Carcinogenic action of 6-chloro-4-nitroquinoline I-oxide on the rat skin. *Gann* **53**, 167—170 (1962).

TAKIZAWA, N., Carcinogenic action of certain quinones. *Proceedings of the imp. Acad.* (Tokyo) **16**, 309—312 (1940).

— Über die experimentelle Erzeugung der Haut- und Lungenkrebse bei der Maus durch Bepinselung mit Chinone. *Gann.* **34**, 158—160 (1940).

— Über die Wucherung des Epithels des Lungengewebes bei der Maus durch die Bepinselung von Chinone. Beiträge zur Histogenese des Lungenkrebses. *Gann* **35**, 327—330 (1941).

TRAININ, N., KAYE, A. M., and BERENBLUM, I., Influence of mutagens on the initiation of skin carcinogenesis. *Biochem. Pharmacol.* **13**, 263—267 (1964).

TRUFFI, M., Lesioni verrucoidi della cute umana da catrame. *G. ital. Derm. Sif.* **65**, 553—562 (1924).

— Sul cancro da catrame nel topo. *G. ital. Derm. e Sif.* **66**, 302—315 (1925).

TRUHAUT, R., Sur l'utilisation des colorants en thérapeutique et les dangers qui peuvent en résulter pour la santé humaine. *Sem. Hôp. Paris* **34**, 902—925 (1958).

— Recherches sur les risques de nocivité à long terme de l'hydroxy-8-quinoleine au cours de son utilisation comme conservateur alimentaire. Comptes-rendus du 5ème congr. internat. de Nutrition Washington 1960, Abstracts, p. 80. Cf. également *Ann. pharm. franç.* **21**, 266 (1963).

TRUHAUT, R., Sur les risques de cancérisation pouvant résulter de l'emploi de certains agents chimiques en thérapeutique. Comptesrendus dela 3ème réunion de l'Association Européenne pour l'étude de la toxicité des drogues, Lausanne, Janvier 1964. *Excerpta med.* (Amst.), *Internat. Congr.-Series,* N° 75, 101—106 (1964).

TUCHMANN-DUPLESSIS, H., and MERCIER-PAROT, L., Malformations of rat embryos produced by trypan blue. *Biol. méd.* (Paris) **48**, 239—251 (1959).

U.S. Food and Drug Administration, Federal Register, 12412, 3 décembre (1960).

VEIEL, F., Teerkrebs beim Menschen. *Arch. Derm. Syph.* (Berl.) **148**, 142—156 (1924/25).

WATANABE, G., and SUGIMOTO, S., Study on the carcinogenicity of formaldehyde. 2nd report. Seven cases of transplantable sarcomas of rats appearing in the areas of repeated subcutaneous injections of urotropin. *Gann* **46**, 365—366 (1955).

WINKLE, W. jr. VAN, and NEWMAN, H. W., Further results of continued administration of propylene glycol. *Food Res.* **6**, 509—516 (1941).

WOODHOUSE, D. L., and IRWIN, J. O., The carcinogenic activity of some petroleum fractions and extracts. Comparative results in tests on mice repeated after an interval of eighteen months. *J. Hyg.* (Lond.) **48**, 121—134 (1950).

Discussion

Schoental: I should be grateful for Professor TRUHAUT's opinion with regard to the carcinogenic hazard from sassafras oil.

Truhaut: Long term toxicological studies in the U.S.A. have shown safrole to be carcinogenic. For this reason the use of safrole and oil of sassafras was discontinued in the U.S.A. by the beverage industry. I have to stress here that safrole has shown carcinogenic action only at high levels in the diet (5000 ppm). By comparison the amounts of sassafras oil used in certain pharmaceutical preparations is small (e.g. 0.5%). This is of the same order as the concentration of safrole in cinnamon and nutmeg, the use of which has not been banned in the U.S.A.

Shabad: I congratulate Professor TRUHAUT on providing us with an excellent introduction to the Symposium which is orientated towards the prevention of cancer.

Frazer: I should like to say how I appreciate the remarks of Professor TRUHAUT regarding the balance between risks and benefits.

Druckrey: I agree with Professor TRUHAUT that every drug should be submitted to long-term tests, including carcinogenicity evaluation, before its use is authorized.

Principles of Methodology Relating to the Potential Carcinogenicity of Medical Drugs

I. Berenblum

Department of Experimental Biology, The Weizmann Institute of Science, Rehovoth, Israel

As you will have gathered from the title of my paper, I shall be dealing with generalities rather than with factual information. Little of what I have to say here is really new; for this is not the first time that I have been called upon to give an account of the principles underlying the work of the UICC Panel on Carcinogenicity.

There is, nevertheless, some justification for reviewing these basic principles from a somewhat new angle, as a contribution towards the eventual integration of the triple attack on the problem of carcinogenesis in man:— (i) the accumulation of knowledge about environmental cancer in man (which is the task of the Committee on Geographical Pathology of the Cancer Research Commission), (ii) the establishment of improved methods and conditions for carcinogenicity testing (which is the function of the Panel on Carcinogenicity of the Cancer Research Commission) and (iii) the prophylactic approach to the problem of human cancer of extrinsic origin (which is the concern of the Committee on Cancer Prevention of the Cancer Control Commission). No one of these three approaches can have much validity in any practical sense without reference to the other two.

My task today is to discuss some of the problems connected with carcinogenicity testing, insofar as these have a direct bearing on the over-all problem of human carcinogenesis.

The principles of methodology referred to here raise 2 separate problems: — (i) what are the most reliable methods and conditions for testing? and (ii) what is the relevance of the results obtained from such animal tests to the actual or potential carcinogenic hazard in man?

The problem of testing methods is essentially technical — having to do with the choice of animal species and strains, the number of species required and the kind and number of tissues on which the test is to be performed, the number of animals per single test, and the kind of controls — e.g. regarding the spontaneous incidence of the particular type of tumour in the particular species, strain and line of animals used, the facilities for accurate histological diagnosis of the lesions elicited, etc.

It may be argued that in a general symposium such as this, there is no need to enter into a detailed discussion of specific techniques. The issue is, however, not quite so simple. It is not as if we were already in a position to agree on what are the optimal conditions for carcinogenicity testing. The existing knowledge is far from sufficient to permit this. All we can do at present is to propose certain minimal requirements, short of which the tests would be of dubious value. But even if optimal conditions for testing were available, one would still not be able to carry them out in a routine fashion, because the amount of effort involved, and the number of animals needed, would be such as to preclude the possibility of coping with more than a few of the many hundreds of substances to be tested. In any event, therefore, the recommended testing system would have to be based on a compromise.

The second issue — concerning the relevance of the results obtained from such animal tests to the actual or potential carcinogenic hazard in man — raises even more difficult problems — of interpretation rather than of technical procedures, though the one is likely to interact on the other. This is a subject which is admirably suited to a general discussion in which a range of experts on widely different aspects of human carcinogenesis can participate.

I propose, therefore, to devote the rest of my talk to this problem, dealing first with carcinogenesis in general, and then with carcinogenesis of medical drugs in particular, in the hope that some of the ideas expressed here will stimulate a fruitful discussion.

Laboratory animals are sensitive to extrinsic carcinogenic action, though each species, and sometimes each particular strain or subline, reacts differently, both in intensity and in relative responsiveness according to organ or tissue. We know, for instance, that responsiveness to local skin carcinogenesis is very pronounced in mice and rabbits, but rather weak in rats and giunea-pigs, while in hamsters, it presents some spe-

cial features; that responsiveness to local subcutaneous carcinogenesis is exceptionally pronounced in rats, but almost nonexistent in the rabbit; and that responsiveness to remotely-acting carcinogenesis, e.g. by acetylaminofluorene, 2-naphthylamine or urethane, varies greatly from one species to another.

Man fits into this confused pattern by also responding to a wide range of carcinogens, though in his case, the latent period is exceptionally long.

The important question, from the viewpoint of using animal tests as a guide to human responsiveness, is which animal species corresponds most closely to man in carcinogenic response. The little we know would indicate that there is no single answer to the question: that it varies according to the carcinogenic system under consideration, that is to say, according to the nature of the carcinogen and the target organ in question. For skin carcinogenesis, the mouse would seem to be closest to man; for urinary bladder carcinogenesis, the dog is closest; while for mammary gland carcinogenesis the mouse, rat and human responses have points of similarities and differences. For gastric carcinogenesis, probably none of the available laboratory animals is suitable; and the same is probably true for lung carcinogenesis, for though the mouse can be made to develop lung tumours through extrinsic action, these tumours are unrelated to those occurring in man. Leukemias in animals also appear to differ in many important respects from those arising in man, so that the results of animal tests for the leukaemias must be interpreted with some reservations.

Fortunately, we are not looking for an absolute correlation between animal and human response to carcinogenic action. A positive response in an animal may not always denote a similar response in man, but it does imply that the substance in question is suspect and, therefore, *potentially* carcinogenic for man. There is, however, a corollary to this, namely, that a negative result in animals does not necessarily exclude the possibility of the substance being carcinogenic for man.

From this, one may conclude that it is possible, on the basis of animal testing for carcinogenicity, to brand a substance as suspect, but not to certify one as safe. (This is, of course, also true for acute and subacute toxicity testing: cf. thalidomide! I could also quote a curious example of our own experience: — A dose of the powerful purgative, croton oil, sufficient to kill a man, can be administered by stomach tube to a mouse without even eliciting the slightest evidence of diarrhoea. Yet, animal testing for acute and subacute toxicity is universally accepted as an essential prerequisite to the introduction of any new drug or other substance for human use.)

Another technical problem with far-reaching implications is that concerned with the dose, concentration and persistence of action of the carcinogen, and related to it is the factor of the age of the responding individual.

For all practical purposes, a carcinogen is, like any other noxious substance, only harmful above a certain critical dose level. For effective carcinogenesis, a cumulative dose, spread over a long period, is more potent than the same, or even a larger dose administered over a very short period. With some carcinogens, newborn animals are much more responsive than adults. The minimal carcinogenic dose may also be influenced by ancillary factors, such as diet, general health, etc.

The question before us is how to apply this information in a rational way towards the prevention of extrinsic car-

cinogenesis in man. Too rigid an application, with the exclusion of all carcinogenic or potentially carcinogenic substances — however weakly-acting they may be in animals, or however restricted their action may be (e.g. only causing tumours at the site of subcutaneous implantation), irrespective of dose, concentration or length of action in man — would be irrational, and in the long run, a self-defeating policy. On the other hand, too complacent an attitude would be dangerous and inexcusable. One cannot even afford the luxury of a wait-and-see policy in doubtful cases, because by the time the carcinogenic hazard expresses itself in man, the population at risk will already have been exposed to the substance for some 10—20 years, with all that this implies.

The problem is particularly important in connection with the introduction of new medicinal drugs, though it applies equally to food additives and to other substances for general domestic use. To suggest that no new product should be accepted for human use until it has been thoroughly tested for carcinogenicity, would be meaningless under existing conditions, since the available laboratory facilities for such testing could not cope with one hundredth of the existing products on the market, let alone the new ones added every day.

Is there, then, any interim solution? Are there certain guiding principles which could, at least, help to avoid major catastrophies, enabling the testing laboratories to set up lists of priorities for urgent testing, on the one hand, and advising the practising clinicians about the conditions under which untested drugs are likely to involve a greater or lesser risk, on the other? Here there is ample scope for debate.

The setting up of lists of priorities for testing has only limited practicability, since the more we learn about chemical carcinogens, the wider the range of compounds found to be capable of inducing tumours. We know that polycyclic aromatic hydrocarbons, azo-dye intermediates, and alkylating agents are, on the whole, more likely to be carcinogenic than other classes of compounds. Epoxides and lactones are generally considered suspect, as well as compounds which are likely to yield, after chemical or metabolic breakdown, reactive radicles. But this does not mean that other types of compounds ought to be neglected. Nor is it possible to predict on *a priori* grounds which, for instance, of the hundreds of dyestuffs and the dozens of intermediates are likely to prove carcinogenic.

Apart from probability based on chemical structure as a guiding factor, high priority for testing should be given to substances likely to be used by large sections of the population, and those likely to be administered for prolonged periods.

This brings us to the role of the clinician in determining the use of a drug which has not been previously tested for carcinogenic action or which is even known to have potential carcinogenic side-effects.

A distinction must surely be made between (a) administering medically useful drugs under careful supervision, for illnesses of short duration, and (b) the indiscriminate use of drugs throughout one's lifetime, without supervision — e.g. as headache pills, contraceptives, etc., where these have not undergone a thorough testing for carcinogenicity. This applies also to medicaments for skin lesions. (The fact that 5—10% of chronic skin diseases tend eventually to undergo malignant change, is hardly surprising when one remembers that such lesions are generally treated by a choice of 3 carcinogenic methods — by application of tar ointments, x-irradiation, or internal administration of arsenic.) The high sensitivity of newborn mice to carcinogenic action might also have relevance to human infants, and allowance should be made accordingly, even if, in this case, the drugs are administered for short periods.

The problem of liver carcinogenesis deserves special consideration. On the one hand, there is the fact that primary carcinoma of the liver is rare in those countries (European and American) where the intake of medicinal drugs of all kinds is very extensive. On the other hand, more and more liver carcinogens are being discovered experimentally, some of them belonging to types of compounds not previously suspected of being carcinogenic, including some actually used in human therapy. The anomaly cannot be attributed to man's inability to respond to liver carcinogenesis, in view of the exceptionally high incidence of liver cancer in Africa and South Asia — presumably caused by as yet unknown extrinsic carcinogens. We can only surmise that we have been very fortunate so far.

I could hardly be expected to end this talk without mentioning the problem of cocarcinogenesis, initiation and promotion, etc. in relation to human carcinogenesis. The suggestion has, for instance, been put forward by several different investigators that tobacco smoke may act as a promoting agent rather than as a complete carcinogen. It is also possible that human leukemia likewise depends on a two-stage process. In theory, the possibility of such factors operating in man exists, and must, therefore, be taken into account in any speculative discussion of human carcinogenic hazards. In practice, we still know very little about promoting action in man, while methods for testing are, except for skin, still very inadequate. To pursue the subject further at this stage would not, therefore, help us very much.

I have tried to describe to you some of the difficulties involved in carcinogenicity testing procedures, and also to draw attention to certain practical benefits to be derived from such services, despite their serious limitations. The potentialities for cancer prevention in man are real; it is our task to remove the obstacles in the way.

Discussion

Roe: The subject of the possible cancer hazard from drugs seems to be made unnecessarily difficult because of the tendency to regard carcinogenicity as an "all or none" phenomenon. As soon as anyone has found a method of producing cancer in any species and under any set of experimental conditions by the administration of a drug, that drug comes to be regarded as carcinogenic. Elsewhere (ROE, 1965), I have suggested a system of "Carcinogenicity Rating" to be applied to drugs. If the assessment is on a 0—100 scale, I would suggest a rating of 50 for substances which have never been tested for carcinogenicity in laboratory animals, but for which there are no a priori reasons for suspecting carcinogenic activity. Ratings between 50 and 1 would apply to substances which have given negative results in experimental and epidemiological studies: the better and more relevant the evidence, the lower the rating. Substances giving rise to positive results in many species (i.e. potent carcinogens) would be given ratings of 100, whilst ratings between 50 and 100 would apply to cases where positive results had been obtained in animals, but only in response to un-realistically high doses or following administration by irrelevant routes.

Such a system takes care of the unpalatable possibility that the only practical distinction to make between drugs in respect of their carcinogenic action is between those which have already been shown to be capable of inducing cancer and those which have not yet been shown to be capable of doing so.

Such a rating system would also be helpful in deciding priorities and how to make best use of the limited facilities available for testing for carcinogenicity.

Reference

ROE, F. J. C., The relevance of preclinical assessment of carcinogenesis. *Clin. Pharmac. Ther.* **7**, 77 (1965).

Rudali: I should like to start a discussion on the sensitivity of newborn animals to carcinogens. It seems from the work of Professor SHUBIK, Dr. ROE, Professor BERENBLUM and my team that the newborn mouse is the animal of choice for testing for carcinogenicity.

Frazer: The object of the studies described by Professor BERENBLUM is to demonstrate possible carcinogenic action, but the problem of the person developing a new drug is to assess any possible cancer risk in man. These two objectives are not synonymous. Many factors come into the picture in assessing the risk in man; for example, the life expectancy of the patient. These matters and the feasibility of carrying out extensive animal studies on every drug will be discussed later.

Those engaged in cancer research are, of course, most interested in substances that are carcinogenic; those concerned with drugs or with food additives are more interested in substances that are not carcinogenic. Is enough attention paid to lack of carcinogenic action? — For example, a substance that is carcinogenic in one species, or by one route of administration, but not by others. The elucidation of the reason for the lack of effect might be illuminating.

Davey: Professor BERENBLUM has made a plea to extend the number of species and strains used in carcinogenic work. I wish to make a plea for more work on methods to study the metabolism of drugs. At present these are difficult and laborious, and simplification is a matter of urgency. Unless we have such methodology we are in danger of wasting much of our work in laboratory animals, at least as it relates to man, because the metabolism of the compound in the species chosen for study might be quite different.

Hueper: Several children developed cancer at the site of poliomyelitis vaccination. This may be due to the presence of mineral oil in the vaccine. It is essential therefore that all drugs intended for administration by the subcutaneous route are first tested by the same route in animals.

Some Aspects of Medical Drug Testing for Carcinogenic Activity

Giuseppe Della Porta

Istituto Nazionale per lo Studio e la Cura dei Tumori, Milan, Italy

Our present knowledge of the mechanism of carcinogenesis is so limited as to make even more difficult than in the field of general toxicology the evaluation of the validity in human terms of any result obtained in tests of medical drugs for possible carcinogenic action. In other branches of toxicology the clinical evidence may come soon to confirm or not the experimental result. This cannot avoid unpleasant happenings which may even reach the dimension of the case of thalidomide, but at least the pharmacologist may have the chance of controlling, sooner or later, the validity of his results. This does not happen with carcinogenesis, where a practical usefulness of epidemiology is at present limited to small groups of population, mostly in the industrial field. The identification of carcinogenic effect induced in man by a drug appears rather problematic because of the long latent period of tumors, of the multiplicity of drugs used and of the many possible other environmental carcinogens. Thus, the results, either positive or negative, offered by the experimental oncologist cannot be confirmed by clinical evidence and are often challenged, and the necessity of testing is often disputed.

The limitation of our knowledge must be recognized not only to encourage research on the subject, but also to discourage drastic positions and useless polemics, which are often based on informations whose apparent soundness can not be scientifically proved. There are some aspects of the problem, however, that should be strongly stressed and defended if we want to maintain a sense to our present experimental efforts, and other aspects that we should be ready to re-evaluate if we want to have better, but simpler and shorter experimental programs.

Medical drug testing for carcinogenic activity follows the same general principles which apply to the testing of food additives, contaminants or components, even if the evaluation of the hazard for man can be different. The first question to which the experiment must give an answer is if the chemical tested is or not carcinogenic to the animal species selected under the experimental conditions used. Then, it is possible to conceive an experimental model which may repeat more closely the situation of the use of the drug in the human consumption.

One specific difficulty is presented by drugs with hormonal activity, whose carcinogenic effect has been proved exhaustively, although other mechanisms than those operating in chemical carcinogenesis are postulated (Mühlbock and Boot, 1959). Natural and synthetic exogenous hormones are able to induce cancer in endocrine and target organs after a long period of treatment, and the same tumors can be obtained with endogenous biological manipulation. The hormonal environment may influence also the spontaneous appearance, or the induction with other carcinogens, of tumors in organs which are not under a direct or specific hormonal control. Moreover, large doses of estrogens have been reported to induce leukemias in mice (GARDNER et al., 1944) and renal tumors in hamsters (KIRKMAN, 1959). It appears that the practical value of the testing of hormones for carcinogenicity is limited and should be mostly directed with a proper experimental design to the study of the possible carcinogenic action on tissues not specifically controlled by hormones.

This paper deals only with a few aspects of the problem of testing, since principles and practical procedures for carcinogenicity tests have been worked out by various committees and frequently discussed in detail, and there is very little to be said that has not yet been said repeatedly.

One of the major difficulties consists in the length of the experiments, that is often disputed by general toxicologists. Waiting for a reliable rapid bioassay method, there is no doubt that an experiment of carcinogenicity must cover the entire life span of the species used. Even a superficial survey of the data available in the literature indicates that chemical carcinogenesis is a long process that may take over a year in mice and about two years in rats before being fully developed. There are exceptions to this rule, where strong carcinogens given at high doses may shorten the process, but usually this happens for special types of carcinogenesis, as skin carcinogenesis, for tumors of particular tissues and organs as, for example, hepatomas in rats, lung ade-

nomas in mice, or thymic lymphosarcomas which may stop to appear after the 30th week of age of the carcinogen-treated mice. In the same experiment, however, other types of tumors may arise from other tissues much later in life. Even the common mammary tumors may start to appear after the 40th week of age in mice and after the 60th week in rats, unless drastic procedures as those introduced by HUGGINS (1959) are used.

A logical approach to the attempts of shortening the experiments, is offered by the study of specific morphological and biochemical lesions which should appear before the onset of tumors and thus give an early indication of the future course of the experiment. The detection of these often unknown early lesions is extremely difficult and may give misleading informations for the difficulty of distinguishing between non specific toxic lesions and preneoplastic lesions, and because their absence is no proof that tumors will not develop later on. With the present methods of investigation, it is questionable, for instance, if differences between the thymic atrophy caused by a carcinogenic polycyclic hydrocarbon or by urethan and that caused by cortisone can be ascertained, although the former compounds will induce a high percentage of thymic lymphosarcomas, and the latter will not; the same consideration applies to the thymic repair and hyperplasia which follow atrophy. However, the study of the kinetics of these changes, may be rewarding (FIORE-DONATI and KAYE, 1964). Similarly, necrotic and regenerative lesions of the liver do not necessarily evolve into hepatomas and are not even obligatory changes for the induction of such tumors (ESCHENBRENNER and MILLER, 1946). On the other hand, cytological abnormalities of the parenchymal liver cells and proliferation of bile-duct cells may be utilized as a good indicator of proliferative disorders in the liver (FARBER, 1963). The relationship in different organs between hyperplastic foci and neoplasia is still undetermined (BERENBLUM, 1954; SHIMKIN and POTISSAR, 1955; FOULDS, 1956; DEOME et al., 1959; CLAYSON et al., 1965), and requires further investigations.

Carcinogenesis certainly involves a series of changes, which may be under different biological and biochemical controls in different organs. In spite of the extensive studies, mostly concentrated on liver carcinogenesis (see in REID, 1962; WEISBURGER and WEISBURGER, 1963; MILLER and MILLER, 1964), it appears that at the present time no biochemical change discovered during the latent period of tumor formation can be assumed as being necessarily relevant to the process of carcinogenesis, but studies in this direction may offer in the future a key solution of the problem.

No short cuts in the length of the experiments can be soundly suggested, but the possibility of shortening the period of treatment may be seriously considered. It is generally suggested that the treatment must be protracted for the entire life span of the species used.

Not too many experiments on dose-response are on record and, naturally, they have been performed with strong carcinogens which in most of the cases are effective even with a single dose, although less so than with repeated smaller doses. With repeated daily doses, it has been established by DRUCKREY (1957, 1959) that within certain limits the carcinogenic effect depends upon the total dose and not on the daily dose which, on the other hand, governs the induction time, in such a way that for very small doses the latent period may exceed the life span of the animal. This means that with the highest possible daily doses the carcinogenic effect will be greater and more rapid. In other words, it is better to adjust the dosage, or at least one of the dosages used, at a level that may cause toxic effect and may compel to a relatively short period of treatment, than to remain on the safe side with a low dose which will permit the experiment to run smoothly for life span.

The stop-experiments of DRUCKREY (1957, 1959) and many other experiments with a single dosing or a brief course of treatment show that in chemical carcinogenesis there is no recovery after the termination of the treatment and that the process which in successive events will end in neoplasia proceeds in absence of the chemical and may take a long time for its full development, with large differences among different species and tissues. It seems likely that a treatment lasting for approximately half the life span of the animal used may be adequate, when followed by an additional observation for the rest of the life. It should be considered that a shortening of the treatment not only makes the experiment less expensive and complicated, but may allow a longer survival of animals in better condition, giving more chances to the possible tumors to develope. Even an undetectable state of chronic toxicity may cause a metabolic alteration or an impairment of general condition which in turn may result in subnormal food consumption and all together affect the development of tumors (TANNENBAUM and SILVERSTONE, 1953).

Another aspect of carcinogenicity testing I should like to discuss is the use of newborn animals. It had been known for some time that young animals are more susceptible to chemical carcinogenesis than older animals, but the report by PIETRA, SPENCER and SHUBIK (1959) demonstrated that mice given a single dose of 30 μg of 7,12-dimethylbenz(a)anthracene when less than 12 hours develop

Table I. *Tabulation of the published data on the occurrence of lymphosarcomas,*

Compound	Strain [1]	Age	Route	Vehicle	Dose μg
7,12-dimethylbenz[a]-anthracene	Swiss	< 24 h	sc-ip	aqueous gelatine	30—60
	Swiss	< 24 h	sc	tricaprylin or olive oil	50—100
	Swiss	< 24 h	it	olive oil	10
	CBA	< 24 h	sc	aqueous gelatine	30
	101	< 24 h	sc	aqueous gelatine	30
	BALB/c	< 24 h	sc	aqueous gelatine	30
	AKR	< 24 h	sc	tricaprylin	100
	C57BL	< 24 h	sc	tricaprylin or olive oil	60—100
	C3Hf	< 24 h	sc	olive oil	60
3-methylcholanthrene	Swiss	< 24 h	sc-ip	aqueous gelatine	30—40
	Swiss	< 24 h	sc	aqueous gelatine	60
	Swiss	< 24 h	sc	olive oil	100
	Swiss	< 24 h	it	olive oil	30
	Sw-germfree	< 24 h	sc	olive oil	100
	Albino	8 d	po	methocel Aerosol OT	1500×10
	Gp/NIH	< 24 h	sc	olive oil	300
	Gp/NIH	< 24 h	sc	olive oil	11—100
	Gp/NIH	7 d	sc	olive oil	100
	Gp/NIH	< 24 h	sc	olive oil	1.2—11.1
	Gp/NIH	< 24 h	sc	olive oil	0.41
	Gp/NIH	< 24 h	sc	olive oil	0.14—0.0051
	C3H	< 24 h	sc	olive oil	100
	C3H	1—2 wks	sc	olive oil	4.5—30
	C57BL	< 24 h	sc	olive oil	100
	C57BL	< 24 h	it	olive oil	30
	AKR	< 24 h	sc	aqueous gelatine	60
	SL	< 24 h	sc	aqueous gelatine	60
benzo[a]pyrene	Swiss	< 24 h	sc	aqueous gelatine	30—40
	Swiss	< 24 h	ip	aqueous gelatine	30—40
	Albino	< 24 h	sc	aqueous gelatine	20—40
dibenz[a, h]-anthracene	Swiss	< 24 h	sc-ip	aqueous gelatine	30—40
	Gp/NIH	< 24 h	sc	olive oil	60—180
	Gp/NIH	< 24 h	sc	olive oil	20

[1] Gp/NIH = General purpose/NIH.

lung adenomas, subcutaneous sarcomas and hepatomas in newborn or infant mice

Lymphosarcomas		Lung adenomas %	Sc. sarcomas %	Hepatomas %	References
%	ALP[2] wks				
19—55	15—19	77—85	0	0	Pietra *et al.*, 1959, 1961; Stick, 1960
27—80	13—15	66—100	7—33	0	Rappaport and Baroni, 1962; Toth *et al.*, 1963; Chieco-Bianchi *et al.*, 1965
55	19	92	0	♂ 67	Chieco-Bianchi *et al.*, 1965
15	26	88	0	0	Roe *et al.*, 1961
20	16	96	0	0	Roe *et al.*, 1961
15	36—43	100	5	0	Roe *et al.*, 1963
60	22	11	16	0	Toth *et al.*, 1962
10—27	21—30	7—23	9—15	0	Baroni and Cefis, 1963; Chieco-Bianchi *et al.*, 1965
53	20	44	19	♂ 88	Chieco-Bianchi *et al.*, 1965
4—16	15—17	88—95	0	4—8	Pietra *et al.*, 1961
6	48	97	38	♂ 23	Nishizuka *et al.*, 1965
6	19	98	53	0	Chieco-Bianchi *et al.*, 1965
48	14	97	0	♂ 28	Chieco-Bianchi *et al.*, 1965
—	—	100	—	—	Pollard and Salomon, 1963
0	—	95	0	♀ 23 ♂ 80	Klein, 1959
16	16—24	100	22	0	Kelly and O'Gara, 1961
0—3	16—24	86—100	11—35	0	Kelly and O'Gara, 1961
0	—	93	20	0	Kelly and O'Gara, 1961
—	—	—	40—42	—	O'Gara *et al.*, 1962
—	—	—	6	—	O'Gara *et al.*, 1962
—	—	—	0	—	O'Gara *et al.*, 1962
0	—	62	42	♂ 54	Kelly and O'Gara, 1961
—	—	—	26—91	—	Saxén, 1953
0—3	—	17—25	29—78	0	Kelly and O'Gara, 1961; Chieco-Bianchi *et al.*, 1965
35	13	16	0	0	Chieco-Bianchi *et al.*, 1965
86	38	22	0	0	Nishizuka and Nakakuki, 1964
0	—	19	31	0	Nishizuka and Nakakuki, 1964
0	—	60	0	3	Pietra *et al.*, 1961
30	43	90	0	0	Pietra *et al.*, 1961
3	30	26—44	0	12	Grant and Roe, 1963
0—5	51	0—26	0	0	Pietra *et al.*, 1961
0—1	—	85—100	13—25	0	Kelly and O'Gara, 1961
0	—	90	0	0	Kelly and O'Gara, 1961

[2] ALP = average latent period.

Table I.

Compound	Strain	Age	Route	Vehicle	Dose µg
dibenz[a, h]anthracene	Gp/NIH	< 24 h	sc	olive oil	2.2—6.7
	Gp/NIH	7 d	sc	olive oil	60
	Gp/NIH	< 24 h	sc	olive oil	6.7
	Gp/NIH	< 24 h	sc	olive oil	0.74—2.2
	Gp/NIH	< 24 h	sc	olive oil	0.083—0.25
	Gp/NIH	< 24 h	sc	olive oil	0.028
	Gp/NIH	< 24 h	sc	olive oil	0.0031 0.0092
	C3H	< 24 h	sc	olive oil	60
	C57BL	< 24 h	sc	olive oil	60
benz[a]anthracene	BALB/c	< 24 h	sc	aqueous gelatine	50
	BALB/c	2—4—8 d	sc	aqueous gelatine	50
ethyl methane sulfonate	BALB/c	< 24 h	sc	water	100
2-naphthylamine	BALB/c	< 24 h	sc	aqueous gelatine	50
2-naphthylhydroxyl-amine	BALB/c	< 24 h	sc	arachis oil	50
dimethylnitrosamine	BALB/c	< 24 h	sc	water	15—30
9-methylanthracene	Swiss	< 24 h	sc-ip	aqueous gelatine	30—40
4-amino-2',3-dimethyl-azobenzene	A	< 24 h	sc	aqueous gelatine	400—700
N-2-fluorenyl acetamide	Albino	7 d	po	methocel Aerosol OT	700 × 10
4-nitroquinoline 1-oxide	A	24 h	sc	aqueous gelatine	40
	A	10 d	sc	aqueous gelatine	100
Urethan	Swiss	< 24 h	sc-ip	water	40
	Swiss	< 24 h	sc-ip	water	1000
	Swiss	< 24 h	sc	water	2000
	Swiss	5 d	sc	water	1000/gbw
	Swiss	2 wks	ip	water	1000/gbw
	CTM	< 24 h	sc	water	1000
	CTM	< 24 h	sc	water	3000
	C57BL	< 24 h— 7 wks	sc	water	1000/gbw × 8
	C3Hf	< 24 h	sc	water	1000/gbw
	C3Hf/Lw	< 72 h	sc	water	1000/gbw

(Continued)

Lymphosarcomas		Lung adenomas %	Sc. sarcomas %	Hepa-tomas %	References
%	ALP wks				
0	—	35—38	0—11	0	KELLY and O'GARA, 1961
0	—	93	0	0	KELLY and O'GARA, 1961
—	—	—	62	—	O'GARA et al., 1962
—	—	—	23—31	—	O'GARA et al., 1962
—	—	—	10	—	O'GARA et al., 1962
—	—	—	0	—	O'GARA et al., 1962
—	—	—	1—2	—	O'GARA et al., 1962
0	—	46	26	0	KELLY and O'GARA, 1961
0	—	9	13	0	KELLY and O'GARA, 1961
2	36—43	46	0	0	ROE et al., 1963
0	—	24—30	0	0	ROE et al., 1963
0	—	53	0	0	ROE et al., 1963
0	—	21	0	1	ROE et al., 1963
0	—	27	0	0	ROE et al., 1963
2	30	21	0	40	TOTH et al., 1964
10	60	7	0	0	PIETRA et al., 1961
11	—	81	0	♀ 18 ♂ 46	NISHIZUKA et al., 1965
0	—	29	0	♀ 1 ♂ 60	KLEIN, 1959
25	36	98	0	0	NISHIZUKA et al., 1964
18	41	95	0	4	NISHIZUKA et al., 1964
0	—	37—46	0	—	PIETRA et al., 1961
20—21	14	71—80	0	—	PIETRA et al., 1961
20—21	15	100	0	♀ 9 ♂ 87	FIORE-DONATI et al., 1961; DE BENEDICTIS et al., 1962; CHIECO-BIANCHI et al., 1963
17	18	100	0	♀ 18 ♂ 70	FIORE-DONATI et al., 1961; CHIECO-BIANCHI et al., 1963
—	—	100	0	—	ROGERS, 1951
8	45	60	0	♀ 32 ♂ 72	DELLA PORTA et al., 1963
29	29	65	0	♀ 34 ♂ 68	DELLA PORTA et al., 1963
100	17	—	0	—	DOELL and CARNES, 1962
♀ 41 ♂ 0	44	40	0	♀ 29 ♂ 96	LIEBELT et al., 1961
0	—	0	0	♀ 75 ♂ 75	LAW and PRECERUTTI, 1963

Table I.

Compound	Strain	Age	Route	Vehicle	Dose µg
Urethan	C3Hf/Lw	< 72 h—3 wks	sc	water	1000/gbw × 4
	C3Hf/Lw	< 24 h	sc	water	2000
	BALB/c	< 24 h	sc	water	2000
	DBAf	< 24 h	sc	water	2000
	AKR	< 24 h	sc	water	1000—2000
	B6AF$_1$	1—6 wks	po	Methocel Aerosol OT	5000 × 15
	B6AF$_1$	1—6 wks	po	Methocel Aerosol OT	2500 × 15

rapidly a high incidence of thymic lymphosarcomas and lung adenomas. This result has been confirmed and extended, and it has been established that by and large newborn or infant mice develop more rapidly more tumors than young adults similarly treated. Very promptly the system has been proposed for testing of new chemicals for carcinogenicity (KELLY and O'GARA, 1961; ROE et al., 1961; KLEIN, 1962) and the suggestion accepted, although with caution (DELLA PORTA, 1964; HUEPER, 1964; WALPOLE, 1964). As a matter of fact there are not enough available informations to warrant the abandonment of the currently accepted use of young adults. In Table I the experiments published and the results obtained in newborn mice are summarized, with the inclusion of infant or suckling animals. A few additional informations are available from experiments in newborn rats and hamsters (TANNENBAUM et al., 1962; HUGGINS and FUKUNISHI, 1963; KELLY et al., 1964; LEE et al., 1963; TERRACINI and MAGEE, 1964; TOTH and SHUBIK, 1963). From the data reported it appears that too few compounds have been tested in this system so far, moreover with a concentrated attention to polycyclic hydrocarbons and to urethan. As for the latter compound, it should be mentioned that LAW and PRECERUTTI (1963) reported inhibition of a viral leukemia in C3H mice injected with urethan at birth, and that in my laboratory an inhibition of the development of mammary tumors was observed in similarly urethan-treated newborn mice (DELLA PORTA et al., 1963). The same compound, however, injected at birth, proved to be highly carcinogenic for the liver with the rapid development of multiple hepatomas. On the whole these results are interesting enough to encourage a more systematic investigation. A number of known non-carcinogenic chemicals and of substances of unknown action should be tested to build up a body of informations apt to assess the validity of a test-system that has undoubtely the advantage of lesser costs and shorter times.

The mechanism of the peculiar reactivity of newborn to carcinogens needs further investigations. From the reports of DOMSKY et al., (1963) for DMBA, and of KAYE (1960), MIRVISH et al. (1964),

(Continued)

Lymphosarcomas		Lung adenomas %	Sc. sarcomas %	Hepatomas %	References
%	ALP wks				
0	—	10	0	♀ 90 ♂ 90	Law and Precerutti, 1963
0	—	17	0	♀ 100 ♂ 100	Trainin et al., 1964
0	—	77	0	0	Trainin et al., 1964
0	—	32	0	♀ 0 ♂ 86	Trainin et al., 1964
37	18	—	0	—	Fiore-Donati et al., 1962
76	21	100	0	10	Klein, 1962
43	21	98	0	♀ 13 ♂ 57	Klein, 1962

and Cividalli et al. (1965) for urethan, it appears that a delayed catabolic pathway of these two carcinogens in newborn or infant mice might be a reasonable explanation. It is known that certain enzymatic and metabolic activities are not completely developed in newborn animals and this may lead to a deficiency of detoxification processes of drugs with retarded elimination and subsequent accumulation. On the contrary, carbon tetrachloride is rapidly excreted by the newborn rat without evidence of liver necrosis (Dawkins, 1963); large amounts of either serine or mercury do not produce renal necrosis in newborn rats (Wachstein and Robinson, 1965); aminopterin causes acute toxicity in the mothers of the injected newborn mice without apparent toxicity in the babies (Toth and Shubik, 1964). Other factors can be thought to be operating in newborn carcinogenesis experiments, as impaired immunological reactions, tissue and cell immaturity and carcinogenic viruses. In this respect, it has to be mentioned that the suceptibility to the induction of thymic lymphosarcoma is very high when irradiation is administered to newborn or infant mice, and declines in older animals (Kaplan, 1948; Upton et al., 1958, 1960).

From the data reported in Table I it appears that already in a few years different techniques of doses, solvents, route of administration have been used. A different procedure is at present used in my laboratory, where 10-day old mice are injected every second day either intraperitoneally or subcutaneously, for five times, and weaned at 30 days. The use of 10-day old animals is more practical since may cut considerably the chance of cannibalism from the mothers; the use of 5 treatments is justified by the desire of overcoming the danger of leakage of a single dose, and by the great enhancement of response. In fact a treatment with 5 doses of urethan 1 mg/g b.w. at 10 days of age increased the incidence of thymic lymphosarcoma to 20% in C3Hf, 50% in C57BL, and 55% in SWR inbred mice from a level of 0 to 5% seen in newborn animals treated only once with 3 mg of urethan. The average latent period for these thymi clymphosarcomas, calculated from the age at death, varied from 20 to 30 weeks, with some appearing already at 10 weeks of age. The incidence of other type of tumors was enhanced also.

Another practical suggestion which may take advantage of the high susceptibility of newborn mice to carcinogens, is the use for carcinogenicity of reproduction experiments for teratogenicity, provided that the treatment is continued during pregnancy and for a few weeks after birth, and the animals are kept under observation for life span.

A third point that I should like to discuss briefly is the selection of animal species to be used. There is not a single scientific evidence that one species is better than another. The animal that appears better suitable for one compound, may not be for the next one and certainly is not for all possible compounds of unknown reactivity which should be tested. Two or three or four species are better than one on a gambling basis only. Even an accurate metabolic and activation study cannot, at the present, give us more valid informations for a sound selection, since it is not known how to correlate with carcinogenesis species differences or similarities. Also the obvious selection of a short-living species is open to criticism. It is difficult to decide, and the decision is made on practical grounds which involve economical reasons (size, number, time), availability and knowledge of the species, low and well known incidence of spontaneous tumors. For practical reasons also, the tests are limited to two species, one rodent and the dog, but this rule is not reinforced, and the final suggestion ends usually in mice and rats (Report UICC Symposium, 1957; Committee on Medical and Nutritional Aspects of Food Policy, 1960; Subcommittee on Carcinogenesis, 1961; Joint FAO/WHO Expert Committee on Food Additives, 1961). One may even suggest to go a little further, even if I am not ready to stand for this suggestion. If practical reasons and minimal requirements (BERENBLUM, 1964) ought to be the guide in this matter, one species might be good enough and I would without hesitation select the mouse. Considering food consumption, space occupied and life span, the mouse is more than 20 times cheaper than the rat. Because of the shorter life span, results may be available at least one year sooner than those obtained from the rat. Certainly the two species are not equally sensitive to the action of the known carcinogens, but it is difficult to find examples of a totally negative response in one of the two species (WALPOLE, 1964; CLAYSON et al., 1965). In many instances a given compound has been used, for basic research, chiefly in one species. For example, 4-dimethylaminoazobenzene is often mentioned for its low carcinogenic activity in the mouse, but it should be noted that out of approximately 200 experiments reported in HARTWELL's (1951) and SHUBIK and HARTWELL's (1957) tabulations, only six were done in mice with oral administration, 5 in stock mice, and 1 in C mice. Over 2000 rats are reported as having been used in experiments with 3'-methyl-4-dimethylaminoazobenzene (SHUBIK and HARTWELL, 1957), while not a single mouse is listed.

One of the advantages of the mouse, is the large number of ready available inbred strains with various incidence of spontaneous tumors. It is well known that there are great differences in reactivity to carcinogens among strains, and often the pattern of induced tumors follows closely that of spontaneous ones (TANNENBAUM, 1961, 1964). It is possible, therefore, to select two or three inbred strains which together with an outbred stock mouse may constitute a better experimental grouping than a single strain of mice and rats, and still be a more convenient method.

At the end of the experiment, we are faced with two problems, the evaluation of the experiment and the evaluation of the hazard for men. In this symposium others will speak on the latter problem which presents different aspects for medical drugs than for food additives, but which is still conditioned by the way the evaluation of the experiments is done and moreover by the way the experiment has been planned and conducted. It should be emphasized once more (Report UICC Symposium, 1957) the importance of collecting and keeping as permanent documents all the experimental data, of complete pathological examinations with every effort to avoid cannibalism and decomposition, and, finally, of proper control groups. In this type of studies false positive results may be more frequent than false negative. This can be avoided only with a perfect knowledge of the species and strains used, with a

perfect control of the breeding and housing conditions and with large control groups run contemporarily with the treated groups. In this matter it is difficult to rely upon thin, statistically constructed differences, particularly when the evaluation involves enhancement and acceleration of tumors which do appear spontaneously.

To conclude, I should like to say that medical drug testing offer some advantages over the testing of other chemicals of the human environment, since their general pharmacological properties are thoroughly investigated and may provide useful informations for the planning of the carcinogenicity studies. Clearly, an essential aspect of the problem rests on the integration of carcinogenicity tests within other toxicity tests (SHUBIK and SICÉ, 1956). This integration is important not only for practical reasons, but because may render better and more understandable results.

References

BARONI, C., and CEFIS, F., A study of the carcinogenic activity of a single injection of 7,12-dimethylbenz(a)anthracene into newborn C57BL mice. *Tumori* **49**, 373—378 (1963).

BERENBLUM, I., Carcinogenesis and tumor pathogenesis. *Advanc. Cancer Res.* **2**, 129—175 (1954).

— The experimental basis for carcinogenicity testing. *Proc. European Soc. Study Drug Toxicity* **3**, 7—14 (1964).

CHIECO-BIANCHI, L., DE BENEDICTIS, G., TRIDENTE, G., and FIORE-DONATI, L., Influence of age on susceptibility to liver carcinogenesis and skin initiating action by urethane in Swiss mice. *Brit. J. Cancer* **17**, 672—680 (1963).

— FIORE-DONATI, L., TRIDENTE, G. e DE BENEDICTIS, G., Ruolo dell' età e di altri fattori condizionanti la cancerogenesi chimica nel topo. *Tumori* **51**, 53—68 (1965).

CIVIDALLI, G., MIRVISH, S. S., and BERENBLUM, I., The catabolism of urethan in young mice of varying age and strain, and in x-irradiated mice, in relation to urethan carcinogenesis. *Cancer Res.* **25**, 855—858 (1965).

CLAYSON, D. B., LAWSON, T. A., SANTANA, S., and BONSER, G. M., Correlation between the chemical induction of hyperplasia and of malignancy in the bladder epithelium. *Brit. J. Cancer* **19**, 297—310 (1965).

Committee on Medical and Nutritional Aspects of Food Policy: Carcinogenic risks in food additives and pesticides. *Mth. Bull. Minist. Hlth Lab. Serv.* **19**, 108—112 (1960).

DAWKINS, M. J. R., Carbon tetrachloride poisoning in the liver of the new-born rat. *J. Path. Bact.* **85**, 189—196 (1963).

DE BENEDICTIS, G., MAIORANO, G., CHIECO-BIANCHI, L., and FIORE-DONATI, L., Lung carcinogenesis by urethane in newborn, suckling, and adult Swiss mice. *Brit. J. Cancer* **16**, 686—689 (1962).

DELLA PORTA, G., The study of chemical substances for possible carcinogenic action. *Proc. European Soc. Study Drug Toxicity* **3**, 29—37 (1964).

— CAPITANO, J., MONTIPÒ, W. e PARMI, L., Studio sull'azione cancerogena dell'uretano nel topo. *Tumori* **49**, 413—428 (1963).

DE OME, K. B., FAULKIN jr., L. J., BERN, H. A., and BLAIR, P. B., Development of mammary tumors from hyperplastic alveolar nodules transplanted into gland-free mammary fat pads of female C3H mice. *Cancer Res.* **19**, 515—520 (1959).

DOELL, R. G., and CARNES, W. H., Urethan induction of thymic lymphoma in C57BL mice. *Nature (Lond.)* **194**, 588—589 (1962).

DOMSKY, I. I., LIJINSKY, W., SPENCER, K., and SHUBIK, P., Rate of metabolism of 9,10-dimethyl-1,2-benzanthracene in newborn and adult mice. *Proc. Soc. exp. Biol. (N.Y.)* **113**, 110—112 (1963).

DRUCKREY, H., Cancer prevention. *Acta Un. int. Cancr.* **13**, 13—19 (1957).

— Pharmacological approach to carcinogenesis. In: *Ciba Found. Symp. on Carcinogenesis*, p. 110 to 130. London: J. & A. Churchill Ltd. 1959.

ESCHENBRENNER, A. B., and MILLER, E., Liver necrosis and the induction of carbon tetrachloride hepatomas in strain A mice. *J. nat. Cancer Inst.* **6**, 325—341 (1946).

FARBER, E., Ethionine carcinogenesis. *Advanc. Cancer Res.* **7**, 383—474 (1963).

FIORE-DONATI, L., CHIECO-BIANCHI, L., DE BENEDICTIS, G., and MAIORANO, G, Leukaemogenesis by urethan in new-born Swiss mice. *Nature (Lond.)* **190**, 278—279 (1961).

— DE BENEDICTIS, G., CHIECO-BIANCHI, L., and MAIORANO, G., Leukaemogenic activity of urethan in Swiss and AKR mice. *Acta Un. int. Cancr.* **18**, 134—139 (1962).

—, and KAYE, A. M., Kinetics of changes, in thymus and other lymphopoietic organs of adult mice, induced by single doses of urethan. *J. nat. Cancer Inst.* **33**, 907—920 (1964).

FOULDS, L., The histologic analysis of mammary tumors of mice. II. The histology of responsiveness and progression. The origin of tumors. *J. nat. Cancer Inst.* **17**, 713—753 (1956).

GARDNER, W. U., DOUGHERTY, T. F., and WILLIAMS, W. L., Lymphoid tumors in mice receiving steroid hormones. *Cancer Res.* **4**, 73—87 (1944).

GRANT, C., and ROE, F. J. C., The effect of phenanthrene on tumour induction by 3,4 benzopyrene administered to newly born mice. *Brit. J. Cancer* **17**, 261—265 (1963).

HARTWELL, J. L., Survey of compounds which have been tested for carcinogenic activity. *PHS Publication No. 149*, U.S. Govt. Printing Office, Washington D.C. 1951.

HUEPER, W. C., and CONWAY, W. D., *Chemical carcinogenesis and cancers*. Springfield (Ill.): Ch. C. Thomas 1965.

HUGGINS, C., BRIZIARELLI, G., and SUTTON, H., Rapid induction of mammary carcinoma in the rat and the influence of hormones on the tumors. *J. exp. Med.* **109**, 25—42 (1959).

—, and FUKUNISHI, R., Mammary and peritoneal tumors induced by intraperitoneal administration of 7,12-dimethylbenz[a]anthracene in newborn and adult rats. *Cancer Res.* **23**, 785—789 (1963).

Joint FAO/WHO Expert Committee on Food Additives, Evaluation of the carcinogenic hazards of food additives. *Wld Hlth Org. techn. Rep. Ser.* No. 220 (1961).

KAPLAN, H. S., Influence of age on susceptibility of mice to the development of lymphoid tumors after irradiation. *J. nat. Cancer Inst.* **9**, 55—56 (1948).

KAYE, A. M., A study of the relationship between the rate of ethyl carbamate (urethan) catabolism and urethan carcinogenesis. *Cancer Res.* **20**, 237—241 (1960).

KELLY, M. G., and O'GARA, R. W., Induction of tumors in newborn mice with dibenz[a,h]anthracene and 3-methylcholanthrene. *J. nat. Cancer Inst.* **26**, 651—679 (1961).

— — GADEKAR, K., YANCEY, S. T., and OLIVERIO, V. T., Carcinogenic activity of a new antitumor agent, *n*-isopropyl-α-(2-methylhydrazino)-*p*-toluamide, hydrochloride (NSC-77213). *Cancer Chemother. Rep.* **39**, 77—80 (1964).

KIRKMAN, H., Estrogen-induced tumors of kidney in the Syrian hamster. *Nat. Cancer Inst. Monogr.* **1**, 1—139 (1959).

KLEIN, M., Development of hepatomas in inbred albino mice following treatment with 20-methylcholanthrene. *Cancer Res.* **19**, 1109—1113 (1959).

— Influence of low doses of 2-acetylaminofluorene on liver tumorigenesis in mice. *Proc. Soc. exp. Biol. (N.Y.)* **101**, 637—638 (1959).

— Induction of lymphocytic neoplasms, hepatomas, and other tumors after oral administration of urethan to infant mice. *J. nat. Cancer Inst.* **29**, 1035—1046 (1962).

LAW, L. W., and PRECERUTTI, A., Inhibition by urethan (ethyl carbamate) of virus induction of leukaemia in C3H mice. *Nature (Lond.)* **200**, 692—693 (1963).

LEE, K. Y., TOTH, B., and SHUBIK, P., Carcinogenic response of the Syrian golden hamster treated at birth with 7,12-dimethylbenz[a]anthracene. *Proc. Soc. exp. Biol. (N.Y.)* **114**, 579—582 (1963).

LIEBELT, R. A., YOSHIDA, R., and GRAY, G. F., Enhancement of liver tumorigenesis in Zb mice injected with urethan at newborn age. *Proc. Amer. Ass. Cancer Res.* **3**, 245 (1961).

MILLER, J. A., and MILLER, E. C., Metabolism of drugs in relation to carcinogenicity. *Ann. N.Y. Acad. Sci.* **123**, 125—140 (1965).

MIRVISH, S., CIVIDALLI, G., and BERENBLUM, I., Slow elimination of urethan in relation to its high carcinogenicity in newborn mice. *Proc. Soc. exp. Biol. (N.Y.)* **116**, 265—268 (1964).

MÜHLBOCK, O., and BOOT, L. M., The mechanism of hormonal carcinogenesis. In: *Ciba Found. Symp. on Carcinogenesis*, p. 83—94. London: J. & A. Churchill Ltd. 1959.

NISHIZUKA, Y., ITO, K., and NAKAKUKI, K., Liver tumor induction by a single injection of *o*-aminoazotoluene to newborn mice. *Gann* **56**, 135—142 (1965).

—, and NAKAKUKI, K., Effect of 20-methylcholanthrene given at birth on tumor development in two high-leukemia strains of mice, AKR and SL. *Gann* **55**, 83—85 (1964).

— —, and SAKAKURA, T., Induction of pulmonary tumors and leukemia by a single injection of 4-nitroquinoline 1-oxide to newborn and infant mice. *Gann* **55**, 495—508 (1964).

— —, and USUI, M., Enhancing effect of thymectomy on hepatotumorigenesis in Swiss mice following neonatal injection of 20-methylcholanthrene. *Nature (Lond.)* **205**, 1236—1238 (1965).

O'GARA, R. W., KELLY, M. G., and MANDEL, N., Induction of fibrosarcomas in mice given a minute quantity of 3-methylcholanthrene or dibenz[a,h]anthracene as newborns. *Nature (Lond.)* **196**, 1220—1221 (1962).

PIETRA, G., RAPPAPORT, H., and SHUBIK, P., The effects of carcinogenic chemicals in newborn mice. *Cancer (Philad.)* **14**, 308—317 (1961).

— SPENCER, K., and SHUBIK, P., Response of newly born mice to a chemical carcinogen. *Nature (Lond.)* **183**, 1689 (1959).

POLLARD, M., and SALOMON, J. C., Oncogenic effect of methylcholanthrene in new-born germfree mice. *Proc. Soc. exp. Biol. (N.Y.)* **112**, 256—259 (1963).

RAPPAPORT, H., and BARONI, C., A study of the pathogenesis of malignant lymphoma induced in the Swiss mouse by 7,12-dimethylbenz[a]anthracene injected at birth. *Cancer Res.* **22**, 1067—1074 (1962).

REID, E., Significant biochemical effects of hepatocarcinogens in the rat: a review. *Cancer Res.* **22**, 398—430 (1962).

Report of symposium on potential cancer hazards from chemical additives and contaminants to food stuffs. *Acta Un. int. Cancr.* **13**, 169—363 (1957).

ROE, F. J. C., MITCHLEY, B. C. V., and WALTERS, M., Tests for carcinogenesis using newborn mice: 1,2-benzanthracene, 2-naphtylamine, 2-naphtylhydroxylamine and ethyl methane sulphonate. *Brit. J. Cancer* **17**, 255—260 (1963).

— ROWSON, K. E. K., and SALAMAN, M. H., Tumours of many sites induced by injection of chemical carcinogens into newborn mice, a sensitive test for carcinogenesis: the implications for certain immunological theories. *Brit. J. Cancer* **15**, 515—530 (1961).

ROGERS, S., Age of the host and other factors affecting the production with urethane of pulmonary adenomas in mice. *J. exp. Med.* **93**, 427—449 (1951).

SAXÉN, E. A., On the factor of age in the production of subcutaneous sarcomas in mice by 20-methylcholanthrene. *J. nat. Cancer Inst.* **14**, 547—569 (1953).

SHIMKIN, M. B., and POLISSAR, M. J., Some quantitative observations on the induction and growth of primary pulmonary tumors in strain A mice receiving urethan. *J. nat. Cancer Inst.* **16**, 75—98 (1955).

SHUBIK, P., and HARTWELL, J. L., Survey of compounds which have been tested for carcinogenic activity, *Suppl. 1, PHS Publication No. 149*, U.S. Govt. Printing Office, Washington D.C. 1957.

—, and SICÉ, J., Chemical carcinogenesis as a chronic toxicity test. A review. *Cancer Res.* **16**, 728—742 (1956).

STICK, H. F., Chromosomes of tumor cells. I. Murine leukemias induced by one or two injections of 7,12-dimethylbenz[a]anthracene. *J. nat. Cancer Inst.* **25**, 649—661 (1960).

Subcommittee on Carcinogenesis, Food Protection Committee, Food and Nutrition Board, National Academy of Sciences-National Research Council: Problems in the evaluation of carcinogenic hazards from use of food additives. *Cancer Res.* **21**, 429—456 (1961).

TANNENBAUM, A., Studies on urethan carcinogenesis. *Acta Un. int. Cancr.* **17**, 72—87 (1961)

— Contribution of urethan studies to the understanding of carcinogenesis. *Nat. Cancer Inst. Monogr.* **14**, 341—356 (1964).

—, and SILVERSTONE, H., Nutrition in relation to cancer. *Advanc. Cancer Res.* **1**, 452—501 (1953).

— VESSELINOVITCH, S. D., MALTONI, C., and STRYZAK MITCHELL, D., Multipotential carcinogenicity of urethan in the Sprague-Dawley rat. *Cancer Res.* **22**, 1362—1371 (1962).

TERRACINI, B., and MAGEE, P. N., Renal tumours in rats following injection of dimethylnitrosamine at birth. *Nature (Lond.)* 202, 502—503 (1964).

TOTH, B., MAGEE, P. N., and SHUBIK, P., Carcinogenesis study with dimethylnitrosamine administered orally to adult and subcutaneously to newborn BALB/c mice. *Cancer Res.* 24, 1712—1722 (1964).

— RAPPAPORT, H., and SHUBIK, P., Accelerated development of malignant lymphomas in AKR mice injected at birth with 7,12-dimethylbenz[a]anthracene. *Proc. Soc. exp. Biol. (N.Y.)* 110, 881—884 (1962).

— — — Influence of dose and age on the induction of malignant lymphomas and other tumors by 7,12-dimethylbenz[a]-anthracene in Swiss mice. *J. nat. Cancer Inst.* 30, 723—741 (1963).

—, and SHUBIK, P., Carcinogenesis in Lewis rats injected at birth with 7,12-dimethylbenz[a]-anthracene. *Brit. J. Cancer* 17, 540—545 (1963).

— — Unexpected acute toxicity of aminopterin. *Nature (Lond.)* 201, 512 (1964).

TRAININ, N., PRECERUTTI, A., and LAW, L. W., Trends in carcinogenesis by urethan administration to new-born mice of different strains. *Nature (Lond.)* 202, 305—306 (1964).

UPTON, A. C., ODELL jr. T. T., and SNIFFEN, E. P., Influence of age at time of irradiation on induction of leukemia and ovarian tumors in RF mice. *Proc. Soc. exp. Biol. (N.Y.)* 104, 769—772 (1960).

— WOLFF, F. F., FURTH, J., and KIMBALL, A. W., A comparison of the induction of myeloid and lymphoid leukemias in x-radiated RF mice. *Cancer Res.* 18, 842—848 (1958).

WACHSTEIN, M., and ROBINSON, M., Neonatal resistence to nephrotoxic renal tubular necrosis in the rat. *Fed. Proc.* 24, 619 (1965).

WALPOLE, A. L., The properties in the laboratory of known carcinogens. *Proc. European Soc. Study Drug Toxicity* 3, 15—27 (1964).

WEISBURGER, J. H., and WEISBURGER, E. K., Pharmacodynamics of carcinogenic azo dyes, aromatic amines, and nitrosamines. *Clin. Pharmacol. Ther.* 4, 110—129 (1963).

Discussion

Saffiotti: The study of the effects of a drug following administration to newborn mice can certainly be of great importance. One must remember however that the significance of tests on newborn animals cannot be properly assessed unless comparable groups of animals of an older age are studied concurrently. Some compounds are metabolized differently by newborn and adult animals and the newborn may be unable to produce the active carcinogenic metabolite that is effective in the adult. Therefore one cannot assume that newborn mice are more susceptible than adults.

The suggestion that agents under test should be administered for one half of the lifespan of the animals is acceptable in most instances. However in the case of some weak carcinogens the induction of tumours may depend on life-long treatment.

Roe: With regard to the sensitivity of newborn animals to carcinogens, I should like to make the following points.

Firstly, we should be quite clear in what we mean by "sensitivity". The word may have a *qualitative* or *quantitative* connotation. Because of their immature state, or for other reasons not yet understood, particular tissues may be capable of a carcinogenic response in the newborn but not in the more mature animal. Examples of such a qualitative difference in susceptibility could be quoted from the literature. In the case of mouse lung, tumours may be induced readily by the administration of carcinogens to older animals. Here differences in sensitivity between newborn and adult are quantitative rather than qualitative. In a recent experiment in which 7,12-dimethylbenz[a]anthracene (DMBA) was administered to newborn (1.5 gramme), suckling (6 gramme) and young adult (18 gramme) mice in doses proportional to body weight, the sensitivity of the newborn animals, as assessed by lung tumour response, was greater than that in suckling or adult mice, but the difference was less than two-fold.

Secondly, it may be of some interest to record that ethyl methane sulphonate (EMS), which, from experiments on adult mice would be regarded as a weak carcinogen, readily gave positive results on injection into newborn animals. Thus the administration of 100 μg EMS daily for 5 days from birth gave rise to multiple lung tumours in 100% of mice in a recent experiment.

Thirdly, I agree with previous speakers that carcinogenicity tests on newborn animals cannot act as substitutes for experiments on older animals. Some undoubted carcinogens, for example, some of the azo dyes, have yet to yield a positive result when tested in newborn animals. However, the potential advantages of using newborn mice, which include (1) possible special qualitative or quantitative susceptibility, (2) the need for much smaller amounts of test material, and (3) the fact that more of the life-span is available for observation, should be borne in mind.

Rudali: I should like to tell Dr. DELLA PORTA about a test which we have often used for the early production of tumours. It involves the administration of carcinogenic substances to newborn mice via the maternal milk. If, for example, one gives 1 mg methylcholanthrene daily for 20 days to mice whilst they are feeding their young, one sees lung tumours in 100 per cent of the progeny by the 3rd month of life.

Schoental: When an animal is treated during pregnancy the foetus may be affected, while the mother remains unscathed.

Druckrey: The use of drugs in pregnancy needs special caution, as illustrated by the following example. Ethylnitrosourea, which has been proposed for therapy in man, given as a single intravenous injection of 60 mg per Kg body weight to pregnant rats, produced teratogenic effects in practically 100 per cent. Furthermore the progeny developed malignant tumours of the brain and nervous system earlier than the mothers (DRUCKREY and IVANKOVIC, not yet published). This indicates the possibility of a relationship between the carcinogenic and teratogenic action and a higher susceptibility of the foetus.

For carcinogenicity tests no strict rules but only certain recommendations should be given. The choice of methods depends on the nature of the substance to be tested and on the conditions of its proposed use and therefore must be left to the scientist responsible for the testing. The use of subcutaneous injections has been and can be useful too. With this method we detected the carcinogenicity of dimethylsulphate, which enabled us to recommend preventive measures for the protection of workers in industries. Later we learned, that some workers died from lung cancer, probably due to exposure to dimethylsulphate vapours.

In testing substances for carcinogenic activity the highest tolerated dosage should be used and the experimentation extended over the whole life span of the animals. For every material to be tested, clear specifications as to identity and purity as well as to the nature and concentration of impurities are indispensable. An observed carcinogenic effect may be due to impurities rather than to the compounds as formulated.

Lacassagne: I recall an early example of the greater susceptibility of young animals to carcinogenic agents. In our first publication on the production of mammary cancer in male mice by means of an oestrogenic hormone (LACASSAGNE, 1932) we obtained a positive result when we used very young mice but not when we used adults.

Reference

LACASSAGNE, A., Apparition de cancers de la mamelle chez la souris male soumise a des infections de folliculine. *C.R. Acad. Sci. (Paris)* **195**, 630 (1932).

Frazer: May I stress the tremendous benefit that modern drugs have conferred on the human community. More than 85% of the drugs used today were not known thirty years ago. The great majority of bacterial infections can now be controlled, in many countries specialist tuberculosis hospitals have ceased to exist, the handling of mental patients has been revolutionised, and many conditions that were inevitably fatal a quarter of a century ago now have a low, or even negligible, mortality. These vast changes are due to new drugs. In the control of any environmental hazard it is necessary to weigh up the benefits and the risks. However, let there be no doubt in any one's mind about the great benefits and incalculable economic gain that has come from the use of modern drugs. There has been reference to isoniazid. This drug has made a major contribution to the relief of disease and suffering, and continues to do so.

Dr. DELLA PORTA mentions newborn animals. Does he think that they should be used for testing for carcinogenicity? Unfortunately, the metabolic status of newborn animals differs greatly from species to species — for example, compare the newborn rat or mouse, which is extremely immature, and the newborn guinea-pig. However, more work on newborn and young animals would undoubtedly be a good thing.

Della Porta: I should like to repeat that I believe that at the present time there is not enough knowledge to justify a brief treatment of newborn animals in substitution of life-span-long treatments in adults. However the advantages offered by the newborn system should stimulate an extensive investigation on its validity and on the mechanisms involved.

A Program for the Investigation of the Possible Chronic Hazards of Drugs

Philippe Shubik

Professor of Oncology, Director, Division of Oncology, The Chicago Medical School, Institute for Medical Research, Chicago, Illinois, U.S.A.

A program of research into the possible chronic hazards, particularly carcinogenicity, of medicaments was begun this year in the Division of Oncology of The Chicago Medical School. This program is a collaborative one with the Field Studies Branch of the National Cancer Institute of the National Institutes of Health and has support for the first year of operation of a contract for * 1 million. It has resulted from the foresight and efforts of Drs. Kenneth Endicott and Paul Kotin. In essence, the program has been divided into two major equal segments. The first segment is devoted to the testing of various drugs in animals: the second to basic research in carcinogenesis. The research segment of the program is designed to assist in better testing of chemicals for carcinogenesis and to gain more insight into mechanisms of action to enable better evaluation of the results to be made.

A series of criteria have been arbitrarily established for the selection of drugs to be tested. These are:

1. Evidence already available that suggests that the compound may be carcinogenic in animals or in man but which necessitates additional confirmatory evidence.

2. Compounds giving rise to other chronic effects in animals or man that suggests further screening for possible carcinogenicity (e.g. induction of blood dyscrasias).

3. Compounds with chemical structures suggesting that they might be carcinogenic.

4. Compounds used in man on a chronic basis for which there is no adequate chronic toxicity data available. (Amongst the large number of compounds in this category it has been decided to accord priority in testing to those in most widespread use).

Testing procedures to be adopted are being tailored to the individual case. In all cases the compound is being tested under conditions most closely approximating the human usage. In the first instance all products are being tested as such without any purification unless certain compounds are common to a series of different preparations. In some special instances both the commercial product and the basic compound are being studied. In all studies detailed chemical analysis of the material to be tested is undertaken. As a preliminary to chronic testing an acute screening procedure is being set up in which LD 50, pathological study of acute findings, hematological study and certain blood chemical determinations are being performed unless such data is available on a reliable basis.

At the present time the following pharmaceuticals are under test in this laboratory:

Diabinese
Fulvicin   Aspirin
Miltown   Isoniazide
Librium   Aminopterin
Leukeran   5,5-diphenyldantoin
Phenylbutazone   Quinophenol
Ethinamate   Isonicotinic acid
Phenacetin   7-iodo-5-cholor-
                  8-OH-quinoline
Banthine   Phenobarbital
Thorazine   Carmurit

These can be seen to cover a large number of diverse types of drug action and I shall not go into the reasons for selecting each one since I believe that it is obvious as to how they fit into the categories of selection outlined previously. I shall discuss certain of the tests which I believe illustrate what was meant by saying that the individual tests were selected on the basis of individual needs. One case in point is a current topic of much discussion, the anti-tuberculosis drug isoniazide. As you are all well aware this drug has been shown to induce lung adenomas in mice in a variety of experiments reported from Hungary, Italy and Japan. Prior to the beginning of our current enlarged program we had wished to repeat these observations and extend them to another species, the hamster. In our initial experiment undertaken with Dr. BELA TOTH we encountered a result which has given us much cause for thought. We did not demonstrate any activity at all in the Syrian hamster although it was our impression that the level of intoxication encountered, even though consistent with a long life span, may have masked any positive results. In the instance of our initial test of this substance in the Swiss mouse we confirmed the findings of others that this substance indeed did give rise to an increased incidence of lung adenomas. However to our astonishment there was a clear cut decrease in the incidence of the other two common tumors in this species, namely lymphomas and mammary tumors. The result was all the more impressive with the mammary tumors since several of the mice developed subcutaneous nodules that we consider to be early mammary tumors and in the treated mice these subsequently regressed. As a result of this initial finding we have extended the test of isoniazide to include several strains of mice. In the first instance we are now testing the compound in C3H mice for their effect on mammary tumor occurrence; on AKr mice for the effects on lymphoma induction. We are repeating the study on the hamster at lower and varied dosages and have also instituted a repetition of the study in rats. It is our feeling that the rat study should be undertaken in view of the toxicity of this drug which will occur in most studies and makes the determination of carcinogenicity most difficult. In addition, we will test INH in dogs and possibly cats. In preliminary findings with AKr mice no lung adenomas are seen; we cannot yet provide information on the inhibitory effects on lymphomas or mammary tumors in these studies but these will be forthcoming. Once again Dr. TOTH is the senior investigator in this study which has been submitted for publication on a preliminary basis. The problem of interpretation of the possible hazards of isoniazide seems to have become a maze of complexity and I welcome the opportunity to have the members of this committee discuss the problem taking into account all these additional facts. It would seem to us that the action of this compound is not only limited but also atypical of carcinogens in general. The only tumor clearly induced is the lung adenoma and no general systemic carcinogenicity appears attributable to this compound. Only carbon tetrachloride seems to approach this compound in the specificity to this action, although it does produce hepatomas in two species, the mouse and the hamster. It is clear once again that we are deficient in information to enable us to generalize about carcinogens. We believe that in the instance of isoniazide no effort should be spared to obtain as much information as possible. This necessitates not only using many species but drawing deductions from preliminary experiments that necessitate the introduction of additional studies that would not be conceived of in a routine type of program.

A considerable proportion of the program in the department is devoted to chemistry and biochemistry under the direction of Dr. WILLIAM LIJINSKY and Dr. KYU LEE respectively. The chemistry program is concerned with methods of chemical analysis of complex carcinogenic materials in the environment and in so far as the drug testing program is concerned, in analysis of products about to be tested, for impurities. The drugs are, of course, tested in the commercial state; however we consider it essential to know the nature of impurities that may occur in advance and, clearly if such impurities turned out to be carcinogenic compounds already known to us we would be saved considerable labor. So far we have been agreeably surprised at the high level of chemical purity of most of the commercial products introduced into this program.

The primary consideration in the organization of this program has been that it should represent a balance between applied and basic research. It is our view, in the first instance, that each test of an untested material is, in fact, a research project. It cannot be treated as a routine matter and still be a satisfactory test. However, in this program each investigator is allowed to devote his time equally to testing the drugs and to basic research. We have a general departmental basic research program in chemical carcinogenesis that has drawn together a series of individuals with essentially similar interests. However, the individual research groups are encouraged to undertake research of an independent nature in chemical carcinogenesis. Dr. LIJINSKY now has a program covering a somewhat wider area both in environmental and basic carcinogenesis. In so far as environmental carcinogenesis is concerned some of our findings are being presented at this meeting by Dr. SAFFIOTTI. These deal with the carcinogenicity of certain petrolatums that have been found to be carcinogenic and involve the much larger question of standard chemical procedures permit Food and Drug officials to determine the suitability of complex mixtures for human usage. Up to this time reasonably good procedures have been devised for limiting the quantities of polycyclic hydrocarbon carcinogens in certain products (mineral oils and waxes); our current studies demonstrate that other possibly related compounds such as heterocyclics may pose a new problem. I am sure that this merely touches upon a much greater problem and that we have been over simplifying considerably as a result of the preoccupation of carcinogenesis workers with coal tar from the inception of the subject. The elucidation of the complete content of carcinogens in any one mixture must be pursued continuously; we still do not have full knowledge of the many carcinogens in coal tar, for example. Taking such materials and determining everything we can of their nature and activity, is essential background information.

I should like to discuss briefly certain other aspects of our basic research program and point out how this continually impinges upon practical matters. In the instance of urethane and related derivatives it is apparent that practical implications will occur continuously. Many tranquilizers are closely related to urethane and it has been drawn to our attention recently that ethyl and methyl urethane are used in quantities in the textile industry. We have been conducting metabolic studies with urethane which are largely concerned with the identification of an alkyl derivative of nucleic acid. However, in the course of these studies it has proved necessary to re-investigate the biological activity of methyl urethane. We have not quite completed this study but I wish to draw attention to it to illustrate certain general points. Methyl urethane was investigated for carcinogenicity some years ago by LARSEN subsequently to his demonstration of the carcinogenicity of ethyl urethane. At that time urethane was known as a limited carcinogen only giving rise to lung adenomas, albeit in several strains of mice. In the past decade it has been found that urethane is a versatile carcinogen inducing mammary tumors, fat pad tumors, lymphomas, and other tumors in mice; this has largely resulted from the careful observations of TANNENBAUM and co-workers who, unlike previous workers, observed the animals to the end of their life span and, additionally performed complete autopsies. In addition, it has been found that urethane can act as a skin initiator in mice, and that it will give rise to an entirely different range of tumors in the hamster including melanocytomas, gastric papillomas, hepatomas, and others. Now when methyl urethane was originally tested it was subjected to limited tests comparing its activity to that of ethyl urethane as a lung

tumor inducing agent. It can be said not to induce lung tumors in the same way as urethane. However, no evidence is at hand at all to suggest whether or not it possesses any of the other biological attributes of the actively carcinogenic carbamate.

I should like to emphasize our view that life time studies and complete pathological examination are the prime requisite of initial testing for carcinogenicity. It is in the instance of many pharmaceuticals, the case that other pathological lesions emerge with some frequency. It would certainly be a major waste if the investigator were not a fully trained pathologist ready to diagnose not only tumors but also other lesions.

It is our continuing desire, of course, to have a better fundamental understanding of the mechanisms of carcinogenesis for it is sure that without this we will not advance too rapidly in environmental cancer studies. However there are clearly certain particular areas of research that are particularly pertinent to testing of compounds for carcinogenesis in the context of human hazard. First and foremost is a better understanding of the metabolic pathways taken by different carcinogens under different biological conditions. Comparative metabolism in different species is a first consideration enabling us to have a logical basis for the selection of the appropriate species. Except possibly in the case of aromatic amines this area has been much neglected. In the second instance, I believe that comparison of metabolic behaviour in the newborn and adult mouse can now provide us with a routine method for distinguishing between carcinogens that act as the original molecule and those that must be metabolized into a "proximate" carcinogen. In some studies of ours with 9,10-dimethyl-1,2-

benzathracene undertaken with Drs. DOMSKY and LIJINSKY it was found that this compound was eliminated much more slowly from the newborn than the adult mouse and that this behaviour correlated with the induction of a higher incidence of malignant lymphomas than seen in the adult. It would seem not unreasonable to infer from this that the intact molecule is, in fact, the "proximate" carcinogen. Similar behaviour on the part of urethan has since been demonstrated by BERENBLUM and his group. Conversely Dr. LEE in our laboratory has shown that the lack of a demethylating enzyme in the liver of mice under 12 hours of age precludes the occurrence of liver tumors by dimethylnitrosamine but that the presence of this enzyme in the kidney at that time favors the development of renal tumors. The nature of the proximate carcinogen and the need for metabolic change of a specific kind or lack of it can certainly be the determining factor in the estimation of a hazard.

Lastly, I should like to make a plea for more electronmicroscopy in carcinogenesis. It would seem to me inconceivable that we should not eventually be able to discern some morphological representation of some of the events specific to carcinogenesis. It may be that we will eventually prove to be as unlucky with the electronmicroscope as we have been with the light microscope. However, I believe strongly that if nothing else the newer techniques of electronmicroscopic radioautography will permit us to localize the precise site of action of carcinogens within the cell and that starting from such studies and correlating behaviour and morphology we stand a much better chance of discovering something than we would by merely studying the ultrastructure of developed tumors. This has been a brief review of our program and some of the reasons behind it. I have not discussed many phases of our work but will be glad to do so in the discussion.

Discussion

Schoental: Could you specify which methylurethane you studied; is the methyl substituent on the nitrogen or in the ester grouping?

Shubik: In the ester grouping.

Boyland: Positive results have been obtained in carcinogenicity tests on isoniazid in some countries but not in others. PEACOCK induced no tumours with it. It is possible that impurities are responsible for the positive results obtained by others. At the present stage, test results should not be made public. The usefulness of the drug is so great that a certain risk has to be taken.

Truhaut: With regard to the potential carcinogenicity of isoniazid I am impressed by the experiments of MORI et al. (1960) and of BIANCI-

FIORI and RIBACCHI (1962) in which mice exposed to the drug in the diet for a prolonged period developed pulmonary tumours in a 100% cases by $7^1/_2$ months.

BIANCIFIORI and RIBACCHI also obtained lung tumours with hydrazine sulphate and the sodium salt of isonicotinic acid. The former observation raises the question as to whether other drugs which may be broken down in the body with the production of hydrazine should be regarded as potentially dangerous.

It is also of interest that PANSA et al. (1962) saw hyperplastic changes in the bronchioles of rats exposed to aerosols of isoniazid or to intraperitoneal injections of isoniazid. They saw no neoplasms in these tests.

References

BIANCIFIORI, C., and RIBACCHI, R., Pulmonary tumours in mice induced by oral isoniazid and its metabolites. *Nature (Lond.)* **194**, 488 (1962).

MORI, K., YASUNO, A., and MATSUMOTO, K., Induction of pulmonary tumors in mice with isonicotinic acid hydrazide. *Gann* **51**, 83 (1960).

PANSA, E., PICCO, A., and GNAVI, M., On the problem of a possible carcinogenic effect of isoniazide. An experimental investigation in the rat. *Minerva med.* **53**, 3162 (1962).

Statistical Approach to the Evaluation and Prediction of Possible Carcinogenic Action of Drugs

RICHARD DOLL, M.D., D.Sc., F.R.C.P., F.R.S.

Director of Medical Research Council's Statistical Research Unit,
University College Hospital Medical School, London, Great Britain

The prediction that a particular drug will produce cancer in man may be made in two ways; either as a result of experiments demonstrating a carcinogenic effect in animals, or by analogy with the effect of a known carcinogen. In the latter case the analogy may be suggested because of a similarity in chemical structure, or because the drug is shown to have a pathological effect associated with cancer induction, such as the ability to damage chromosomes. Both types of prediction depend for their correctness on an adequate understanding of biological mechanisms. In the first instance, one has to be able to extrapolate from one animal species to another; in the second one has to know how cancer is produced at the molecular level. In the absence of such knowledge either type of prediction is hazardous and no refinement of statistical technique will make it reliable.

That is not to say that statistics has nothing to contribute. Valid and efficient methods of experimental design (FISHER, 1960; COX, 1961) and of analysis of experimental results (IRWIN, 1946; PIKE and ROE, 1963) will help to eliminate false predictions based on statistically inadequate evidence. Such methods are widely used in other fields of biological research, but they still have to make their full impact on experimental oncology. They can, however, do nothing to overcome the major difficulties in the way of prediction that have been referred to previously.

Evaluation

Simple Situations

The problem of recognizing and evaluating a risk in man is, in contrast, largely dependent upon adequate statistical methodology. That is not to say that a quantitative analysis is always necessary. If the site in which the cancer occurs, or its histological picture, is extremely unusual, the observation of a handful of cases in a group of persons with a common exposure may be sufficient to demonstrate a causal relationship, without further detailed examination. It did not need many cases of cancer of the palm of the hand in patients who had been given medicinal doses of arsenic, of haemangio-endothelioma of the liver in patients who had been given thorotrast, or of erythro-leukaemia in benzene workers to suggest that these conditions could be produced respectively by inorganic arsenic, thorium and benzene. And it needed only two cases of ethmoid cancer among nickel workers in the village of Clydach to alert an intelligent general practitioner to the possibility that the refining of nickel might be a cause of the disease. In all these instances a comparison with the expected incidence in the absence of specific exposure is implied, but the diseases are normally so rare that quantitative comparison is unnecessary. Confidence in the causal nature of the relationship was, moreover, increased by the demonstration that it was biologically plausible; that is, the disease had occurred some years after first exposure so that the "induction period" was of the order of duration that is commonly observed with human cancer and in some instances there was also evidence that the substance had other pathological effects on the tissue in which the cancer occurred. Cancer of the skin of the palms was, for example, always associated with arsenical pigmentation and keratoses, and erythroleukaemia was often associated with evidence of a previous marrow aplasia.

In the same way, it should not be difficult to recognize a relationship between connective tissue sarcomas and the injection of Imferon — if the drug is indeed capable of producing tumours in man in the doses normally given. One case has been reported at the site of a previous injection (Robinson, Bell and Sturdy, 1960), but even if the histological diagnosis had not been denied (Golberg, 1960) this case alone could not carry much weight. Few people, however, would need to see more than three or four cases to be convinced that the drug was carcinogenic.

Quantitative Analysis

In other circumstances, the problem is much more difficult, and the fact that a drug is carcinogenic to man can be shown with confidence only as a result of a detailed quantitative study. Four features in particular complicate the assessment. First, few human cancers, other than leukaemia, occur within ten years of first exposure to the carcinogenic agent. It is probable that most types of cancer can occur as soon as five years after first exposure; but the usual induction period for all cancers other than leukaemia is likely to be much longer. Secondly, we have to be concerned with very small effects as well as with large ones. A risk[1] of fatal cancer of one per cent, would weigh heavily against the use of any drug that was not life-saving and, with many drugs, a risk of 1 in 1,000 would be a serious contra-indication to their use. Thirdly, it has to be remembered that drugs are not usually given to healthy individuals, but to patients with illnesses that may themselves be associated with the development of cancer (for example, ulcerative colitis with colon cancer, chronic bronchitis with lung cancer and pernicious anaemia with gastric cancer). Fourthly, drugs are not given in isolation, but as part of a scheme of investigation and treatment, that may include exposure to other carcinogenic agents — for example, X-rays — and the effect of one treatment has to be distinguished from the possible effects of other aspects of medical intervention.

Two general methods of investigation are possible: the retrospective, in which we start from patients with cancer and inquire into their past history of drug taking; and the prospective, in which we start from persons who are known to have taken the drug and follow them to determine the number who develop cancer.

---

[1] The risk of developing a particular disease depends not only on the strength of the disease producing agent, but also on the strength of the other forces that may kill the subject before the disease has a chance of appearing. For the purposes of this report, this complication has been ignored.

Retrospective Studies

Of these two methods, the retrospective is the simpler to organize and carry out; but it cannot always be relied on to detect a carcinogenic effect when one exists. The first difficulty is that it may not be possible to obtain an adequate history of drug usage. This may be avoided if the use of the drug produces some other marker condition, as in the case of arsenic, and it may not arise if the use of the drug is associated with some dramatic medical event, as was the case with thorotrast. The history may also provide no great difficulty if the drug is in common use and can be readily recognized by the patient. These circumstances enabled BOYD and DOLL (1954) to use the retrospective method to demonstrate a weak relationship between cancer of the gastro-intestinal tract and the prolonged use of liquid paraffin as a laxative. Many patients, however, are unable to provide a clear lead to the drugs they have taken — and certainly not to those taken more than 10 years previously — and the retrospective method can then be used only if it is possible to get independent evidence of the drugs to which they have been exposed. BEAN (1960), for example, was able to obtain details of the previous us of butazolidine in patients with leukaemia from departmental records, by studying only men in receipt of war pensions and entitled to a free medical service.

Provided evidence of drug usage can be obtained, there is not likely to be any great difficulty in making a control estimate of the expected frequency of use in the absence of any carcinogenic effect. National figures from the pharmaceutical industry or governmental sources provide a useful check on the order of magnitude that may be expected; but the only truly comparable figure is one obtained in the same way as for the cancer patients under study — that is, from an appropriate control group of other subjects. In my experience, the most suitable control group is likely to be provided by patients with other types of cancer diagnosed over the same period in the same area (BOYD and DOLL, 1954; WOODLIFF and DOUGAN, 1964).

A much greater difficulty results from the fact that a drug is likely to be only one of many causes of a particular cancer and responsible for only a small proportion of the total cases. Consider, for example, the situation in which a drug that is given to 1 in 100 young or middle-aged men doubles the risk of gastric cancer, increasing it from (say) 3 per cent to 6 per cent. In these circumstances, inquiry into the past history of drug taking of 500 patients with gastric cancer would be expected to reveal 10 who had taken the drug, whereas if it had had no carcinogenic effect the expected number would be 5. Since retrospective histories, however well taken, are never completely accurate, the actual difference observed between the cancer and the control patients would be smaller and it might be necessary to investigate several thousand gastric cancer patients before any serious evidence was obtained to incriminate the drug. The situation would, of course, be different if the drug was used more widely, and particularly if the cancer produced was normally less common. If, for example, the same drug had produced primary cancer of the liver in 3 per cent of persons, a history of taking the drug might well be obtained in 10 out of 20 patients with the disease, whereas a control group of the same size would probably fail to give a positive history in any.

One way in which a retrospective study may be made more efficient is, therefore, to limit it to a selected group of cancer patients in whom the common causes of the disease are known not to have been involved. If, for example, the drug is suspected of producing cancer of the lung, the study may be limited to non-smokers or ex-smokers of (say) more than 20 years duration — thus effectively studying patients with a rare type of cancer instead of those with a common one. It may be noted, in this respect, that Robson and Jelliffe's (1963) report of 6 cases of bronchial carcinoma in patients with skin changes due to medicinal arsenicism suggested that arsenic might be a cause, primarily because the sex ratio and smoking habits of the patients were so unusual: — 4 of the 6 patients being women, 3 being non-smokers, and 1 of the 2 men being a light pipe smoker.

There remains the problem of interpreting the results. This is never easy in a retrospective study, but it should not be more difficult in relation to the use of a drug than in relation to many other aetiological agents. The general principles have been discussed in many recent papers (for example, Doll, 1964; Hill, 1965) and there is no need to review them further here.

Prospective Studies

In contrast to retrospective studies, prospective studies can be relied on to demonstrate the effects of a drug, if they are of any importance — provided only that enough time and energy are devoted to them. The amount required may, however, be so oppressive that it is impractical to carry out the study unless there is some over-riding reason for doing it. A study of the long-term effects of ionizing radiations, for example, required the compilation of records on 15,000 patients and their individual follow-up over a period of 10 years, before it could be shown that the substantial doses of X-rays that had been given were liable to increase the risk of developing the com-

mon epithelial cancers by about 60 per cent (Court Brown and Doll, 1965).

In favourable circumstances, it may be possible to reduce the work in two ways. First, the length of time required to complete the study may be shortened if records exist which enable patients who took the drug in the past to be identified, without introducing bias due to knowledge of what happened to them subsequently. If the treatments were given sufficiently long ago, enough time may already have elapsed for cancers to have been induced and all that remains to be done is to discover the fate of the individual patients. This, however, may be difficult, and if a large proportion of the patients are not traced it will be possible to recognize only those effects that are relatively large in comparison with normal risks. With a follow-up that was 50 per cent complete, Horta, Abbatt, da Motta and Roriz (1965) could confirm the large risk of haemangio-endothelioma of the liver in patients who had been given thorotrast and demonstrate a risk of leukaemia, but they were unable to adduce significant evidence in regard to other cancers. Pochins' (1960) follow-up of patients treated with radioactive iodine for thyrotoxicosis was, in contrast, so incomplete that it was impossible to reach any definite conclusion about the possible leukaemogenic effect of the treatment — save only that it was unlikely to be large.

Secondly, it may be possible to reduce the labour by studying only patients who have been given very large doses. In this case, it may be relatively easy to demonstrate that the drug is qualitatively carcinogenic and, on the assumption of proportionality between dose and effect, to set down some sort of limits to the size of the effect that may be expected from lower doses. It must be recognized, however, that extrapolation from large to smaller doses involves assumptions that may lead to either of two types of error. If there is a threshold dose below which no effect is produced, it may not be recognized and small doses may be unjustifiably incriminated. Alternatively, large doses may so damage a tissue that cancer induction is actually inhibited and an effect that would be produced by smaller doses may be overlooked. In this way, X-ray treatment for thyrotoxicosis or for cancer of the cervix uteri may be proportionally less likely to produce cancer of the thyroid and leukaemia than smaller doses given to the same parts of the body for other purposes (International Commission for Radiological Protection, 1966).

When these difficulties are overcome there remains the problem of interpreting the results. Suppose, for example, that a large group of tuberculous patients were treated with isoniazid and their mortality from different types of cancer recorded over the subsequent 20 years. Suppose, moreover, that their mortality from lung cancer was found to be $2^1/_2$ times 'normal' (as was found for tuberculous patients in Australia by CAMPBELL, 1961) and their mortality from leukaemia was found to be twice 'normal' — after having made allowance for the sex and age distribution of the patients, the calendar years of observation and possibly also the patients' social class. What would the results mean? Isoniazid can produce pulmonary tumours and leukaemia in mice (though not apparently in rats nor hamsters), but it does not necessarily follow that the excess mortality from lung cancer and

leukaemia in the tuberculous patients is due to the drug[1]. The patients will have been X-rayed repeatedly and this may have contributed to the excess leukaemia, and the tuberculous process itself may have contributed to the excess lung cancer. To distinguish between these alternative interpretations with certainty it would be necessary also to study a similar group of patients who had been X-rayed equally frequently but not treated with isoniazid. In existing conditions, however, this may not be possible and the best one could do would be to collect a large amount of data and analyse the results in detail, trying to define the time and dose relationships between the use of isoniazid and the appearance of the excess mortality from cancer. If these made 'biological sense', on the assumption of a causal relationship between the use of the drug and the excess mortality, the evidence to incriminate the drug would be greatly strengthened. Fortunately, however, in this particular case such a complicated and difficult study may not prove necessary. A large-scale study is being carried out in the U.S.A. in which isoniazid is being given prophylactically for a year to a randomly selected half of a group of persons at high risk of developing tuberculosis, and it will be possible to make a direct comparison between the isoniazid-treated group and another group which was truly comparable in all other respects — at least at the start of treatment.

---

[1] In fact, isoniazid cannot have been responsible for the excess mortality in CAMPBELL'S (1961) series, as only 6 of the 24 patients who developed lung cancer had received chemotherapy.

Conclusion

Prospective studies provide the best way of recognizing the carcinogenic effect of a drug and, despite the difficulties,

they should be carried out routinely when new drugs of any importance are introduced. Not only would they provide a check that the drug is not qualitatively carcinogenic, but they would also provide the quantitative evidence that alone allows a balance to be struck between the beneficial and the harmful effects. I stress however, that they should be carried out routinely. Cancer induction is not the only harmful long-term effect that may be produced by drugs and there are many reasons why new drugs should be kept under observation for some years after they are first introduced. It is wasteful in time and energy to organize special studies for each drug, and there should be national schemes whereby the effect of each new drug is routinely kept under review.

The 'early warning' system of recognizing adverse reactions, which has been introduced in some countries, depends solely on the initiative of doctors in reporting what they suspect to be an unwanted effect. This is highly inefficient for the detection of cancer induction and, I suspect, worse than useless for the detection of some other effects. Modern systems of record linkage, that have been made practicable by the development of electronic computers, have, however, revolutionized the situation and by their use a semi-automatic method of detecting a carcinogenic effect should be possible — at least in countries where there is a national system of medical provision. Once a system for linking medical records has been introduced, the additional work required to enable the carcinogenicity of drugs to be detected is relatively small.

References

BEAN, R. H. D., Phenylbutazone and leukaemia: a possible association. *Brit. med. J.* **1960** II, 1552—55.

BOYD, J. T., and DOLL, R., Gastro-intestinal cancer and the use of liquid paraffin. *Brit. J. Cancer* **8**, 231—37 (1954).

CAMPBELL, A. H., The association of lung cancer and tuberculosis. *Aust. Ann. Med.* **10**, 129—36 (1961).

COURT BROWN, W. M., and DOLL, R., Mortality from cancer and other causes following radiotherapy for ankylosing spondylitis. *Brit. med. J.* **1965** II, 1327—1332.

COX, D. R., *Planning of experiments*, second ed. New York: John Wiley & Sons, Inc., 1961.

DOLL, R., *Medical surveys and clinical trials*, second ed., p. 64. London: Oxford University Press 1964.

FISHER, R. A., *The design of experiments*, seventh ed. Edinburgh: Oliver & Boyd 1960.

GOLBERG, L., Hazards of iron-dextran. *Brit. med. J.* **1960** II, 1598—99.

HILL, A. B., The environment and diseases: association or causation. *Proc. roy. Soc. Med.* **58**, 295—300 (1965).

HORTA, J. DA S., ABBATT, J. D., DA MOTTA, L. C., and RORIZ, M. L., Malignancy and other late effects following administration of thorotrast. *Lancet* **1965** II, 201—205.

INTERNATIONAL COMMISSION FOR RADIOLOGICAL PROTECTION. The evaluation of risks from radiation. ICRP Publication 8. Oxford: Pergamon Press 1966.

IRWIN, J. O., Statistical treatment of measurements of the carcinogenic properties of tars (part I) and mineral oils (part II). *J. Hyg. (Lond.)* **44**, 362—419 (1964).

PIKE, M. C., and ROE, F. J. C., An actuarial method of analysis of an experiment in two-stage carcinogenesis. *Brit. J. Cancer* **17**, 605—610 (1963).

POCHIN, E. E., Leukaemia following radio-iodine treatment of thyrotoxicosis. *Brit. med. J.* **1960** II, 1545—50.

ROBINSON, C. E. G., BELL, D. N., and STURDY, G. H., Possible association of malignant neoplasm with iron-dextran injection. *Brit. med. J.* **1960** II, 648—50.

WOODLIFF, H. J., and DOUGAN, L., Acute leukaemia associated with phenylbutazone treatment. *Brit. med. J.* **1964** I, 744—46.

Discussion

Roe: As a general rule, in the course of testing chemical agents for carcinogenicity, one is most likely to achieve a positive result by administering the test substance at doses close to the maximum compatible with longevity. However, there are many instances, especially where the effect of the test substance is spent mainly on a non-vital tissue, of carcinogenic action being optimal at doses less than the maximum tolerated. Thus it is possible to apply a carcinogenic substance to the skin in such a high dose that there is widespread destruction of tissue. The yield of tumours may then be less than with lower doses.

Schoental: The hepatotoxic and hepato-carcinogenic pyrrolizidine alkaloids are a good example of compounds which are less likely to be effective as carcinogens, when the dosage is increased above the optimal. While in our experiments a single dose of about LD_{30} induced hepatomata in some of the rats which survived longer than 2 years, atrophic livers and no tumours were produced in rats by BULL and DICK (1959) by the repeated administration of 0.1 of LD_{50} resulting in a total dosage, about $2 \times LD_{50}$ or more.

A necrotic cell cannot divide or produce a tumour.

Reference

BULL, L. B., and DICK, A. T., The chronic pathological effects on the liver of the rat of the pyrrolizidine alkaloids heliotrine, lasiocarpine, and their N-oxides. *J. Path. Bact.* **78**, 483 (1959).

Higginson: In addition to the methods indicated by the speaker, namely prospective and retrospective studies, would it be possible to get an approximation of risk by comparing two geographically different populations, one exposed to a drug in high concentration, and the other in low concentration? If no difference in incidence of the relevant form of cancer were seen could this be taken as evidence of carcinogenic safety?

Taylor: In our experience we can count on the accuracy of mortality records for some types of cancer, e.g. breast cancer, but not on those for rarer forms of cancer e.g. bone cancer.

Doll: Differences between cancer incidence in different parts of the world are so great and so many factors are likely to contribute to them,

that it will usually be very difficult to test the effect of a given drug by comparing the different incidences of cancer in countries that use it in different amounts. I agree with Dr. HIGGINSON, however, in believing that such comparisons can sometimes be of great value. It is notable, for example, that cancer of the thyroid in children was commoner in the U.S.A. than in many other countries, corresponding to the greater use of radiotherapy for a supposedly abnormal enlargement of the thymus in infants. We may note also that cancer of the liver is common only in populations that do not use drugs extensively, so that this condition is unlikely to be commonly iatrogenic. Similarly, as the incidence of gastric cancer falls in the U.S.A. it becomes increasingly unlikely that sophisticated food additives are an important cause.

I agree with Professor SHUBIK in thinking that long-term studies ought to be made of the incidence of cancer in women taking oral contraceptives. Cancer of the breast is such a common condition that an increase of, say, 20 per cent in incidence would be of substantial importance; it would, however, be extremely difficult to recognize in the absence of a planned prospective study. If an increase in cancer is produced it will be necessary, also, to measure its effect against the beneficial effects of family limitation.

Dr. POEL stressed the need for precise definition of terms. In my paper, I must admit that I used 'carcinogen' loosely to include all agents that contributed in any way to an increased cancer incidence. I agree, of course, with his point that we need to study the effect of a drug on the whole life span and not just on the frequency of occurrence of a particular disease.

I agree with Dr. TAYLOR that death certificate information may be unreliable as medical evidence of the cause of death. The degree of unreliability, however, varies from cause to cause and for some causes vital statistics data can be very useful — certainly in those countries which could entertain the idea of introducing a national system of record linkage. Any such system should also include the information obtained by cancer registration (if available) as well as that obtained by death certification.

Quantitative Aspects in Chemical Carcinogenesis

H. Druckrey

Forschergruppe Praeventivmedizin am Max Planck-Institut für Immunbiologie, Freiburg i. Br., Deutschland

A proper scientific judgement of the potential risks which may arise from carcinogenic substances — wherever they may be present in human environment — as well as of the possible and necessary measures for cancer prevention presumes the knowledge of the pharmacological laws, governing the carcinogenic action. This applies especially to the dose-response relationships.

Some problems are of special importance: The persistence and accumulation of carcinogenic effects, the reversibility or irreversibility of the specific changes on the cellular level, the efficiency of very small doses at continuous exposure, the existence or non-existence of sub-threshold doses, which can be considered harmless for human health even at continuous exposure to several carcinogens, and the specificity of carcinogenic actions.

A thorough investigation of these fundamental problems is only possible in systematic *animal experiments* in which the objects are fully uniform, the causal agent, the dosage and experimental conditions are determinable at will, and the entire process can be surveyed from the beginning. Moreover, a true advance can only be expected from quantitative results that are expressible in measurement and number and thus available to criticism.

Our own work to be reported here in comparison to results of other investigators covers a time of more than 25 years and embraces an animal material of about 10000 rats, in which some 3000 malignant tumours of several organs like liver, oesophagus, forestomac, kidneys, urinary bladder, skin, lungs, nasal cavity, brain, spinal cord and peripherical nerves have been induced, mostly selectively and some of them for the first time in investigations of almost 100 partly new carcinogenic compounds of various groups. The histology was done almost exclusively by H. Hamperl and C. Thomas (Bonn).

The first studies of dose-response relationships we carried out with *4-dimethyl-aminobenzene* (4-DAB) given continuously in the diet of BD III — rats (Druckrey, 1943) [5]. Within the range of daily dosages from 3 to 30 mg per rat the induction time (t) up to the appearance of liver cancers was inversely proportional to the daily dose (d)

$$t = \frac{k}{d}. \tag{1}$$

(Table I): By plotting the dependency of t on d in a double logarithmic network linearity resulted [5]. This will be discussed lateron (compare Fig. 9).

According to equation (1) the product of the daily dosage and the induction time is constant

$$dt = k \tag{2}$$

corresponding to the sum of all individual doses or the total dose (D) administered, which was practically 1000 mg in these dosage groups (Table I).

Table I. *Induction of liver cancer in rats by 4-DAB in the daily diet. Dependency of induction time and carcinogenic total dose upon daily dosage* (Druckrey and Küpfmüller, 1948) [10]

d daily dosage mg/rat	t induction time days	D total dose mg/rat
30	34	1.020
20	52	1.040
10	95	950
5	190	950
3	350	1.050
1	700	700

span of the rats summing up to final tumour manifestation. Accordingly the carcinogenic action (A) is to be considered as a function of the sum of all consecutive doses

$$A = f(\textstyle\sum d). \qquad (4)$$

Therefore the term *"summation action"* was proposed and defined theoretically on the basis of molecular pharmacology (Druckrey and Küpfmüller, 1948, 1949). [10, 11].

The apparent dangerousness of carcinogenic substances and the fact, that 4-DAB has been used as colouring matter for food made it necessary to re-

Table II. *Production of liver cancer in rats with 4-dimethylaminoazobenzene. Treatment discontinued after certain total doses. Dependency of the latent period and the tumour yield upon total dose administered* (Druckrey, 1951) [6]

d daily dosage mg/rat	t_1 exposure time days	$D = d \cdot t_1$ total dose mg/rat	t_2 latent period days	yield liver carcinomas %
5	200	1000	0	81
5	140	700	110	80
5	100	500	240	49
5	60	300	280	26
5	40	200	320	20

With the lowest dosage of 1 mg per day, however, the total dose up to tumour appearance was only $D = 700$ mg and thus significantly smaller, although the induction time of 700 days was extremely long. Therefore the time apparently makes a contribution to the action and the total process of cancer production would be more accurately described by modificating the formula (2) into

$$d t^n = k \qquad (3)$$

with $n > 1$. This has later proved to be appropriate [see equations (6) and (7)].

These results indicated, that the primary carcinogenic effects of all individual doses, even the smallest persist and remain irreversible over the whole life

commend practical measures for cancer prevention (Druckrey, 6. International Cancer Congress, Paris 1950)[1].

To investigate the *time factor* in carcinogenesis further feeding experiments with 4-DAB were carried out on young rats in which the daily dosage was kept constant (5 mg/rat) but the duration of treatment and hence the total dose administered were varied. Five groups of rats have been used. The treatment was discontinued after reaching a total dose of 200, 300, 500, 700 and 1000 mg per rat respectively ("stop-experiments"). The results are given in Table II.

---

[1] „Vorschlag zu einer internationalen Zusammenarbeit für den Schutz der Bevölkerung vor carcinogenen Agentien", publ. in: Acta Unio intern. Canc. IX, 277, 1953.

Although the 4-DAB is metabolized or excreted in a few days, the typical liver cell- and bile-duct carcinomas developed lateron in 268 rats of all groups. The latent period was the longer — up to 800 days after the "stop" of the treatment — and the tumour yield the lower, the smaller the total dose administered (Druckrey, 1951) [6]. Corresponding experiments of Glinos and Bucher

strict control. Furthermore it was to be investigated whether the findings made in the case of 4-DAB are reproducible also with other types of carcinogens and in the production of cancer of other organs.

In the next series of experiments we used *4-dimethylaminostilbene* (4-DAST), a more potent carcinogen which produces carcinomas in the ear-duct of rats, as first shown by Haddow et al. (1948 [22].

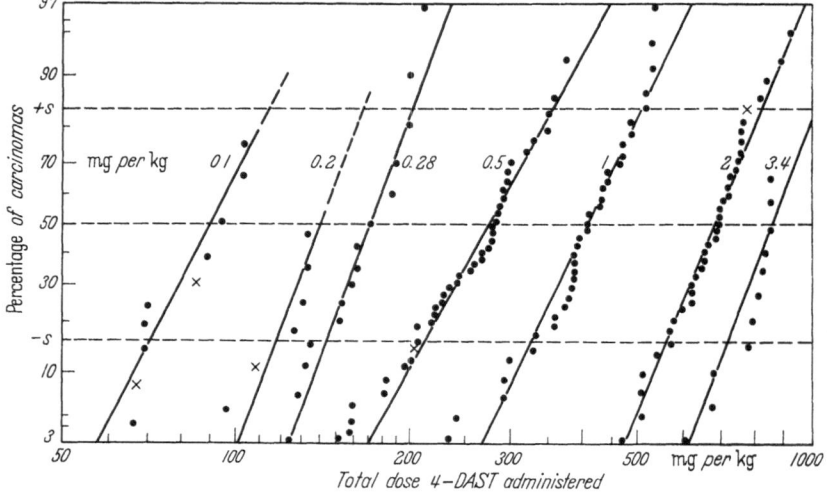

Fig. 1. Incidence of carcinomas in dependence on the sum of doses 4-dimethylamino-stilbene (4-DAST) administered in BD II rats for 7 separate dosage groups, ranging from 0.1 to 3.4 mg per kg b.w. respectively, given in the daily diet. Continuous treatment up to tumor appearence. Dots: rats with ear duct carcinomas, crosses: mammary cancer. — Ordinate: Percentage of carcinoma incidence, probits. Abscissa: total dose, mg per kg b.w., 5 fold elongated

(1951) [21] and of Hecht (1952) [23] produced similar results.

These results proved that the carcinogenic action is not only irreversible but progresses with time although the causal agent is no longer present.

The experiments with 4-DAB had already led to some valuable information. They could however only be regarded as a first approach. For a more far-reaching quantitative evaluation a much greater accuracy must be aimed at. Therefore in the following experiments inbred strains of rats [7] have been used and the dosage given in mg per kg body weight under

BD II — rats (cPah) [7] have been treated with 4-DAST, given in a standard diet in seven dosage groups, about 40 animals each, with the following doses: 3.4; 2.1; 1.0; 0.5; 0.28; 0.2 and 0.1 mg per kg body weigth per day. As soon as the development of a carcinoma was observed, the total dose of 4-DAST absorbed and the length of the induction time was determined for each individual animal. Practically all surviving rats developed carcinomas of the ear duct (Druckrey et al., 1963) [17].

The entry of the increasing percentages of carcinomas produced (dots) in a probit-network gave a clear linear dependence on the logarithm of the total dose in all groups, corresponding to a normal distribution as presented in Fig. 1. This proves that the carcinogenic action of 4-DAST also is a function of the total dose, the sum of all individual doses administered ("summation action").

Fig. 1 shows already that the straight lines of the individual dosage groups move the more to the left into the range of smaller total doses, the smaller the

The plotting of the results in a double logarithmic system of coordinates (Fig. 2) showed a definite linear relationship between the medium total dose D 50 (left ordinate) or the medium induction time t 50 (right ordinate) and the daily dosage (d) (abscissa). Even in the case of the lowest dosage of only 0,1 mg/kg per day no deviation from the linear course is recognizable, although the ear-duct carcinomas developed only on the 900th day of treatment, i.e. after 1,000 days of

Table III. *Dose-response relationships for the production of ear-duct carcinomas in BD II-rats by 4-dimethyl-aminostilbene, given in the daily diet* (DRUCKREY, SCHMÄHL and DISCHLER, 1963) [17]

d daily dosage mg/kg	yield carcinomas survivors numbers	D 50 total dose mg/kg	t_{50} induction time days	s standard deviation %
3.4	11/18	852	150	17
2.0	37/38	680	340	20
1.0	36/37	407	407	25
0.5	42/44	275	550	25
0.28	15/16	170	607	18
0.2	6/12	140	700	18
0.1	9/12	90	900	24

daily dosage was. This falling off is significant and constant.

The quantitative relationships were determined by calculating the medium total doses D 50 and the medium induction times t 50 up to tumour appearance in 50 per cent of the treated rats for each of the seven dosage groups. The results are contained in Table III. They show for the total doses a decrease from 852 mg/kg in the case of the highest daily dosage to only 90 mg/kg in the lowest, i.e. almost to a tenth part. From this it appears very clearly, that the total dose needed to produce cancer with small daily doses over a long period ist not greater but significantly smaller. Thus the carcinogenic action goes considerably beyond a pure "summation action" and increases with the time.

life. Since this is the highest age for our rats, with lower dosage the manifestation of tumours would no longer be experienced. Accordingly the limiting factor lies solely in the limited expectation of life. There is no evidence of a sub-threshold dose.

The ascertained linearity of the dose-effect relationships in Fig. 2 permitted a more precise evaluation. The slope of the straight line for the logarithmic dependence of the induction time t to the appearance of 50% carcinomas (= constant) on the daily dosage d corresponds to an angle of 71.5° and tangens = 3. Therefore is

$$\log d = \log k - 3 \log t \qquad (5)$$

or

$$d \, t^3 = \text{const.} \qquad (6)$$

According to equation (6) the carcinogenic action of 4-DAST at continuous oral administration of constant doses proceeds with the third potency of the time. It thus corresponds to a *"reinforcing action"* (Verstärkerwirkung) or an accelerated process (Druckrey, Schmähl and Dischler, 1963) [17].

Since this type of action was new in pharmacology and with regard to some cially attacking N 7 of guanine has been first demonstrated by Farber and Magee (1960) [29] with dimethylnitrosamine given in the diet of rats. The induced changes of genetic informations most probably are to be regarded as the primary carcinogenic process on the cellular level [26].

DENA was administered in the daily drinking water to BD II rats. [7]. In this

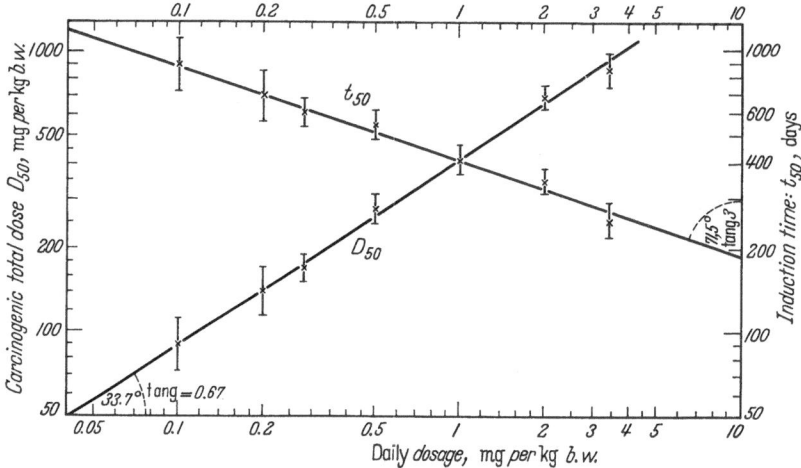

Fig. 2. Linear dependence of the medium carcinogenic total dose D_{50} and of the medium induction time t_{50} on the daily dosage of 4-dimethylaminostilbene, feeding experiments in BD II rats. Columns: 3ε ($P = 0.01$). Ordinate left: sum of all doses administered up to 50 per cent tumor appearance, right: medium induction time

criticism [20, 31], further experiments seemed to be necessary. For this purpose we used *diethylnitrosamine* (DENA), a potent liver carcinogen for rats [15]. This compound is readily soluble in water and has the great advantage that its biochemical mechanism of action is far better explained than that of other carcinogens [29].

Dialkynitrosamines are quickly hydroxylated and dealkylated by microsomal ("drug metabolizing") enzymes, contained preferentially in the liver [27]. The resulting diazoalkanes are highly unstable and powerful alkylating agents. Alkylation of intact nucleic acids especially strain the rate of spontaneous malignancies is very low, less than 5 per cent at an age of 2 years. Nine groups of rats have been used, the dosage ranging from 14.2 to 0.075 mg per kg body weight per day. As a whole 273 malignant tumours were observed, mostly carcinomas of the liver, at low dosages also of the oesophagus and in some cases of the nasal cavity. Even at the lowest dosage of only 0.075 mg per kg, corresponding to 1/4,000 part of the acute LD 50, all five surviving rats developed carcinomas after more than 800 days of treatment (Druckrey, Schildbach, Schmähl, Preussmann and Ivankovic, 1963) [15].

The most striking result of these experiments was the extraordinary precision with which the tumours appeared. The introduction of the cumulative tumour appearance dependent on the logarithms of the total dose administered into a probit network, where each dot represents a rat with carcinoma, yielded clear linear and unusual steep regressions (Fig. 3, abscissa 5 fold elongated). The

calculated tangens values were 25 to 80 corresponding to ascending angles of 89°. This goes far beyond the accuracy of dose-action relationships hitherto attained in pharmacology.

Fig. 3 shows again that the carcinogenic total dose of DENA does not increase when spread at lower dosage over a longer time, but actually becomes considerably smaller, falling from 1,000 to

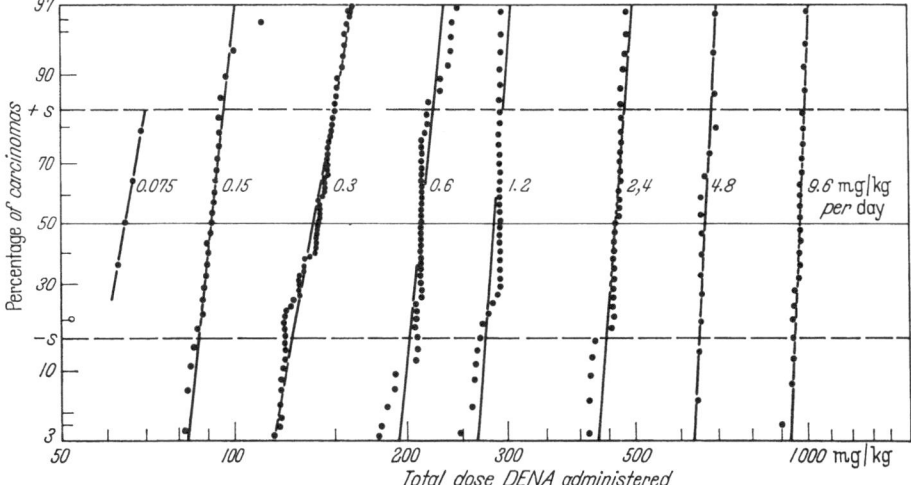

Fig. 3. Dose-response relationships for the carcinogenic action of diethylnitrosamine (DENA) in BD II rats. 8 dosage groups, ranging from 0.075 to 9.6 mg per kg body weight, given in the daily drinking water. Each dot corresponds to an individual rat with carcinomas. Normal distribution over the total dose administered = sum of all daily doses. Abscissa 5-fold elongated

Table IV. *Medium total dose and induction time dependend on daily dosage in diethylnitrosamine carcinogenesis (mg per kg body weight, BD II-rats)* (DRUCKREY et al., 1963) [15]

d daily dosage mg/kg	yield carcinomas survivors number	D 50 total dose mg/kg	t 50 induction time days	s standard deviation %
14.2	5/5	1000	68	8
9.6	25/25	963	101	1
4.8	25/25	660	137	3
2.4	34/34	460	192	4.7
1.2	36/36	285	238	6.5
0.6	49/49	213	355	7.1
0.3	67/67	137	457	8.9
0.15	27/30	91	609	6.3
0.075	5/7	64	840	—
1:200	273/278	1:15	1:12	

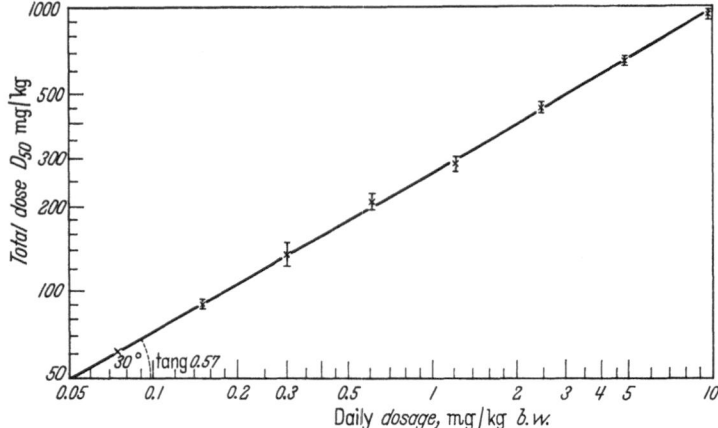

Fig. 4. Linear dependency of the carcinogenic total dose (D_{50}) diethylnitrosamine upon the daily dosage plotted on log-log coordinates. 8 groups, daily dosage: 0.075; 0.15; 0.3; 0.6; 1.2; 2.4; 4.8 and 9.6 mg per kg b.w. respectively. BD II-rats, columns: 3 s ($p = 0.01$)

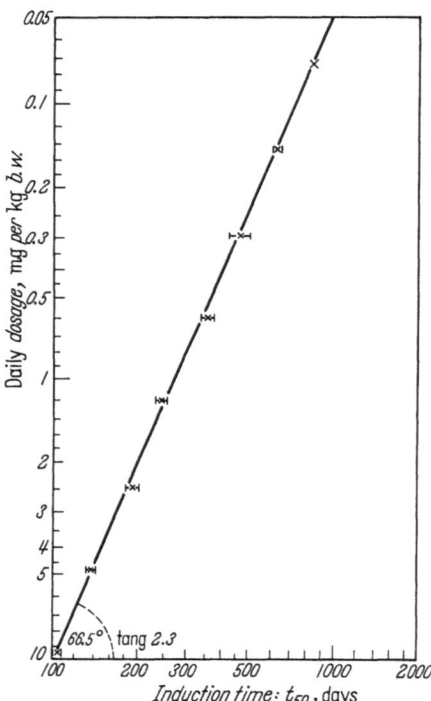

Fig. 5. Linear dependency of the medium induction times (t_{50}) upon the daily dosages diethylnitrosamine, plotted on log-log-coordinates. 8 groups, dosage ranging from 0.075 to 9.6 mg per kg

only 64 mg per kg. Thereby the former results with 4-DAST (Fig. 1) are confirmed.

The medium values of the total doses (D 50) and of the induction times (t 50) for the various dosage groups are assembled in Table IV.

For their dependence on the daily dosage (d) a striking linearity was found in the double logarithmic network. This is shown for the *total doses* in Fig. 4. Again, as in Fig. 2, even in the case of the lowest dosage groups no deviation from the linear course is recognizable. Correspondingly there is no indication for the existence of a "subthreshold dose".

The straight line for the *induction times* is presented in Fig. 5. The angle to the abscissa is 66.5° and the corresponding tang. = 2.3. Thus, analogous to equation (6)

$$d\, t^{2,3} = \text{const.} \tag{7}$$

and a "reinforcing action" is to be assumed.

Similar results have been obtained in quantitative experiments with many other dialkylnitrosamines, mostly producing cancer selectivily in a certain organ like liver [15], oesophagus [12], urinary bladder [13], nasal cavity [8] or brain [9] of rats. In all cases the appearance of cancers in dependence on the total dose administered and on the induction time corresponded clearly to a normal distribution.

Surprisingly this was also observed with such compounds, which produced cancer in several organs. Two examples

groups. The medium values observed for the induction time (t) dependend on daily dosage (d) corresponded fairly well to formula (7). Therefore, the values of the constants have been calculated as *"indices of carcinogenic dosage"*

$$d \, t^{2,3} = \text{index} \qquad (8)$$

the daily dosage d expressed in [m Mol] per kg body weight, to have a direct comparability. Accordingly, a low "in-

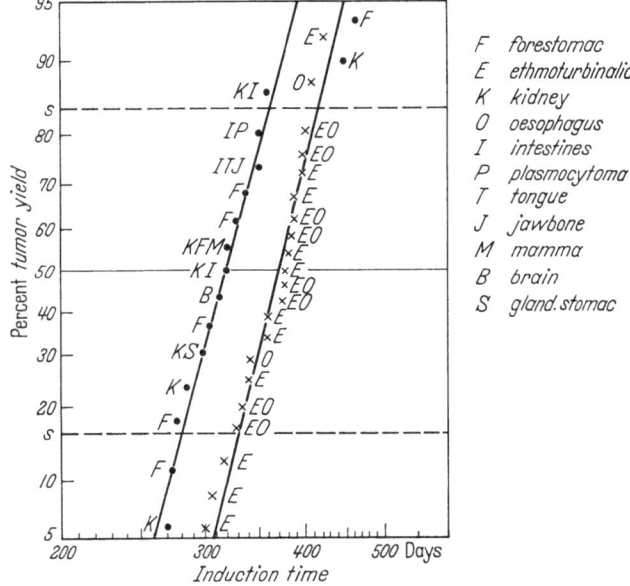

Fig. 6. Normal distribution of the induction times in carcinogenesis, independent upon the variety of organs of tumor development in BD-rats. left: methylnitrosourea, single i.v. injection, 70 mg/kg. right: N-nitrosopiperidine, 10 mg/kg, s.c. twice a week

are given in Fig. 6. Although many organs are involved, the individual cases fit strikingly into the same straight line for normal distribution. Furthermore in spite of the variety of the tumour types, of the two compounds investigated, and of the experimental conditions, both streight lines are practically parallel. This indicates, that lastly a similar mechanism of action has to be assumed (compare Fig. 10).

With some dialkylnitrosamines the experiments included several dosage

dex" corresponds to low dosage and therefore to high carcinogenicity. For better convenience the figures are divided by 10,000 in the following graphs.

As a first example the "indices" of the homologous group of dialkylnitrosamines dependend on the number of C-atoms per chain are presented in Fig. 7. It shows, that diethylnitrosamine surprisingly is more potent than the dimethyl-compound and with higher alkylchains the carcinogenic potency decreases in a strikingly linear order, indicating the reliability of the results obtained.

As a more heterogeneous group, some alkyl-ethylnitrosamines are compared in Table V.

Here, the ethanol-(2)-ethyl-compound, which is practically non toxic in acute experiments, seems to be a relatively weak carcinogen, but it produced liver-carcinomas in all treated rats within less

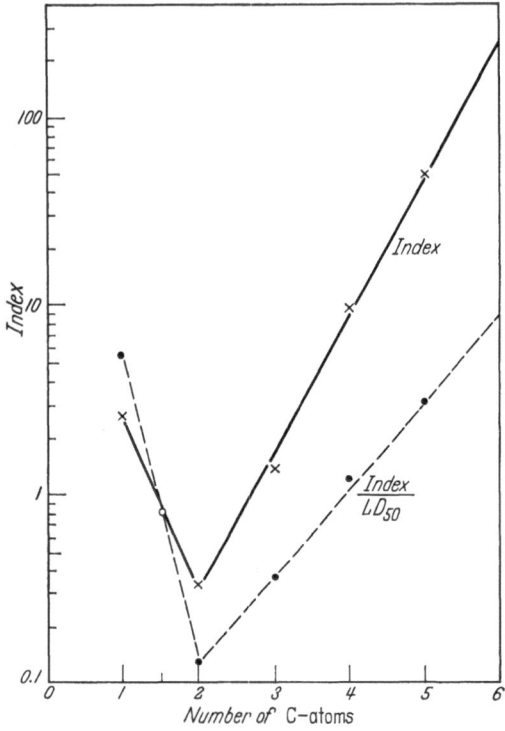

Fig. 7. "Index of carcinogenic dosage" of symmetric dialkylnitrosamines, dependend on the number of C-Atoms in each chain. Index: $dt^{2,3} = $ konst [mMol · 10⁴]; $d = $ daily dosage, oral administration, BD-strain rats, LD$_{50}$ in mMol per kg body weight, $t = $ med. induction time 1 = dimethyl-; 1.5 = methyl-ethyl-; 2 = diethyl- up to; 5 = diamyl-nitrosamine

Table V. *Acute lethal doses and "Indices of carcinogenic dosage" of several alkyl-ethyl-nitrosamines, given in the daily diet of BD-strain rats. Index: $d \cdot t^{2,3} = $ const. [mMol] · 10⁻⁴, $d = $ daily dosage, $t = $ med. induction time*

R\\ >N—N=O C₂H₅/	LD 50		carcinogenic dosage	
	mg/kg	mMol/kg	Index	Index LD 50
R = methyl	90	1	0.81	0.81
ethyl	280	2.8	0.35	0.13
vinyl	88	0.88	0.4	0.45
ethanol	8000	60.0	5.0	0.08
iso-propyl	1100	9.5	8.5	0.9
n-butyl	380	2.9	0.9	0.31
tert. butyl	1600	12.0	not carcinogenic	

than 12 months, this however only at relatively high dosage (unpublished).

This raises the question, how to judge "weak" and "potent" carcinogens. Four criteria are applicable: 1) the dosage needed, 2) the length of the induction time, 3) the percentage of tumour yield, and 4) the malignancy of the tumours induced. All these factors are included in formula (8). But there is an other point to be considered.

anol-ethyl-nitrosamine for example is still effective with 0.025 "units" (percent of LD 50) and benz(a)pyrene (DRUCKREY and SCHILDBACH, 1963 [14], the dosage calculated per day) with only 1 "milli-unit" is the most powerful and specific acting carcinogen in this group.

The declaration of the effective dose or dosage in percent of the acute LD 50 as "units" has been proposed first in cancer chemotherapy for comparison of

Table VI. *Relative potency of several carcinogenic substances. Relationships between the lowest dosage (per day) producing cancer in more than 50 percent of treated rats, and the acute LD 50. Carcinogenic dosage in percent of the LD 50 = "carcinogenic range" or "carcinogenic units"*

Compound	acute LD 50		lowest carcinogenic dosage per day	
	mg/kg	route	mg/kg	percent of LD 50
systemic action				
4-dimethylamino-azobenzene	175	oral	6.0	3.5
4-dimethylamino-stilbene	70	oral	0.1	0.14
diethylnitrosamine	280	oral	0.1	0.03
N-ethyl-N-ethanol-nitrosamine	8000	oral	2	0.025
Local action				
3,4-benzopyrene	100	subcut.	0.001	0.001

When the "indices" are calculated in relation to the acute LD 50 (last column in Table V), results are obtained which pharmacologically seem to be more correct and permit at the same time a proper judgement of the "carcinogenic range" and therefore of the specificity of the carcinogenic action. Under these circumstances ethanol-ethyl-nitrosamine appears as a very potent and highly specific carcinogen.

As a more simple method the comparison of the lowest daily dosage producing a 50 percent tumour yield at continuous treatment, to the acute LD 50 may be used as a first approach. If this is expressed in percentages of the LD 50, as presented in Table VI for various compounds then the figures obtained can be used as "carcinogenic units". Eth-

drugs acting at very different dosage levels (DRUCKREY et al., 1963) [18] but it is generally applicable in pharmacology and toxicology. Even as the time factor is not respected to, this simple calculation provides valuable and obvious information as to the "range" and "specificity" of the action considered.

The striking conformity of the results obtained with carcinogens of such chemical variety as 4-DAB, 4-DAST, DENA and several other nitrosamines, suggested a comparison with the dose-response relationships reported by other investigators. They concern mainly higher *aromatic hydrocarbons,* which have a predominantly local action.

The first quantitative experiments by BRYAN and SHIMKIN (1943) [3] with 1,2,5,6-dibenzanthracene, benzopyrene and methylcholanthrene, given as a single subcutaneous injection to about 1,000 C3H-mice had already shown a normal distribution for the incidence of the tumours produced in dependence of the

Table VII. *Dose-effect relationships for the carcinogenic action of methylcholanthrene on the skin of the mouse with continuous treatment. According to the results of* HORTON *and* DENMAN *(1955) [24]*

Dosage	Induction period	Total dose
mg/week	weeks	mg
0.132	30.3	4.0
0.225	23.8	5.3
0.27	21.3	5.8
0.45	18.1	8.1
0.516	16.1	8.3
1.04	11.1	11.5
2.07	7.3	15.1

um induction period in the experiments of HORTON and DENMAN and of POEL. The results are presented in Tables VII and VIII. They show in complete agreement with our own results (Tables III and IV) that with smaller individual doses and hence longer induction time the total dose decreases considerably. This is particularly clear in the experiments by POEL (Table VIII) which embrace a large range of dosage. The carcinogenic total dose falls here from 21.5 mg in the case of the highest dosage to only 0.47 mg in the lowest, although the production of carcinomas still amounts to 65 percent of the animals.

The introduction of the calculated *total doses* in a double logarithmic network yielded a linear dependence on the

Table VIII. *Dose-effect relationships for the tumorigenic and carcinogenic action of 3,4-benzpyrene in painting experiments on mice with continuous treatment. Dosage in mcg per mouse three times weekly. According to the results of* POEL *(1959) [32]*

Dosage	Tumors (Total)			Carcinomas		
	Produc-tion	Induction time	Total dose	Produc-tion	Induction time	Total dose
mcg	%	(days)	mcg	%	(days)	mcg
0.38	20	392	64	4		
0.75	13	322	103	7		
3.8	84	252	410	65	287	470
19	100	136	1030	97	175	1400
94	100	112	4500	100	147	5900
188	86	91	7400	71	133	10700
376	100	77	12800	86	133	21500

logarithm of the dose below the limit of saturation. Similar results have been reported by HORTON and DENMAN (1955) [24] and by POEL (1959) [32] in extensive studies on the dose-effect relationships of several aromatic hydrocarbons, regularly painted to the skin of mice up to tumour appearance.

Since according to our findings the carcinogenic action is a function of the sum of all individual doses, the effective total doses (D 50) have been calculated from the individual doses and the medi-

individual dosage. As an example the data of POEL (Table VIII, last column) are presented Fig. 8 in comparison to these obtained with 4-DAST and DENA. It shows the relative high efficacy of small doses at continuous exposure. Quite similar results are reported by HUEPER [25]. This proves, that the carcinogenic effects even of very small doses remain irreversible and sum up beyond a mere additive manner.

On the basis of our results reported here, the dependence of the medium *in-*

duction time on the dosage seemed to be especially important. This mode of evaluation is also possible, when the carcinogen was given only in a single dose, as in the fundamental experiments of BRYAN and SHIMKIN (1943) [*3*]. If the values obtained by several authors and

ed and the tumour types produced, the dose-effect and induction-time relationship in chemical carcinogenesis can be expressed most satisfactory by the same formula (10). The only difference apparently lies in the value of the tangens n, which at the same time is characteristic

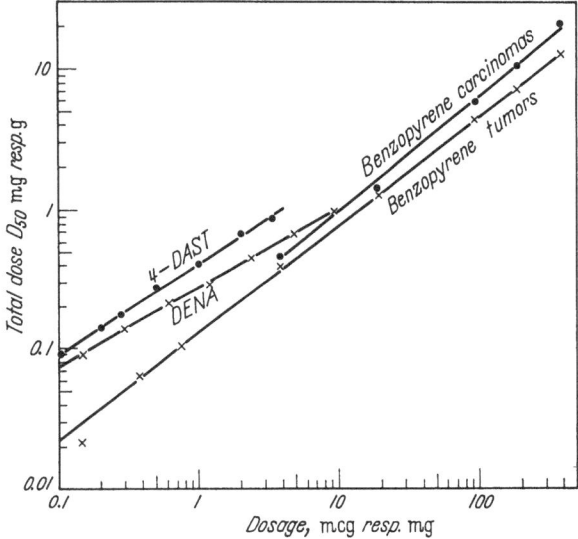

Fig. 8. Linear dependency of the carcinogenic total dose (D_{50}) upon the dosage, plotted on log-log coordinates. Continous treatment. benzopyrene, skin painting of mice, 3 times weekly, abscissa: mcg, ordinate: mg, POEL, 1959; 4-dimethylaminostilbene, orally on rats, abscissa: mg per kg b.w. ordinate: g per kg, DRUCKREY, SCHMÄHL and DISCHLER, 1960; diethylnitrosamine, orally in rats, daily dosage: mg per kg body weight, ordinate: g per kg, DRUCKREY, SCHILDBACH, SCHMÄHL a.o. 1963

by ourselves (Tables I, III, IV, VII and VIII) are represented graphically on logarithmic coordinates, straigth lines resulted in all cases [*16*]. This is demonstrated in Fig. 9. The course of the straight lines correspond to the general formula (9)

$$\log d = \text{const.} - n \log t \quad (9)$$

or

$$d\,t^n = \text{const.} \quad (10)$$

where d is the dosage, t the induction time up to 50 percent tumour appearance (constant) and n indicates the tangens of the slope.

These results proved, that in spite of the variety of the compounds investigat-

for each individual carcinogen and therefore can be considered as the decisive parameter. Formula 10 has a wide applicability in quantitative pharmacology. In contrast to all other actions known up to now, however, carcinogenesis is distinguished by the condition: $n > 1$[1].

---

[1] Recently, a quantitative study on "Experimental tumorigenesis in the Hamster Checkpouch", induced by single injection of 3,4,9,10-dibenzopyrene has been published by J. WODINKY, A. HELINSKI and C. J. KENSLER in Nature 1965, 207, 771. Using the reported data, plotted on log coordinates again a linear relationship between dose and induction time was obtained, corresponding fo formula (10) with $n = 4.1$.

In order to test the applicability of formula (10) and to determine the respective values of n, quantitative experiments have been performed with several other nitrosamines, producing carcinomas of genic action at continuing exposure is to be considered as an accelerated process or a reinforcing action (Verstärkerwirkung).

Similar results have been reported by Blum (1950, 1959) [2] in the production

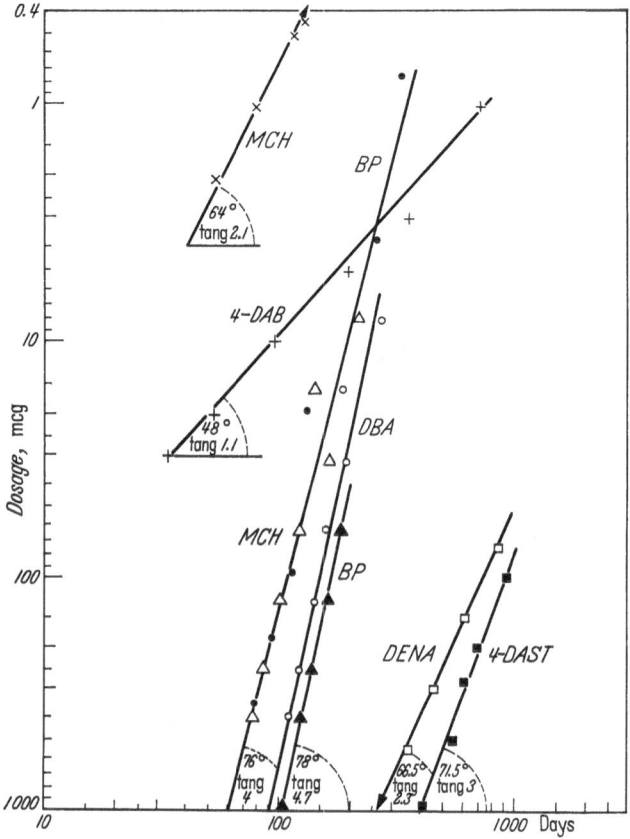

Fig. 9. Linear dependency of the medium induction times (t_{50}) upon dosage, plotted on log-log-coordinates for several carcinogens. × methylcholanthrene, mice skin, 3× weekly, Horton and Denman, 1955; ∓ 4-dimethylaminoazobenzene, rats, daily diet, Druckrey et al., 1943/48 (dosage ×1000); ● 3,4-benzopyrene, mice skin, 3× weekly, Poel, 1955; △ methylcholanthrene, mice, single s.c. inj. Bryan and Shimkin, 1943; ○ 1,2,5,6-dibenzanthracene single s.c. inj. Bryan and Shimkin, 1943; ▲ 3,4-benzopyrene single s.c. inj. Bryan and Shimkin, 1943; □ diethylnitrosamine, rats, daily drink. water, Druckrey et al., 1963; ■ dimethylaminostilbene, rats, daily diet, Druckrey, Schmähl et al., 1963

the liver, oesophagus and urinary bladder in rats. The results of all experiments are combined in Table IX. It shows that in most cases $n > 2$ and ranges up to $n = 4.7$ with benzopyrene and dibenzanthracene as the most powerful carcinogens. Correspondingly the carcino- of skin cancer in mice by U.V.-light. The comprehensive quantitative experiments on a uniform population lead to the formula (11)

$$d\,t^2 = \text{const.} \qquad (11)$$

and accordingly to the conclusion, that the carcinogenic action at regularly re-

Table IX. *Slope of the linear regressions for the relationships between dosage and induction times, plotted on log-log-coordinates, and values of the respective tangens = n, according to equation d · t^n = konst for several carcinogens, type of exposure and target organ of cancer development*

compound	species	administration per week	route	angle (o)	n tang.	tumors	authors
continuous exposure							
4-dimethylaminoazobenzene	rats	7	diet	48	1.1	liver	DRUCKREY (1943, 1948)
di-n-butylnitrosamine	rats	7	diet	55	1.4	bladder	DRUCKREY et al. (1962)
20-methylcholanthrene	mice	3	skin	64	2.1	skin	HORTON and DENMAN (1965)
di-n-propylnitrosamine	rats	7	drink	65	2.2	liver	DRUCKREY et al. (1961)
di-ethylnitrosamine	rats	7	drink	66.5	2.3	liver	DRUCKREY et al. (1963)
N-nitroso-sarcosinester	rats	7	drink	68	2.5	esophagus	DRUCKREY et al. (1963)
4-dimethylaminostilbene	rats	7	diet	71.5	3.0	ear duct	DRUCKREY et al. (1963)
3,4-benzopyrene	mice	3	skin	76	4.0	skin	POEL (1959)
ethyl-butyl-nitrosamine	rats	7	drink	77	4.3	esophagus	DRUCKREY et al. (1963)
single dose injection							
20-methylcholanthrene	mice	1	subcut.	76	4.0	sarcomas	BRYAN and SHIMKIN (1943)
1,2,5,6-dibenzanthracene	mice	1	subcut.	78	4.7	sarcomas	BRYAN and SHIMKIN (1943)
3,4-benzopyrene	mice	1	subcut.	78	4.7	sarcomas	BRYAN and SHIMKIN (1943)

peated irradiation increases with the square of the time and therefore must be interpreted as a constantly accelerated process.

On the basis of experiments with carcinogenic hydrocarbons Berenblum

results from epidemiological data of lung cancer in heavy smokers. At chronic exposure the incidence showed a continuous increase again with the fifth or sixth power of time, dependent on the number of smoked cigarettes.

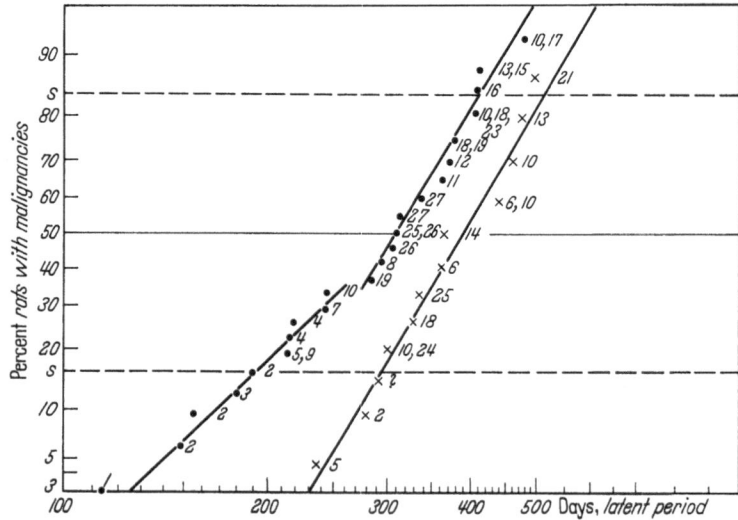

Fig. 10. Carcinogenesis induced by a single dose of methyl-nitroso-urea, given intravenously to BD-strain rats. two dosage groups; ● = 90 and × = 64 mg per kg body weight. *1* spleen, lymphosarcoma; *2* lymphatic leucemia; *3* thymoma; *4* myeloic leucemia; *5* odontoblastoma; *6* jaw, osteoma; *7* abdominal sarcoma; *8* abdominal carcinoma; *9* rectum, adenocarcinoma; *10* bowels, adenocarcinoma; *11* intestines, adenocarcinoma; *12* gland. stomach, sarcoma; *13* forestomach, squam. carcinoma; *14* parotis carcinoma; *15* ear, cholesteatoma; *16* ethmoturbinalia, squam. carcinoma; *17* branchiogenic tumor; *18* nephroblastoma; *19* mamma carcinoma; *20* vagina, myxosarcoma; *21* skin, squameous cell carcinoma; *22* lungs, alveol. cell carcinoma; *23* lungs, adenocarcinoma; *24* brain, reticulosarcoma; *25* brain, polymorph. glioma; *26* spinal cord, spongioblastoma; *27* spinal cord, malign. neurinoma

(1945) [*1*] already proposed an empirical formula (12)

$$G = 16 - 6.5 \log t \qquad (12)$$

which corresponds to $t^{6,5}$. In evaluating the cancer statistics of *men* in England, France, Norway, and the U.S.A., Nordling (1953) [*30*] came to the conclusion, that the death-rate increases with the sixth power of age, and accordingly a practically linear dependence was obtained by plotting the data on double logarithmic coordinates. More recently Doll (1963) [*4*] reported quite similar

This proves that carcinogenesis at continuous exposure in animal experimentation as well as with human beings corresponds to the same dose-effect and time relationships as explained by the general formula (10)

$$d \, t^n = \text{const.} \qquad (10)$$

with $n > 1$. The numeric value of n therefore can be considered as an indicator for the potency of the carcinogen.

If in fact carcinogenesis is to be regarded as an accelerated process or an "reinforcing action", then it should be possible to start the carcinogenesis with only one "impulse" of adequate strenght, and thus to produce cancer with a single dose, even with such carcinogens which are destroyed in the body or excreted within a few hours. This does actually occur. MAGEE and BARNES (1959) [28] with a single dose of 30 mg dimethyl-nitrosamin succeeded to produce cancer of the kidney in rats, as confirmed by DRUCKREY et al. (1964) [19] with several nitrosamines.

This has been most convincingly shown in experiments with methyl-nitroso-urea. Although this highly reactive compound decomposes very rapidly in the organism, a great variety of malignant tumours and leukemias were produced in rats by a single intravenous injection [19].

The results of a second series of quantitative experiments (DRUCKREY, IVANKOVIC and STAHL, 1965, unpublished) are presented in Fig. 10. Practically all rats treated with a single injection of 64 and 90 mg methyl-nitroso-urea per kg body weight respectively, lateron developed tumours. On the whole 27 different types of malignancies in nearly all organs including the brain and spinal cord have been observed. In spite of this extraordinary variety, the time of the individual tumour appearance fits strikingly into the same straight lines for normal distribution, which are practically parallel in both dosage groups. Therefore a similar mechanism of action is to be assumed. However the leukemias and lymphatic tumours, considerably preceding the appearance of carcinomas at the higher dosage, make an exception. Here the straight line unequivocally is broken and a different normal distribution occurs. This indicates that in the production of leukemias a different mechanism of action may be involved.

The apparent linearity and parallelism of the relationships for the induction of solid tumours in both groups (Fig. 10) prove, that carcinogenesis in fact can result from a single "impulse" as it had to be expected according to formula (10), and therefore cannot be considered alone on the basis of the "chronic irritation theory". If the products of the dose (64 and 90 mg per kg) and the respective medium induction time $t\,50$ (380 and 300 days) are calculated, then even a smaller value is obtained with the lower dose (24,000 against 27,000) indicating its relatively high carcinogenic efficacy.

Conclusions

In *conclusion,* the results of the quantitative experiments presented here conformingly show that also in carcinogenesis at continuous exposure with all substances tested and without regard to the organ of tumour development, clear dose-effect and time relationships exist, which are explained by the general formula

$$d\,t^{n} = \text{const.} \qquad (10)$$

with $n > 1$. Accordingly on logarithmic coordinates linear regressions are obtained. Even in the range of very small doses d no deviation from linearity is recognizable. There is no indication for the existence of a "subthreshold dose" as far as the primary effects on the cellular level are considered.

Formula (10) proved to be valid not only in animal experimentation but also in human cancer statistics as demonstrated by NORDLING (1953) and by DOLL (1963). The numeric value of n, however, differs considerably with different carcinogens, ranging from 1.1 up to 6.5 and thus can be considered as an indicator for the carcinogenic activity of the individual compound.

According to formula (10) the carcinogenic action at continuous exposure increases with a higher power of time and must be interpreted as an accelerated process („Verstärkerwirkung"). From this the possibility to produce cancer by a single "impulse" was to be expected and has been demonstrated experimentally on several examples.

For a proper judgement of the relative potency of a carcinogen and of the specificity of its action a few simple methods are proposed. The values abtained with a great variety of compounds range in the order of 1 : 10 millions. This naturally has to be respected to in the toxicological judgement of carcinogens and their potential risk.

References

[1] BERENBLUM, I., System of grading carcinogenic potency. *Cancer Res.* 5, 561 (1945).

[2] BLUM, H. F., *Carcinogenesis by ultraviolet light.* Princeton, New Jersey: Princeton University Press 1959.

[3] BRYAN, W. R., and SHIMKIN, M. B., Quantitative analysis of dose-response data obtained with three carcinogenic hydrocarbons in strain C3H male mice. *J. nat. Cancer Inst.* 3, 503 (1943).

[4] DOLL, R., Interpretation of epidemiologic data. *Cancer Res.* 23, 1613 (1963).

[5] DRUCKREY, H., Quantitative Grundlagen der Krebserzeugung. *Klin. Wschr.* 22, 532, (1943).

[6] — Experimentelle Beiträge zum Mechanismus der carcinogenen Wirkung. *Arzneimittel-Forsch.* 1, 383 (1951).

[7] — DANNENBERG, P., DISCHLER, W., u. STEINHOFF, D., Reinzucht von 10 Rattenstämmen (BD-Stämme) und Analyse des genetischen Pigmentierungssystems. *Arzneimittel-Forsch.* 12, 911 (1962).

[8] — IVANKOVIC, S., MENNEL, H. D., u. PREUSSMANN, R., Selektive Erzeugung von Carcinomen der Nasenhöhle bei Ratten durch N,N'-Di-Nitrosopiperazin, Nitrosopiperidin, Nitrosomorpholin, Methyl-allyl-,Dimethyl- und Methylvinyl-nitrosamin. *Z. Krebsforsch.* 66, 138 (1964).

[9] — — u. PREUSSMANN, R., Selektive Erzeugung maligner Tumoren im Gehirn und Rückenmark von Ratten durch N-Methyl-N-nitrosoharnstoff. *Z. Krebsforsch.* 66, 389 (1965).

[10] —, u. KÜPFMÜLLER, K., Quantitative Analyse der Krebsentstehung. *Z. Naturforsch.* 3b, 254 (1948).

[11] — — *Dosis und Wirkung.* Aulendorf: Ed. Cantor 1949.

[12] — PREUSSMANN, R., u. SCHMÄHL, D., Carcinogenocity and chemical structure of nitrosamines. *Acta Un. int. Cancer* 19, 510 (1963).

[13] DRUCKREY, H., PREUSSMANN, R., IVANKOVIC, S., SCHMIDT, C. H., MENNEL, H. D., u. STAHL, K. W., Selektive Erzeugung von Blasenkrebs an Ratten durch Dibutyl- und N-Butyl-N-butanol (4)-nitrosamin. *Z. Krebsforsch.* 66, 280 (1964).

[14] —, u. SCHILDBACH, A., Quantitative Untersuchungen zur Bedeutung des Benzpyrens für die carcinogene Wirkung von Tabakrauch. *Z. Krebsforsch.* 65, 465 (1963).

[15] — — SCHMÄHL, D., PREUSSMANN, R., u. IVANKOVIC, S., Quantitative Analyse der carcinogenen Wirkung von Diäthylnitrosamin. *Arzneimittel-Forsch.* 13, 841 (1963).

[16] —, u. SCHMÄHL, D., Quantitative Analyse der experimentellen Krebserzeugung. *Naturwissenschaften* 49, 217 (1962).

[17] — — u. DISCHLER, W., Dosis-Wirkungsbeziehungen bei der Krebserzeugung durch 4-Dimethylaminostilben bei Ratten. *Z. Krebsforsch.* 65, 272 (1963).

[18] — STEINHOFF, D., NAKAYAMA, M., PREUSSMANN, R., u. ANGER, K., Experimentelle Beiträge zum Dosisproblem in der Krebs-Chemotherapie und zur Wirkungsweise von Endoxan. *Dtsch. med. Wschr.* 88, 651 (1963).

[19] — PREUSSMANN, R., u. IVANKOVIC, S., Erzeugung von Krebs durch eine einmalige Dosis von Methyl-nitroso-harnstoff und verschiedenen Dialkylnitrosaminen an Ratten. *Z. Krebsforsch.* 66, 1 (1964).

[20] ERDMANN, W., Referat vom Dtsch. Pharmakologen Kongr. 1957 in Freiburg. *Dtsch. med. Wschr.* 82, 1447 (1957).

[21] GLINOS, A. D., BUCHER, N. L. E., and AUB, I. C., The effect of liver regeneration on tumor formation in rats fed

4-dimethylaminoazobenzene. *J. exp. Med.* **93**, 313 (1951).

[22] HADDOW, A., HARRIS, R. J. C., KON, G. A. R., and ROE, E. M., The growth-inhibitory and carcinogenic properties of 4-aminostilbene and derivatives. *Phil. Trans.* B **241**, 147 (1948).

[23] HECHT, G., Zur Wirkung von Dimethyl-aminoazobenzol. *Naunyn-Schmiedebergs Arch. exp. Path. Pharmak.* **215**, 610 (1952).

[24] HORTON, A. W., and DENMAN, D. T., Carcinogenesis of the skin. A Re-examination of methods for the quantitative measurement of the potencies of complex materials. *Cancer Res.* **15**, 701 (1955).

[25] HUEPER, W. C., Environmental carcinogenesis and cancers. *Cancer Res.* **21**, 842 (1961).

[26] LEE, K. Y., LIJINSKY, W., and MAGEE, P. N., Methylation of ribonucleic acids of liver and other organs in different species, treated with C^{14}- and H^3-di-methylnitrosamines in vivo. *J. nat. Cancer Inst.* **32**, 65 (1964).

[27] MAGEE, P. N., Toxic liver injury. The metabolism of dimethylnitrosamine. *Biochem. J.* **64**, 676 (1956).

[28] —, and BARNES, J. M., The experimental production of tumours in the rat by dimethylnitrosamine. *Acta Un. int. Cancr.* **15**, 187 (1959).

[29] — and FARBER, E., Toxic liver injury and carcinogenesis; methylation of rat-liver nucleic acids by dimethylnitrosamine in vivo. *Biochem. J.* **83**, 106, 114 (1962).

[30] NORDLING, C. O., A new theory on the cancer-inducing mechanism. *Brit. J. Cancer* **7**, 68 (1953).

[31] OETTEL, H., Zur Frage der Gesundheitsgefährdung durch Kunststoffe im täglichen Leben. *Arch. Toxikol.* **16**, 381 (1957).

[32] POEL, W. E., Effect of carcinogenic dosage and duration of exposure on skin-tumor induction in mice. *J. nat. Cancer Inst.* **22**, 19 (1959)

Discussion

Saffiotti: On the question of the induction time of internal tumours, I should like to ask Professor DRUCKREY whether the diagnoses were made by pathologists, and how the day of appearance of these tumours was determined. Were the clinical diagnoses made by people who knew the nature of the experiment? Were any experiments done to establish the relationship between the first clinical symptoms and the size and pathology of the tumour at that time? How often was the clinical diagnosis verified at the same time by sacrifice and pathological examination of the animal? Certain internal tumours are indeed very difficult to detect clinically, for example lung cancers.

Druckrey: I quite agree that lung cancers are very difficult to detect clinically. For this reason, the quantitative data presented do not apply to lung tumours. The histological diagnoses of all tumours were made by Professor HAMPERL in Bonn, without knowledge of the design of our quantitative experiments.

Rudali: Could Professor DRUCKREY tell us how he diagnoses the presence of cancers by the clinical examination of animals. I accept that the careful and regular palpation of the liver often permits the early diagnosis of liver tumours, but for other cancers, such as those of the oesophagus, or the plasmocytomas, the thing seems to me to be much more difficult.

Druckrey: The clinical signs and symptoms are quite characteristic.

Kreyberg: How did you decide the starting point of tumour formation in your studies, presumably this is necessary for the measurement of the induction period?

Druckrey: By palpation we are able to detect a variety of tumours whilst they are still small. Liver tumours tend to grow very rapidly so that only a few days elapse between when they are first palpated and when the animal dies.

Kreyberg: Each neoplasm has a minimum development time to manifest itself to naked eye observation or microscopic diagnosis. This minimum development time is characteristic for each tumour type. After application of carcinogens with different potencies, the number of individuals developing a tumour at a certain time will increase with increasing potency, only if the number of individuals is large enough. The earliest tumours will be found at the minimum development time, even after application of the lowest doses.

Roe: May I ask you, Professor DRUCKREY, how did you take into account incidental deaths in your experiments? How did they figure in your calculations?

Druckrey: In all experiments incidental deaths are liable to occur. Our calculations are based on the assumption that the probability that an animals which dies during an experiment would have developed cancer is the same as that for animals which did not die. In this way the intermittent deaths are eliminated.

Frazer: With increasing dosage, was there a corresponding increase in absorption and half-life of the substance in the animals? Some of the effects you describe might be accounted for by changes in amounts absorbed. No doubt, you studied this point.

Druckrey: This is a very important question. Changes in absorption can be expected only below the saturation level. Therefore we tested the saturation in body fluids, first by testing the solubility of the compound, and secondly the excretion of the compound in the faeces. I can definitely state that with all these compounds absorption was complete.

Schoental: I would expect diethylnitrosamine (DENA), which is watersoluble, to be excreted, if at all, in the urine and not in the faeces.

Druckrey: The faeces are only examined to ascertain whether or not the compound was completely absorbed. In the case of DENA administered in the drinking water no nitrosamine is detectable either in the faeces or in the urine. Only in the case of higher homologues that are hydroxylated and possibly combined with glucuronic acid are appreciable concentrations found in the urine.

Druckrey to Higginson. Nitrosamines produced carcinomas in our experiments by oral as well as by parenteral administration and by inhalation.

Druckrey to Frazer. The length of the induction time depends on dosage. With low dosage tumours develop only in old age. With still lower dosage, animals die before tumours appear, nevertheless carcinogenic effects of the cellular or molecular level are present, and their presence can be revealed by exposure to tumour-promoting agents as shown by Professor Berenblum.

Druckrey to Doll. According to our experimental results young or newborn animals and especially embryos are more susceptible to carcinogenic activity than old animals. With regard to the time factor in carcinogenesis, it is appar-

ently not the age of the animals, that contributes to cancer development, but the persistence and progression of carcinogenic changes at the cellular level. Most probably these involve the loss of genetic information essential for organ specific functions, and the progressive release of cells from homeostatic control.

Druckrey Summarizing. In discussing the quantitative aspects in carcinogenesis, we have to differentiate two processes, namely

1. the primary carcinogenic effects at the cellular or molecular level, responsible for the conversion of normal cells into cancer cells, and

2. the subsequent multiplication of the cancer cells so induced to the point at which a malignant tumour is manifest.

Both processes are in theory irreversible and progress with time. With regard to the first process, no threshold dose is demonstrable. For the development of a growing tumour, however, threshold doses exist. The values of these threshold doses differ in the order of 1 to a million with different carcinogens, as shown in my report. In experimental animals as well as in human beings it is now accepted that the smaller the dose, the longer is the induction time, so that the age at which exposure takes place is vitally important. Thus with children who have a long life-expectancy special caution is mandatory. With very low dosage the induction time can be longer than the life-expectancy, which apparently is the limiting factor in carcinogenesis. Every assessment of the potential risk of carcinogenesis, therefore, must take into account both factors: dose and time. Since a real zero tolerance for carcinogens is not always practicable and is scientifically objectionable, I think that the results of our quantitative studies offer the basis for a better approach. As a basis for future discussions it is proposed, that 1 per cent of the lowest dosage, which, given daily over the whole life span to susceptible experimental animals, produces cancer only at the end of the life span, can be considered as the maximum tolerable dose for human beings. This, however, only in such cases, in which a complete exclusion from human environment is not feasible.

Carcinogenic Hazards from Arsenic and Metal Containing Drugs

W. C. Hueper

Chief, Environmental Cancer Section,
National Cancer Institute,
Bethesda 14, Md., U.S.A.

1. General Considerations

Among the numerous non-radio-active metalloids and metals and their inorganic and organic compounds used in the modern industrial economy some have displayed carcinogenic properties when introduced into man and/or animals by various routes (table I). While the bulk of the evidence incriminating some of these chemicals as human carcinogens has been obtained from studies of occupational cancer hazards, arsenicals have elicited cancers in man also when employed as drugs. For the other members of this group of carcinogens (cobalt, selenium, zinc, iron, lead, nickel, chromium), cancerous effects from their use in medicinal preparations and in prosthetic implants have remained so far only suspected of possible sequelae. The experimental evidence incriminating gold and mercury as experimental carcinogens is at present rather tenuous, while it is dubious or absent for other medicinally used metals, such as silver, copper, thallium, bismuth, gold, aluminium, tantalum, molybdenum, cadmium, and manganese.

A critical evaluation of the data available on actual or potential cancer hazards related to the incorporation of arsenic and metals in medicinal preparations re-presents an essential segment of a general assessment of cancer hazards associated with the administration of drugs.

2. Arsenic

a) Historical Data. An occupational exposure to arsenical dust and fumes was incriminated as the cause of cancers of the scrotal skin in tin miners and smelter workers of Cornwall as early as 1822 (Paris). It was not until 1887 that Hutchinson related a prolonged medicinal use of arsenic to the subsequent development of cutaneous cancers in 5 patients treated for psoriasis. When about 10 years later Geyer reported an excessive incidence of cancers of the skin and viscera among the inhabitants of Reichenstein among whom symptoms of chronic arsenic poisoning were frequently noted because of the consumption of drinking water polluted with arsenic, the dietary source which is the third principal type of exposure to arsenicals was placed on record.

Despite the fact that during subsequent decades numerous additional observations on the development of cancers of the skin and viscera following an occupational, dietary and medicinal contact with arsenic have incriminated this chemical as a potent human car-

Table I. *Cancers in man and animals exposed to arsenic and metals*

Agents	Human Evidence				Animal evidence		
	Cancer in man	Target organs	Route of exposures	Types of exposures	Species	Target organs	Routes of exposures
Arsenicals inorganic	pos.	Skin, lung, esophagus, liver, larynx, nasal sinus, etc.	Oral, respiratory, cutaneous	Occupational, dietary, medicinal, environmental	Mouse? rat? rabbit?		Oral, cutaneous parenteral
organic	pos.?	Skin? viscera?	Parenteral	Medicinal	Mouse? trout	Breast, liver	Parenteral, oral
Asbestos	pos.	Lung, pleura, perioneum, intestine?	Respiratory	Occupational, environmental	Rat, mouse?	Viscera lung	Parenteral, respiratory
Chromates	pos.	Lung, nasal, sinus, larynx, skin?	Respiratory cutaneous	Occupational, environmental, medicinal	Rat, mouse	Lung, connective tissue	Respiratory, intrapleural, parenteral
Nickel and nickel compounds	pos.	Nasal, sinus, lung	Respiratory	Occupational, environmental, medicinal	Rat, mouse, guineapig	Lung, connective tissue	Respiratory parenteral
Beryllium and compounds	pos.?	Lung	Respiratory	Occupational environmental	Rat, rabbit, monkey	Lung, bone	Respiratory, parenteral
Iron, iron oxide	pos.?	Lung	Respiratory	Medicinal, occupational, environmental	Rat, mouse	neg. neg.	Parenteral
Iron-polymer complex	pos.?	Connective tissue	Parenteral	Medicinal	Mouse, rat, hamster, rabbit	Connective tissue	Parenteral
Cobalt	neg.	Lung	Respiratory, oral	Occupational, dietary, medicinal	Rat	Connective tissue	Parenteral
Selenium	neg.	Liver	Respiratory, oral	Occupational, dietary, medicinal, environmental	Rat	Liver, thyroid	Oral
Cadmium	neg.	Lung	Respiratory	Occupational, dietary	Rat	Connective tissue	Parenteral
Lead and Lead compounds	neg.	Lung, kidney	Respiratory, oral, parenteral	Occupational, dietary, medicinal environmental	Rat	Kidney	Oral
Zinc compounds	neg.	Skin	Cutaneous, respiratory	Occupational, medicinal	Rooster	Testis	Parenteral
Mercury	neg.	Skin, kidney, lung, intestine	Cutaneous, oral, resp.	Occupational, dietary	Rat	Connective tissue	Parenteral

cinogen, some medical and industrially interested parties have persisted in denying the validity of this impressive human evidence by pointing to the repeated failure of producing cancers in experimental animals given arsenicals by various routes. In further support of this disclaimer, they have advanced the speculative allegation that the cancers observed in arsenic workers were not induced by arsenic but by selenium or cadmium simultaneously present (FROST). The real scientific merits of such commercially inspired contentions are apparent from the fact that some representatives of the nickel industry have attempted to remove from nickel the onus of being a human carcinogen and of being responsible for the production of cancers of the nasal sinuses and lung among nickel refinery workers by claiming that these cancers are induced by contact with arsenic formerly present in the sulfuric acid employed in the processing of nickel matte, although such workers have not exhibited any symptoms of arsenic poisoning.

The fundamental fallacy of such arguments against a carcinogenic action of arsenic has become increasingly apparent in recent years by the rapidly growing evidence which established medicinal, occupational and dietary exposures to arsenicals as the cause of cancers of the skin and of various viscera. The in part epidemic-like occurrence of arsenic cancers is closely associated with the remarkable rise in the use of inorganic and organic arsenicals for a variety of purposes and the thereon dependent increased and intensified exposure of large portions of the general population to arsenicals contained in medicinal preparations, pesticides, herbicides, wood preservatives, feed additives, and industrial chemicals and present as contaminants of foodstuffs, tobacco, air, water and soil.

The scope of this development is indicated by the remarkable rise in the production of inorganic and organic arsenicals in the United States from 1,500 short tons in 1910 to 10,800 short tons in 1955. The consumption of arsenicals in this year in the United States, on the other hand, stood at more than 18,000 tons. The bulk of these arsenicals was used in the form of pesticides and wood preservatives. The remainder went into weed- control programs on non-farming lands and in bodies of water and into public health and medical uses for combatting diseases. During the last decade, large amounts of benzene arsonic acid compounds (arsanilic acid; 3-nitro-4-hydroxyphenyl arsonic acid; 4-nitrophenyl arsonic acid; arsenosobenzene) have been incorporated into poultry and cattle feeds for promoting egg production and weight increase (FROST and SPRUTH). In 1963, more than 4 million, pounds of arsanilic acid have been used as a feed additive in the United States alone. This rather recently introduced practice of employing arsenicals as biologic stimulants in the food animal production industry resembles in many respects the former, now well discredited, use of these chemicals as general tonics in human medicine.

b) Medicinal uses. Inorganic arsenicals employed in medical preparations are as a rule trivalent arsenic compounds, such as potassium arsenite in FOWLER's solution, arsenic iodide in DONOVAN's solution, arsenious acid in Asiatic pills, arsenic sulfide in escharotic ointments. Several pentavalent organic arsenicals (sodium cacodylate, Solarson) are metabolically converted in the body into inorganic arsenic compounds, such as arsenic oxide. Other organic arsenicals of the aromatic variety are either trivalent arsenicals, such as mapharsen, arsphenamine, or are pentavalent, such as atoxyl, tryparsamide, acetarsone, carbasone and treparsol. In these compounds the arsenic is attached directly to the benzol ring from which it is not readily liberated in the body.

An approximate appraisal as to the relative amounts of inorganic arsenicals still used in modern medical practice can be made from the statement of DAMBOLT and FOSS who, in their search of determining the role which medicinal arsenicals play in the induction of lung cancer in Norway, estimated that an average of 50 kg. of arsenic have been sold yearly by druggists in Norway during the last 20 years.

Inorganic and organic arsenicals have been and still are administered by cutaneous, oral and parenteral routes for a variety of human diseases (anemia, debility, chorea, bronchial asthma, alopecia, acne, eczema, epilepsy, rheumatic fever, psychoneuroses, psoriasis, amebiasis, trypanosomiasis, syphilis, cancer of the skin, leukemia, etc.). In veterinary medicine, arsenicals, particularly several organic arsenicals, have widely been used, often given as additives in feeds, for the control of a number of parasitic diseases in fish, poultry and livestock (amebiasis, coccidiosis, blackhead, bluecomb, nonspecific and hemorrhagic enteritis, spirochitosis, scours) and for counteracting dietary selenium poisoning (Arsenic Development Committee; FROST, OVERBY and SPRUTH; WAHLSTROM, KAMSTRA and OLSON; FROST; FROST and SPRUTH).

Inorganic arsenicals have belonged to the medical armamentarium for many centuries. Hippokrates (466—377 B.C.) recommended an ointment containing arsenic sulfide for the treatment of ulcers of the skin. The medicinal use of organic arsenicals started soon after the turn of the last century and has progressively increased since, especially for the control of several parasitic diseases (Buchanan), including intravaginal infections with trichomonas vaginalis (acetarsol) (BOWEN, LEWIS and EDWARDS).

c) *Acute and Chronic Toxic Reactions and Cancers.* The various acute and chronic toxic reactions observed in man by arsenical drugs are identical with those produced by the same or similar arsenicals upon occupational, dietary or environmental contacts. Some of the chronic toxic manifestations, such as hyperkeratoses, cutaneous warts, BOWEN's disease, cirrhosis of the liver and chronic bronchitis, represent precursor reactions to subsequent and delayed cancerous developments. These preparatory stages in the cancerization process belong to the precancerous portion of the arsenic cancer syndrome. They are, however, not obligatory phases in the chain of events, since arsenical epitheliomas may develop in a skin which has not undergone a previous keratotic change (CURRIE). The high incidence of epitheliomas in psoriatic individuals after treatment with arsenicals (PUTMAN; NEUBAUER; SCHWENZNER and WALTHER; SOMMERS and McMANUS; UNNA et al.; WILLIAMSON; BILTZ) as well as the appearance of cancers on the hands, the back of fingers, on the neels and toes, where hyperkeratotic lesions are commonly found as symptoms of chronic arsenicosis, on the other hand, indicate that such keratotic responses favor the development of cancerous changes. They have been observed in about 80% of individuals with medicinal arsenic cancers of the skin.

Similar limitations apply to the interpretation of quantitative analytic tests for arsenic in nails, hair, urine, blood, liver and other tissues as evidence of a previous exposure to this chemical. Although arsenic is accumulated in such tissues and products and is retained there for many months, it is ultimately mobilized and excreted (NEUMANN and SCHWANK). The "standard" values of these biologic materials moreover fluctuates considerably with the living habits and the relative degree of arsenic contamination of the environment in which a particular individual has been living. It is therefore often not possible to ascribe the total amount of arsenic demonstrated in human tissues or excreta to the arsenic contained in the drugs taken. While the majority of investigators (GRAHAM *et al.*) noted an excessive arsenic content of the skin and epitheliomatous tissue in persons who received arsenical medication, Domonkos claimed that there is no significant difference in the amount of arsenic present in arsenic epitheliomas and in epitheliomas of patients without an arsenic history.

The diagnosis of medicinal arsenic cancers of the skin and of internal organs depends on a critical evaluation and integration of the following data:

A. The demonstration of a more or less prolonged or repeated intermittent medication with inorganic or organic arsenicals is important for establishing the specific etiologic background. Whenever such information cannot be obtained from the medical records or from the patient, it should be attempted to secure suggestive circumstantial evidence indicating whether the patient has suffered in the past from a disease or diseases for the control of which arsenicals are or were customarily administered.

B. Special inquiry should be made whether the past medical history contains information on the occurrence of an attack of acute arsenic poisoning or of transitory symptoms characteristic of chronic arsenic poisoning which developed after some known or undetermined medication was received and which would represent specific exposure stigmata. A similar significance has the demonstration of excessive arsenic values in the hair, nails, urine, blood and liver.

C. Medicinal arsenic cancers like arsenic cancers of the skin of occupational and dietary genesis exhibit a topographical distribution which in many respects is etiologically specific and which differs from that seen with cancers of the skin of unknown causation as well as those induced by contact with coal tar and pitch, mineral oil, paraffin oil, and solar radiation. While cutaneous cancers of the latter origin affect mainly the exposed parts, especially the head (KOELSCH), the majority of arsenic cancers involves the trunk and extremities including the fingers and toes, heels and hands (48% cancers of fingers, feet and trunk; 23% cancers of arms and hands; 23% cancers of scrotum, penis, head, face, neck, eye, eyelids; 8% cancers in other parts) (NEUBAUER; SOMMERS and McMANUS; ARHLEGER and KREMEN).

D. Synchronic and heterochronic multiplicity of arsenic cancers of the skin is common. NEUBAUER noted in his analysis of over one hundred cases of medicinal cancers that a single carcinoma was present in only 29% of the cases, while over 10 separate lesions were seen in 24%. The remaining cases had between 2 to 9 cancers each. Although multicentric cancers of the skin are frequent also in individuals exposed to solar radiation, coal tar, mineral oil and ionizing radiations, these tumors involve mainly the specially exposed parts of the skin and thereby differ from arsenic cancers. It is significant that the scrotal skin is rarely the site of a medicinal arsenic cancer. Scrotal cancers are relatively frequent, on the other hand, after occupational exposures to arsenicals as well as of coal soot, crude paraffin oil and shale oil.

E. About 50% of the medicinal arsenic cancers of the skin are squamous cell carcinomas, some 30% are basal cell carcinomas and the rest are of mixed cell type. The induction of melanomas has been attributed only very exceptionally to medicinal, occupational or dietary exposures to arsenicals despite the fact that melanoderma represents a common symptom of chronic arsenicosis (NEUBAUER; UNNA, MEMMESHEIMER and HERZBERG). Intraepidermal superficial epitheliomatosis of the Bowen type, on

the other hand, is so common that arsenic is regarded by many investigators as an important cause of this lesion (SCOTT; GRAHAM and HELWIG; GRAHAM, MAZZANTI and HELWIG; PETERKA, LYNCH and GOLTZ; ANDERSEN). The existence of such relations is supported not only by the fact that the arsenic content of such manifestations is often excessively high and that a medical history of a medicinal exposure to arsenic can frequently be elicited for patients exhibiting such lesions, but that cancers of the internal organs are unusually often associated with BOWEN's disease (PETERKA, LYNCH and GOLTZ; GRAHAM and

Table II. *Occupational arsenic cancers of the Lung, larynx and paranasal sinuses*

Sites and numbers					Exposure Period	Occupation	Author, year
Lung	Larynx	Nares and nasal sinuses	Coexisting keratoses	Skin cancers			
7						Copper smelter worker	SNEGIREFF and LOMBARD, 1951
19			1			Gold ore miner	OSBURN, 1957
	1			5		Pesticide producer	DEROBERT and HADENGUE, 1952
9			9	4	17	Vineyard worker	BRAUN, 1958
1					36	Cobalt smelter worker	KRUG, 1959
19	1	2	19	9		Vineyard worker	ROTH, 1956, 1958
2						Arsenic smelter worker	SCHMORL, 1928
1				1		Farmer	MONTGOMERY and WAISMAN, 1941
1					43	Arsenic worker	CURRIE, 1947
2					37	Pesticide worker	BRIDGE et al., 1939
17					20	Copper ore miner	AKAZAKI, 1960
8			6		3—8	Vineyard worker	HESS, 1956
45			45		8—45	Nickel-cobalt ore smelter worker	ROCKSTROH, 1959
5	1					Pesticide producer	HILL and FANING, 1948
2						Sheep-dip producer	HENRY, 1934
4					37—43	Sheep-dip producer	MEREWETHER, 1944
1			1	1		Vineyard worker	v. PEIN, 1943
1				1		Vineyard worker	LIEBEGOTT, 1950
1						Vineyard worker	KOELSCH, 1958
8						Furrier	FROMMEL, 1927
2			1	1		Pesticide sprayer	HUEPER, 1961
3			3			Vineyard workers	GALY et al., 1963

Table III. *Chronic arsenicism and cancers among vineyard workers of the moselle valley* FERD. ROTH

Cases	Cause of death	Coexisting cancers	Total number of cancers
16	Lung cancer with cirrhosis of liver	2 Cases with 1 skin cancer 1 Case with 2 skin cancers 1 Case with 3 skin cancers 2 Cases with 4 skin cancers	31
2	Double lung carcinomas	1 Case with 1 larynx cancer 1 Case with 1 skin cancer	7
1	Cholangiocarcinoma	1 Case with Lung carcinoma	2
6	Sarcomas of the liver with cirrhosis	1 Case with 2 skin cancers	8
5	Esophageal carcinoma with 2 cirrhosis of liver	1 Case with carcinoma of tomgue 1 Case with 3 skin cancers	9
8	Cirrhosis of liver	1 Case with 5 skin cancers	5
1	Arsenicosis	1 Case with 5 skin cancers	5
1	Chronic bronchitis	1 Case with 5 skin cancers	5
40			72

HELWIG). Such combinations were noted in 80% of the cases of BOWEN's disease which either came to autopsy or which were surgically explored (GRAHAM and HELWIG). In one third of the cases, they appeared at an average of 6 to 10 years after the initial diagnosis of BOWEN's disease and involved the lungs, prostate, breast, colon, vulva, liver and gallbladder.

Following the initial observation of HUTCHINSON regarding the occurrence of a cancer of the lung in a patient suffering from chronic arsenicosis and medicinal arsenic cancer of the skin, similar cases of heteroorganic multiplicity of medicinal arsenic cancers have been recorded particularly during recent years. NEUBAUER collected in 1945 from the literature 9 cases of visceral arsenic cancer affecting the lungs, stomach, mouth, breast, esophagus, tongue, ureter, bladder and uterus. Among the additional observations placed on record since then, the lung and liver were most often the sites of such visceral cancers (KOELSCH).

SOMMERS and McMANUS added 9 new cases of their own to the 8 they collected from the literature. Their visceral medicinal cancers were located in the lungs, tonsil, esophagus, pancreas, colon, kidney, bladder, breast, prostate and chestwall. Similar observations were reported by SANDERSON (lung), ROSSET (liver), CALMAN (lung), WILLIAMSON (2 cases, lung), RUSSELL and KLABER (lung), DAMBOLT and FOSS (12 cases, lung), RUSSELL (20 cases involving mainly lung), ROBSON and JELLIFFE (6 cases, lung). It is now widely recognized that arsenic favors the development of cancers of the skin as well as of internal organs (KOELSCH; MINKOWITZ; SOMMERS and McMANUS). This general principle has received during the last 20 years strong support from observations reported from several countries on the occurrence of visceral cancers after occupational and dietary exposures to arsenicals (ROTH; KOELSCH) (tables II and III).

Primary arsenic cancers of the liver may exhibit different histologic structures (hepatocarcinoma, cholangiocarcinoma, hemangioendothelioma, reticulum cell sarcoma (KOELSCH; ROTH; ROSSET). Similar variations in histologic structure prevail for arsenic cancers of the lung. Among 47 such cancers, 19 were squamous cell carcinomas, 24 were undifferentiated round cell carcinomas, and 4 were adenocarcinomas.

In analogy with the interval of several years which elapsed between the appearance of lesions of BOWEN's disease and that of the associated visceral carcinomas, it was noted that the latent period of medicinal visceral cancers, like that of their occupational and dietary counterparts, was by 5 to 20 years longer than that of the cutaneous cancers (ROTH; SOMMERS and McMANUS; WILLIAMSON). This organ-dependent multiphasic type of chemical carcinogenesis has been seen with other occupational and experimental cancers (HUEPER; HUEPER and CONWAY).

The evidence presented leaves little doubt concerning the actual existence of medicinal visceral cancers induced by arsenicals, and thereby refutes the recent contention of DINMAN that all claims concerning the occurrence of extracutaneous cancers after an ingestion of arsenicals are untenable. The available data contradict also the statement of KOELSCH that lung cancers have been observed only after occupational or dietary exposures to arsenicals but not following their medicinal introduction into man. The growing recognition that arsenicals possess pluripotential carcinogenic properties is in accord with the recent discovery that such qualities are rather common with various human and experimental carcinogens (HUEPER and CONWAY).

F. No worthwhile data exist concerning the frequency and incidence of medicinal arsenic cancers. This deficiency in epidemiologic information is mainly due to the fact that as a rule physicians omit to inquire into the environmental causal background of the cancers for which they assume therapeutic care. Whatever evidence is on hand on this particular aspect of medicinal arsenic carcinogenesis underestimates doubtlessly the role which arsenicals probably play in the production of cancers. DAMBOLT and FOSS stated that a history of arsenic medication could be elicited in 12 of 74 cases of lung cancer surviving operation, while similar data were obtained from 19 out of 248 cases of skin cancer surviving over 20 years the arsenic medication received earlier in life. ARHELGER and KREMEN saw within 2 years among 110 cases of skin cancer 9 cases attributable to medicinally administered arsenicals. Such data, together with those recently published by ROTH on the frequency of occupational and dietary arsenic cancers among German vintners, suggest that the role which arsenicals seem to play in the induction of cancers in man is distinctly more serious than this was suspected in the past.

G. Since the large majority of reported medicinal arsenic cancers followed upon the administration of inorganic arsenicals an even more marked uncertainty regarding the frequency of such effects exists for medicinal organic arsenic cancers. Although the possibility of such sequelae was first mentioned by HUTCHINSON concerning salvarsan, NEUBAUER in his tabulations over thirty years later could list only four cases in which arsphenamine was incriminated as the cause of subsequently appearing cutaneous cancers (LEVIN; FRANSEEN and TAYLOR), carcinoma of the oral mucosa (ROSEN) and fibrosarcoma at the site of injection in the subcutaneous tissue (HARBITZ). Cannon, in a discussion of the paper of MONTGOMERY on medicinal arsenic cancers, reported his observation of several cases of multiple basal cell epitheliomas in syphilitics given treatments with arsphenamine. ROTHMAN and FELSHER observed arsenical dermatitis, hepatic degeneration, hemorrhagic encephalitis and malignant melanoma in a syphilitic patient. The melanoma appeared 18 months after the dermatitis and the injection of neoarsphenamine. The occurrence of signs of arsenic poisoning, such as dermatitis, melanosis and keratosis following the injection of arsphenamine, was noted by AYRES and ANDERSON; HELLER, PHILIP and EBERT.

It has been suggested moreover that the excessive frequency of cancer of the tongue in syphilitic males (BELOTE; ROSAHN) and of cancer of the uterus in syphilitic women (WOJEWODZK) might causally be related to the therapeutic use of organic arsenicals (HARDING; ROJEL; GROSSE). DÖRKEN called attention to the highly excessive frequency of cancer of the lung in syphilitic women and proposed that the arsenobenzol treatment administered might account for this phenomenon. The possibility of a transplacental carcinogenic effect of oxyphenarsine hydrochloride given to a syphilitic women 2 years prior on the birth of a baby with congenital multiple fibrosarcoma (WILLIAMS and SCHRUM) presents another intriguing aspect of this problem. For elucidating further these suggestive relationships, it seems to be profitable in future studies on the association of syphilis and cancer to shift their emphasis from the syphilitic infection as a possible cause of cancer to the arsenic treatment administered for its control.

Because of the far reaching similarity between the toxic manifestations elicited by organic and inorganic arsenicals (EP-STEIN; BUTZENGEIGER; DÖLLE et al.), it is likely that they do not differ in their carcinogenic action, although the evidence supporting such an effect by organic arsenicals is at present merely suggestive. Distinct and comprehensive efforts should be made for obtaining definite evidence on the point in view of the growing use of organic arsenicals in medical practice, as well as their wide use as feed additives, pesticides and veterinary medical preparations used therapeutically and prophylactically in food animals.

The at present rather surprisingly scanty data on a carcinogenic action of organic arsenicals despite their extensive therapeutic use on large numbers of patients for over 50 years may indicate that organic arsenicals are indeed carcinogenically less potent than inorganic ones. Such variations in the relative carcinogenic effectiveness of the two types of arsenicals may be due to differences in their metabolic activity, in their rates of retention and excretion and in their affinity to specific cellular components. On the other hand, it is also possible, that they merely reflect a lack of adequate medical curiosity and alertness as far as the occurrence of long delayed sequelae of the administration of organic arsenicals is concerned.

H. It is suprising that, despite the ample and adequate human evidence establishing arsenicals as human carcinogens, the many attempts at duplicating these observations by administering orally and cutaneously inorganic arsenicals to experimental animals (mice, rats, rabbits) have yielded occasionally equivocal results and were mostly failures (CURRIE; HUEPER; HUEPER and PAYNE; LEITCH and KENNAWAY; LEITCH LIPSCHUTZ; RAPOSO; BOUTWELL; CHOLDIN; CHOLEWA; MAISIN; VOLLMANN; BARONI; VAN ESCH and SAFFIOTTI). The significance of the tumors produced in chickens, mice and rats by the implantation of embryopulp and arsenic (WHITE; McJunkin and Cikrit; Collier and Hartnack) is likewise uncertain, since chicken tissue not infrequently may contain a carcinogenic virus which may have been activated by the experimental conditions used. The tumors induced in the uterine horns of rats implanted with the mixture were teratomas, while those obtained in mice were only granulomas. The induction of a singular sarcoma in a rabbit at the site of repeated subcutaneous injections of potassium arsenite requires confirmation on large series of animals before being acceptable as positive evidence (Cholewa).

Despite these discouraging results obtained in planned experiments, the occurrence of symptoms of chronic arsenic poisoning (baldness, hyperkeratoses, malformed antlers) and of one cutaneous horns (in a deer) in wild and domesticated animals (deers, hares, foxes, cattle, horses, goats and hogs) living within the fume zone of arsenic smelters on the contaminated vegetation indicate that this situation is not hopeless (Prell). Nieberle in fact suggested that the endemic adenocarcinomas of the ethmoid found in a flock of sheep grazing in the same general region might be attributable to the arsenic inhaled by these animals with the smelter fumes polluting the general atmosphere.

It appears from these observations that a continued search for a suitable species and for proper experimental conditions may ultimately lead to a successful production of inorganic arsenic cancers in experimental animals and thereby provide that final piece of evidence so insistently demanded by some industrial interests before they are ready to accept the fact that inorganic chemicals are human carcinogens (Vallee,

Ulmer and Wacker; Pinto and Bennett).

Attempts to produce cancers in mice fed or painted with various organic arsenicals (arsanilic acid, phenarsazines) have so far yielded equally disappointing results (Boutwell; Lacassagne; Buu-Hoi; Royer and Rudali). The recent observation of Mego and McQueen that an azoalbumin-As^{74} complex prepared from arsanilic acid is accumulated in the liver and kidney of mice may be of methodologic importance, because rainbow trout given carbasone with their feed developed hepatomas in about 5% of the fish thus treated (Halver).

I. The latent period of medicinal arsenic cancers ranged from 3 to over 40 years (Neubauer; Arhelger and Kremen; Sommers and McManus; Robson and Jeliffe; Williamson). While keratotic lesions appeared from 1 to 20 years (average 8.8 years) after the start of the arsenic medication, an additional 1 to 23 years (average 9.6 years) elapsed from this event until cancers became manifest (Neubauer).

J. The exposure time varied greatly ranging from a few weeks to over 30 years (Neubauer; Russell and Klaber; Sommers and McManus). It was in general considerably shorter than the latent period.

K. Similarly marked variations were observed in the total dose of arsenic administered to patients with arsenic cancers (range from 0.19 gm. of As_2O_3 to 121 gms.) (Neubauer; Russell and Klaber). These data indicate that it is not possible to calculate or even vaguely estimate a "minimal carcinogenic dose" of arsenic, quite apart from the fact that exposure to arsenic from various sources has become so universal that the adoption of such a dose would provide a false sense of security.

L. The manifestation age of medicinal arsenic cancer is younger than that of occupational arsenic cancer (HUEPER) and of skin cancers of unknown etiology (NEUBAUER). While these make their first appearance usually after 40 years of age and reach their peak of frequency after 60 years of age, 25% of all medicinal arsenic cancers affect individuals less than 35 years old (PYE-SMITH), one third of the cases is not older than 40 years and two thirds are not older than fifty years. This shift into younger age groups is especially noticeable among females (NEUBAUER). It is likely that this extraordinary type of age distribution of medicinal arsenic cancers is closely related to the fact that the individuals affected received arsenic medication at a rather early age. Thus multicentric epitheliomas of the skin were observed in a person 21 years old, who had been given arsenicals between the age of 7 to 10 years (MINKOWITZ). Similar shifts in the age distribution have been recorded for several occupational cancers (scrotal cancers of chimney sweeps (HUEPER) and bladder cancers of aromatic amine workers (GOLDBLATT and GOLDBLATT), for which the manifestation age depended on the relative age at entrance in the trade by the individuals affected.

M. NEUBAUER reported a sex distribution of medicinal arsenic cancers which favored the male sex by a ratio of 2.3 to 1 (131 cases). A similar ratio (2.4 to 1) was obtained when a total of 56 subsequently reported medicinal arsenic cancers was analyzed.

Conclusions

A medicinal administration of inorganic arsenicals has been the direct cause of cancers of the skin and of various internal organs, among which the lungs and liver were most prominent.

The existence of similar causal connections is at present less certain for organic arsenicals. Because of a growing use of organic arsenicals in medical practice for a variety of mainly parasitic diseases, this problem deserves serious consideration.

The marked differences in the total dose of arsenic administered in cases of medicinal arsenic cancers, as well as the distinct variations in the length of exposure time and preparatory period, prevent the establishment of a maximal tolerance dose and of a minimal carcinogenic dose.

The total number of medicinal arsenic cancers is in all probability considerably larger than this is indicated by the published cases. Members of the medical profession therefore should be made aware of the cancer risks connected with the administration of arsenicals.

Medicinal arsenic cancer hazards form an important segment of the total cancer risks to the general population related to the rapidly growing and rather indiscriminate use of arsenicals in the human economy, particularly its food supply.

Because of the demonstrated cancer risks, the future use of arsenicals in medicine might well be restricted to the treatment of those diseases for the control of which no other effective therapeutic measure is available.

Patients who received arsenical remedies, especially when administered in appreciable amounts and over considerable times, should be kept under medical surveillance for a period of several decades.

The evidence presented indicates that arsenicals represent unsuitable means for a prophylactic control of diseases in man. Their use in veterinary medicine should be limited for such a purpose to animals not furnishing food to the human population.

3. Metals

Among the various metals and metal compounds used in medical practice in drugs and prosthetic materials, only chromium and nickel are recognized human carcinogens (Hueper; Tietz, Hirsch and Neyman). Some epidemiological evidence suggests that iron oxide and various iron-carbohdyrate complexes also may be carcinogenic to man. For all other metals incorporated into medicinal preparations only observations made on experimental animals justify a suspicion of such effects. The pertinent information on hand on these metals is included in the discussion because past experiences with several carcinogens (thorium dioxide, Bergius hydrogenated coal oils, beryllium) have shown that the discovery of a carcinogenic action on man by such agents may follow upon a primary demonstration of their carcinogenic potency in animals, once the medical profession has been alerted to such possible risks. The fundamental importance of observations made in experimental animals for human carcinogenesis is moreover demonstrated by the fact that, with few exceptions, it has been possible to elicit in animals cancers with all known chemical carcinogens capable of producing cancers in man.

Finally, it must be emphasized that it is scientifically unsound to consider any carcinogen which has demonstrated its potency for man upon occupational contact to be innocuous upon medicinal exposure. The record established on this point by arsenicals, ionizing radiations, petroleum waxes and coal tar militates definitely against the adoption of a philosophy of escapism and complacency by the medical profession.

a) *Chromium.* Epidemiological and clinical observations made on the occurrence and incidence of cancers of the lungs in workers of chromate and chrome pigment producing plants in Germany, England, the United States, France and Italy establish firmly chromium and chromates as human carcinogens (Alwens, Bauke and Jonas; Gross; Spannagel; Gross and Koelsch Machle and Gregorius; Mancuso and Hueper; Baetjer; Fisher; Brinton, Frasier and Koven; Gafafer et al.; Bidstrup and Case; Newman; Vigliani and Nicola; Imprescia; Portigliattu-Barbos; Renard et al.). Confirmatory evidence on the carcinogenic action of various chromates, including pigments, on different tissues, including the lungs, has been obtained in experimental animals (mouse, rat) following a parenteral administration of these chemicals (Schinz; Hueper; Hueper and Payne; Payne). Attempts to elicit pulmonary cancers in mice and rats by the inhalation of dust of several chromates were unsuccessful (Hueper and Payne; Worth and Schiller; Baetjer).

Chromium alloys (stainless steel; vitallium) have been implanted into human tissue for prosthetic purposes in traumatic and orthopedic surgery and have been employed in dental repair work (Oppenheimer et al.; Bascom et al.; Täge). While implants of powdered metallic chromium deposited into the thigh muscle and into the pleural cavity of rats did not induce cancers (Hueper), Oppenheimer et al. reported the development of sarcomas in 5% of 25 rats with 50 embeddings of vitallium foil (an alloy of chromium, cobalt, and molybdenum). Since cobalt alone has elicited under such experimental conditions sarcomas in rats (Heath), it is doubtful whether chromium participated in any way in the causation of the tumors obtained by OPPENHEIMER *et al.* Similar doubts must be entertained regarding the significance of the role which chromium may have played in the production of sarcoma around foil of stainless steel implanted into rats (OPPENHEIMER *et al.*).

The occasional occurrence of cancers developing many years after a bone nailing or bone plating of fractures (STRUPPLER; MCDOUGALL; LUBINUS) and around shell fragments following similar long periods of delay (BLUMLEIN) deserve consideration as possible manifestations of chromium metal cancers in man.

Cancerous reactions apparently have not followed upon a topical application of chromic acid ointment to benign lesions, such as verruca, botryomycosis, and chronic cervicitis (FRANKLIN; KIRKLAND; PETGES) and to laryngeal papillomas (COLBERT). Cancerous responses to chromic acid are not likely to occur because comprehensive experiences with the ultimate fate of chronic ulcerative defects of the skin and nasal mucous membrane frequently seen in workers having occupational contact with chromic acid mist and chromates indicate the extreme rarity of such sequelae (WELZ). Equally negative in these respects is the evidence associated with the subcutaneous introduction of green chrome oxide in tattoos. Foreign body granulomas occasionally exhibiting sarcoid features were seen around such deposits (LOEWENTHAL). The risk of cancerous complications from a medicinal use of chromic acid and chromates therefore appears to be negligible.

Whether the growing use of radioactive chromium (Cr^{51}) given either as a chloride or as a sodium chromate for the determination of circulating red cell volume entails any cancer hazards related to the metal as such remains to be seen (GRAY and FRANK; STERLING and GRAY;

FRANK and GRAY; KRAINTZ and TALMADGE; MEYER). This diagnostic method has been introduced too recently for permitting the appearance of cancerous reactions. Since Cr^{51} penetrates with the maternal erythrocytes the placental barrier (ZAROU, LICHTMAN and HELLMAN), the possibility of an untoward effect upon the fetus represents another possibility. While cancer hazards from a medicinal use of chromium and chromates appear possible, they are not likely.

b) Nickel. Adequate evidence obtained in nickel refining plants of England, Canada, Norway and the USSR attest to the carcinogenic action of nickel and its compounds on the respiratory organs (lung, nasal sinuses) of the workers employed in these establishments (AMOR; MORGAN; MEREWETHER; DOLL; WILLIAMS; LOKEN, ZNAMENSKII). A respiratory as well as parenteral (intramuscular, subcutaneous, intrapleural, intrapulmonary) introduction of metallic nickel powder and of several nickel compounds, including nickel carbonyl and nickel sulfide has induced sarcomas and carcinomas in the lungs, muscle tissue and connective tissue of mice, rats, and guinea pigs (HUEPER; HUEPER and PAYNE; SUNDERMAN; SUNDERMAN and SUNDERMAN; GILMAN and HERCHEN; HERCHEN and GILMAN; GILMAN and RUCKERBAUER; JASMIN; NOBLE and CAPSTICK; HEATH and DANIEL).

Alloys of nickel, like those of chromium, have been employed in traumatic surgery and in dental practice in prostheses. Dental fillings made from such materials have been suspected as a cause of oral leukoplakia and oral cancer (MELCZER and KISS; MACDONALD; LAIN; REINHARD and SALOMON). MITCHELL, SHANKWALKER, and SHAZER who tested various dental materials for carcinogenicity through implantation into rats noted the development of sarcomas around nickel metal implants, while such manifestations were not observed around vitallium (chrome-cobalt-nickel alloy). These findings are, in the opinion of these investigators, of potential significance since nickel is also used for the bleaching of gold fillings and because implantation techniques (implant dentures; metals placed in root apexes, implants for fracture fixation) are becoming increasingly popular.

The evidence on hand indicates that metal implants which contain nickel and which remain over long periods in human tissues might create delayed potential cancer hazards to their recipients. It is important that, according to observations made in experimental animals, the physical form in which nickel is implanted does not affect or modify the process of nickel carcinogenesis (Hueper; Gilman and Herchen).

c) Cobalt. Cobalt has repeatedly been accused in the past of being an occupational human carcinogen and especially of being the principal or an important contributory factor in the causation of the lung cancers afflicting the cobalt ore miners of Schneeberg, Saxony. There exists, however, at present no valid epidemiologic and clinical evidence in support of this allegation. Experimental studies, on the other hand, have shown that metallic cobalt or its sulfide and oxide, when deposited intramuscularly, intrathoracically and intrafemorally into mice, rats, and rabbits, induce sarcomas (Schinz; Schinz and Uehlinger; Heath; Gilman and Ruckenbauer; Gilman; Heath and Daniel; Hatem).

The potential significance of these findings to the medicinal use of cobalt in man relates mainly to the presence of cobalt in alloys (vitallium) employed for prostheses (Bascom *et al.*). So far clinical observations suggesting such complications have not been reported. However, because of the long latent period for such reactions to develop, patients who received such implants should be kept under proper medical surveillance for several decades.

Because of the strongly suspected connection between the action of goitrogenic chemicals (Hueper) to a subsequent development of malignant thyroid tumors in man and animals, the recently recorded occurrence of thyroid hyperplasia in children given a cobalt-iron preparation deserves attention (Kriss, Carnes and Gross; Gross, Kriss and Spaeth; Weaver, Kostainsek and Richards; Gairdner, Marks and Roscoe). Although Jaime and Those, as well as Holly, failed to substantiate these findings, some caution seems to be advisable when cobalt containing preparations are to be administered over prolonged periods and in considerable cumulative amounts.

Since cobalt is present as an active principle in vitamin B_{12}, its repeated oral and parenteral administration may entail a local as well as thyroid-related hazard. Medicinal preparations containing cobalt which are widely employed because of their erythropoiesis stimulating action in the treatment of anemic conditions (Glass *et al.*; Rohn and Bond; Holly) may possible be involved in precipitating abnormal proliferative reactions of the blood forming tissues. Experiments on rats, rabbits, guinea pigs, dogs, cats and ducks have demonstrated that a repeated and prolonged introduction of cobalt containing preparations elicits the development of an erythrocytosis or polycythemia (Klipstein; Browning; Bech, Kipling and Heather; Catelli and Varetto; Davis, McCullough and Rigdon; Davis; Mascherna; Schubmehl *et al.*; Orten *et al.*; Ritini and Messina; and others). Considering the facts that cobalt is a carcinogen for several species, that some of the anti-anemic cobalt preparations become effective through a depot action, that cobalt is able to induce an erythrocytosis through an overstimulation of the bone marrow, that a primary anemic stage has been observed to precede the development of a final leukemic phase in occupational benzol leukemia and radiation leukemia, and that polycythemia exhibits an unusual tendency to coexist with or to be followed by leukemia, there is sufficient reason for using cobalt preparations with some discrimination and restraint especially when given over long periods and in maximal therapeutic doses.

d) Iron. Iron has recently been incriminated as a carcinogen to man and experimental animals. It is remarkable that such claims have been made not only in connection with an excessive occupational and medicinal introduction of iron, but also in relation to a deficient intake of dietary iron. While LINDBLOM blamed a dietary sideropenia for the occurrence of cancers of the hypopharynx in women of northern Sweden, WARREN and DRAKE proposed that the excessive iron content of the liver in hemochromatosis was responsible for the unusually high liability of such livers to develop primary hepatocarcinomas. Recent epidemiologic studies on the frequency of lung cancers among hematite miners. foundry workers, metal polishers, and boiler scalers often affected by pulmonary siderosis have provided additional evidence implicating iron as a cause of cancer in man (STEWART and FAULDS; DREYFUSS; VORWALD and KARR; SIMONS; FAULDS; DUNNER and HICKS; DUNNER and HERMON; MCLAUGHLIN and HARDING; HARDING and MASSIE; FAULDS and NAGELSCHMIDT; FAULDS and STEWART; BRAUN *et al.*; MONLIBERT and HAYANGE; HUEPER; GERNEZ-RIEUX *et al.*).

These observations suggesting a carcinogenic action of iron in man have received during the last few years support from reports on the induction of sarcomas at the site of repeated subcutaneous injection of various iron-carbohydrate complexes (iron-dextran, iron-dextrin, iron-sorbitol, iron-polymaltose) into mice, rats, and rabbits (RICHMOND; HADDOW and HORNING; HADDOW; GOLBERG; BAKER, GOLDBERG, MARTIN and SMITH; LUNDIN; KUNZ, SHAHAB, HENZE and DAVID; FIELDING; ZOLLINGER). HADDOW and HORNING, as well as RICHMOND, proposed that the iron in such complexes represented the carcinogenic factor active in the production of the cancers induced by these medicinal preparations.

At the present time there does not exist any reliable human evidence duplicating these observations made in experimental animals. The ultimate significance of two observations made in man, one of which referring to the appearance of a tumor diagnosed as a sarcoma at the site of repeated iron-dextran injections in a woman and the second one reporting the development of a transitory leukemoid state in an infant similarly treated, remains undetermined or controversial (ROBINSON, BELL and STURDY; SAMUELS). They nevertheless deserve serious consideration because various iron-carbohydrate complexes, as well as numerous inorganic and organic iron compounds (iron oxide, iron sulfate, iron gluconate, iron glutamate, iron citrate, iron carbonate, etc.), are extensively used and officially approved as therapeutic agents mostly used in the treatment of several forms of anemia (COUNCIL; ZOLLINGER).

In assessing the claim that iron is a carcinogenic agent, the following additional information on the relation of iron to cancer in man and experimental animals is of value. None of the several comprehensive studies of the severe and probably dietary siderosis frequently found in South African Bantus associates this conditions with the excessive incidence of primary carcinoma of the liver prevailing in the same population group (BRADLOW, DUNN and HIGGINSON; BOTHWELL and BRADLOW; HIGGINSON, GERRITSEN, and WALKER; MENDEL). There is likewise no published evidence indicating that the siderosis of the liver existing in individuals with COOLEY's anemia creates such a liability (ELLIS, SCHULMAN and SMITH).

The reports on the occurrence of occupational siderosis in German ochre miners are equally silent concerning the existence of any special abnormal liability of such miners to cancer of the lung (OTTO; EHRHARDT and HEIDEMANN; MÜLLER and EHRHARDT). The possibility that some other carcinogenic factor is inhaled together with iron oxide and is responsible for the development of lung cancer in English and French hematite miners appears probable.

Although CAMPBELL noted that mice exposed to the inhalation of iron oxide dust displayed a significant increase in the number of lung adenomas over that seen in the controls, HUEPER and PAYNE failed to induce cancers in rats intramuscularly and intrapleurally implanted with pellets of finely powdered pure iron precipitated from iron carbonyl. The claim of MÜLLER and EHRHARDT that iron is not carcinogenic because mice intraperitoneally injected with iron oxide did not develop tumors, on the other hand, is not acceptable as valid evidence because of an observation time of only five months. Of definite value are the negative results obtained by GILMAN in rats intramuscularly injected with FeS and observed for 627 days. A partial solution to this contradictory evidence is perhaps offered by the recent investigations of SAFFIOTTI et al. When these investigators injected intratracheally a suspension of powdered iron oxide after 3,4-benzpyrene had been adsorbed to the surface of its particles, they obtained squamous cell carcinomas in the lungs of hamsters. The iron oxide particles retained intracellularly and extracellularly in the bronchial tree seemed to prolong the action of the carcinogen adsorbed to the surface of the particulate. There is a distinct likelihood that iron particles may act in this capacity in facilitating the process of chemical carcinogenesis.

Iron may assume such a role also in potentiating the carcinogenic action of the various carbohydratic polymers by delaying their resorption from the site of injection. This explanation is in accord with the fact that various water-soluble polymers of this type have displayed carcinogenic properties when repeatedly subcutaneously injected into rats (HUEPER; LUSKY and NELSON; TURNER; JASMIN) (dextran, carboxymethylcellulose, polyvinyl pyrrolidone).

Since it is uncertain at present whether any carcinogenic hazards may be connected with a medicinal use of iron preparations, it may be wise to avoid for the time being the production of any iron depots.

e) Selenium. Exposure of man and animals to selenium and its compounds has mainly been associated in the past with the ingestion of selenium contained in vegetable matter grown on seleniferous soil (MOXON and RHIAN; SMITH; FRANKE and WESTFALL) and with occupational contacts sustained in various industries (DRINKER and NELSON; KINNIGKEIT; BUCHAN; Editorial; Current Comment; MANVILLE). Only during recent years have selenium compounds been introduced into medical practice.

After having been used for a period in the treatment of cancers in man and animals (COENEN and SCHULEMANN; BOUGEANT), selenium sulfide has become the active ingredient in medicinal preparations employed against seborrhoic dermatitis, seborrhea sicca (dandruff), seborrhoic blepharitis and related skin disorders (COUNCIL; BERESTON; COHEN; SLINGER and HUBBARD; SAUER; ORENTREICH). The addition of selenium compounds to animal feed has recently been recommended to counteract arsenic poisoning and dietary hepatic necrosis in sheep (SCHWARZ; FROST). Selenium has found biological use as a miticide.

While chronic selenium poisoning (alkali disease) has often been observed in animals feeding on seleniferous vegetation, the occurrence of such manifestations among members of populations living in areas with seleniferous soil where chronic selenium poisoning is endemic among animals has not been established. Acute and chronic selenium poisoning has been noted after an occupational exposure to selenium chemicals in industry. Selenium poisoning characterized by loss of hair has been reported also following the use of selenium sulfide containing hair shampoo (GROVER). Degeneration and cirrhosis of the liver has been a symptom commonly met in dietary, occupational and experimental selenium poisoning (MOXON and RHIAN; CAMERON; LILLIE and SMITH; FITZHUGH, NELSON and CALVERY). It is important moreover that selenium is excreted with the milk and that it may produce congenital malformations in the embryo after having penetrated the placental barrier (GRUENWALD; McCONNELL).

When ammonium potassium selenide and sodium selenate was fed to rats, it induced not only necroses and cirrhosis of the liver but also adenomas and carcinomas of the liver (NELSON, FITZHUGH and CALVERY; TCHERKES, APTEKAR and VOLGAREV; TCHERKES, VOLGAREV and APTEKAR). When SEIFTER et al. administered to rats bis-4-acetamino-phenyl-selenium dihydroxide, these animals developed adenomas of the liver and thyroid.

There do not exist at present any acceptable observations on selenium cancer of any source in man. It may be noted, however, that FROST claimed a selenium genesis for the scrotal cancers reported by Paris to have occurred among tin miners and millers in Cornwall, which are usually attributed to an occupational exposure to arsenic containing smelter fumes. More recently, MARCKS proposed that the development of multiple basal cell carcinomas of the face in a worker might have been induced by his exposure to selenium oxide dust and fumes.

In view of the definite experimental evidence on the carcinogenic potency of selenium and its compounds, it seems to be wise to refrain from administering selenium containing medicinal preparations in the treatment of chronic disease conditions which do not justify any potential risk of cancer. The administration of such medicines to pregnant women appears to be contraindicated, because of a possible special hazard to the fetus.

f) Zinc. Zinc metal and zinc compounds find wide use in industry and in consumer goods. Various compounds of zinc represent also active ingredients in a number of medicinal preparations. Zinc oxide, a mild antiseptic, is a constituent of powders, pastes and ointments. Zinc stearate is employed in baby powders as a substitute of talc, although it has some irritating action when introduced parenterally (HARDING). A zinc-insulin complex is an important antidiabetic drug. Zinc chloride, a powerful escharotic, is the active principle in ointments and pastes used for the chemosurgical treatment of cancers of accessible sites (skin, penis, breast, vagina, etc.) (Mohs; Ackerman and Eberhard). Zinc peroxide is applied to ulcerative carcinomas for controlling exudation and foul odor (Freeman).

Although it is widely used in metallurgical and chemical industries, zinc has not given rise, as far as this is known, to occupational cancer hazards. Several recent studies on the relation between chemical constituents of soil and drinking water supplies and the relative frequency of cancer in different region have revealed statistical associations between a high zinc content of soil and drinking water and an excessive frequency of cancer of the stomach and of other internal cancers in man and mice, respectively (Stocks and Davies; DeSzilvay).

Numerous experimental investigations have shown that an intratesticular injection of zinc chloride, zinc sulfate and zinc nitrate into roosters when performed during the spring, while the proliferative activity of the testicular epithelium is high, results in extensive testicular necroses followed by the development of teratoid tumors (Michalowsky; Anissimova; Falin and Gromzewa; Bagg; Kahlau; Carleton; Friedman and Bomze; Guthrie; Smith and Powell; and others). Zinc stearate and zinc acetate proved to be ineffective (Guthrie). While Rivière et al. obtained testicular tumors (seminoma, interstitial cell tumors, chorioepithelioma) when rats were injected into the testes with zinc chloride, Elwi and El-Katib were unsuccesful in this respect when they injected zinc sulfate. This apparent failure of Elwi and El-Katib, however, may be attributable to the fact that they observed their animals for only 285 days, while none of the testicular neoplasms

seen by Rivière et al. became manifest before 15 months had elapsed from the start of the experiment.

None of the various explanation proposed regarding the tumors induced connects their appearance to a definite carcinogenic action of zinc. Cornil and Schachter, for instance, suggested that the teratomas might be a reaction of the testicular epithelium to the necrotizing action of the zinc compounds and therefore represent a nonspecific response. Guthrie speculated on the possibility that the large amounts of iron pigment accumulating in the necrotized testicular tissue as a secondary reaction might represent the causal factor. This proposal has few merits, since iron pigment accumulations are a phenomenon common to traumatized tissue in which the development of benign or malignant tumors is not the rule. Smith tested the theory of germ cell misplacement associated with the chemical injury to the testis by explanting testicular tissue into the muscle tissue of roosters, but failed to obtain any teratoid tumors. While Guthrie was unsuccessful in finding any histological evidence supporting the view that the teratoid reactions might be attributable to a stimulation of the production and action of gonadotropic hormone in the hypophysis resulting from the partial chemical castration (Valleee), Bagg succeeded in the induction of teratomas in roosters after spring had passed when he combined the injection of zinc chloride with the simultaneous administration of gonadotropic hormone. Despite their close histologic similarity with teratomatous carcinomas seen in human testes, these zinc teratomas elicited in roosters have not produced metastases. Whether the observed accumulation of zinc in testicular tissue after a parenteral injection of this chemical into rats supports the concept that such zinc deposits favor neoplastic responses remains undetermined (GUNN, GOULD and ANDERSON). The existence of such an association appears to be unlikely, however, because the zinc levels are depressed in prostatic cancer (SCHRODT et al.; KERR et al.).

The evidence on hand does not encourage any suspicion that a medicinal use of zinc and its compounds creates a cancer hazard.

g) *Copper*. Copper has been used in the human economy since early historical times. During more recent periods, copper compounds, especially copper sulfate, have enjoyed a moderate popularity as medicinal agents in the treatment of trachoma, cholera, malaria, and schistosomiasis (cupri-bis-(8-hydroxy-quinoline-5-diethylaminosulfonate) as well as of cancer (DAVENPORT; HIEGER; CHATTERJI; WEIL; LÖWENSTEIN; SHARPLESS; PEDERO and KOZELKA; HAHN). Lately, copper compounds are mainly employed for their antianemic action as nutrients and food additives (GUBLER; Conferences; Editorial; Council on Foods and Nutrition). Additional biological uses of copper compounds are in the form of insecticides, fungicides and molluscicides (DAVENPORT).

While copper poisoning has occurred as the result of occupational exposures as well as of ingestion of water and food kept in or cooked in copper vessels, there are recorded no observations so far which implicate copper as a human carcinogen upon occupational, dietary or medicinal exposure. Cancers of the skin and lung found in copper miners and millers which have been attributed to copper are actually due to the arsenic present in varying but often appreciable amounts in copper ore.

Since hemochromatosis, which exhibits a tendency toward the development of liver carcinoma, has been attri-

buted by MALLORY and PARKER to the toxic action of copper (PEDRO and KOZELKA), could not be produced in animals given copper by FLINN and VON GLAHN as well as POLSON, also such an indirect carcinogenic effect of copper in man lacks substance in reliable facts. Hypercupremia moreover is not only found in some cancers, but also in thyrotoxicosis, mononucleosis, various acute and chronic infections, and pregnancy (PIRRIE). The subcutaneous implantation of powdered copper oxide and of cuprous and cupric sulfide into rats also did not induce sarcomas at the site of deposition of the copper compounds (GILMAN). Contrasting with this essentially negative evidence on a carcinogenic potency of copper is the successful production of teratoid tumors, seminomas and interstitial cell neoplasms in testes of mice, rats and roosters injected with copper sulfate solution (FALIN and ANISSIMOVA; ISAKA; BRESLER).

When criticaly assessing the significance of positive and negative observations concerning the carcinogenicity of copper and its compounds, there does not seem to exist any valid reason for suspecting that medicinal copper preparations constitute a cancer hazard to the recipients of such drugs.

h) *Aluminum*. It is only since the turn of the last century that metallic aluminum and several of its compounds have widely been used in medicinal preparations. Aluminum hydroxide and aluminum phosphate gels taken orally have become accepted remedies for the control of gastric ulcers and hyperacidity. Dry powdered aluminum hydroxide, alumina and metallic aluminum are administered by inhalation for preventing and arresting silicosis. Colloidal aluminum hydroxide and aluminum acetate are being incorporated into preparations used in the treatment of dermatitis, wounds, fissured nipples and cutaneous sores. Aluminum foil and powdered metallic aluminum are applied to burns. Potassium and ammonium aluminum sulfate are contained in antiperspirant preparations and antideodorants. Various halogenated aluminum salts had found accasional uses in the therapeutic management of gonorrhea and in the maintenance of vaginal hygiene. The adsorptive qualities of aluminum hydroxide are being utilized in preparation employed for the control of digestive disturbances induced by certain antibiotics (CAMPBELL, CASS, CHOLAK and KEHOE; BROWN and VAN WINKLE; FRIEDMAN; COUNCIL; MEIKLEJOHN).

Despite a large scale industrial production of aluminum and its compounds and despite a wide use of these products in industry, the home and medical practice during the past five decades, no acceptable evidence has been placed on record which incriminates aluminum and its compounds in the development of cancers of the skin, alimentary system and respiratory tract. Although aluminosis of the lungs has been observed in an appreciable number of workers exposed to the inhalation of aluminum dust (SWENSSON et al.; DOESE), there is no indication that this occupational dust disease of the lungs creates any excessive liability to cancer of the lung similar to that related to pneumoconioses induced by other metals (beryllium; iron; chromium, nickel) or minerals (asbestos).

The widely accepted suspicion that aluminum is a carcinogen is based on the often repeated allegation that the traces of aluminum related from aluminum cooking utensils during the preparation of foods may cause cancers in the consumers of such foodstuffs (BETTS; ODIER). Apart from the fact that no valid and reliable epidemiologic and clinical data support such claims (BLUMENTHAL), BERTRAND and SERBESCU

failed to produce cancers with aluminum in experimental animals.

There is no reason for assuming that aluminum containg medicinal preparation carry any cancer hazards.

i) Tantalum. Tantalum is used as a surgical implant in the repair of cranial defects and of ventral and inguinal hernias (FULCHER; SCHOLER). OPPENHEIMER et al. reported that 2 out of 25 rats which received 2 subcutaneous implants each of tantalum discs had sarcomas at the site of these metal deposits after 844 days of observation. This is a relatively low tumor yield when compared with that seen with implants of nickel, silver, selenium, cadmium, and chromates.

As with other surgical implants of this type, no reports are available concerning an occurrence of cancerous responses from such implants in man.

j) Silver and Gold. Drugs containing inorganic and organic silver and gold compounds are used for the treatment of infections of the skin and mucous membranes, chronic arthritis, lupus erythematosus, cutaneous tuberculids and syphilis. In dental practice alloys of the two metals serve for fillings and dentures.

NOTHDURFT reported that sarcomas were formed around subcutaneous implants of thin discs of silver, gold and platinum in rats and mice. They were seen in 32 per cent of the rats with silver discs. While rats which were subcutaneously injected with a colloidal gold solution did not develop any tumors at the site of injection, rats which received by injection colloidal silver solutions showed cancers at such locations in 6 out of 26 rats (SCHMÄHL and REITER).

There are no reports concerning an occurrence of cancers in man following a medicinal use of silver and any of its compounds. IRGANG, on the other hand, mentioned the development of keratoderma and melanoderma of the plantar surfaces in three patients treated with a gold preparation. He commented on the similarity of these reactions to those seen with arsenic medication. Silver and gold preparations have been employed in medical practice for many years and many of the patients thus treated have remained under close and prolonged medical surveillance for decades, such as the arthritics, without having exhibited a noticeable tendency to develop cancers. Hence it is most doubtful that these two metals and their compounds create any extraordinary cancer risk when employed in medicinal preparations. Observations on an occupational causation of cancers from contact with gold and silver are lacking and thereby support this conclusion.

k) *Mercury*. Metallic mercury and its inorganic and organic compounds are extensively used in industry and in various consumer goods, such as fungicides, and medicinal preparations, such as antiseptics, diuretics, antisyphilitics, and dental amalgams. Although DRUCKREY, HAMPERL, and SCHMÄHL observed sarcomas in rats which developed after an intraperitoneal introduction of metallic mercury, there does not exist any acceptable evidence from all sources that would indicate or suggest a carcinogenic hazard from a medicinal use of medicinal preparations containing mercurial compounds.

l) *Lead*. Exposure to lead and its compounds is connected mainly with their industrial production, commercial use and environmental dissemination through plant effluents and automobile exhaust. Drugs containing a lead compound have found scanty application. Solutions of lead acetate thus were used in the treatment of tuberculous colitis and various organic lead compounds were rather popular for a few years in the treatment of cancer where they gave

rise not too infrequently to severe plumbism (GERAGHTY).

Exposure to lead has been associated not only with the development of congenital malformations (BUTT, PEARSON and SIMONSEN), but also with that of cancers in experimental animals and possibly also in man. Although KEHOE asserted, according to JECKLIN, that the literature does not contain any reference on a carcinogenic action of lead and specifically on the occurrence of lung cancer in lead workers, recent reports are distinctly less certain on these aspects.

Already BLACK had pointed out in 1943 that lead might be the inciting factor in bronchiogenic carcinoma in lead workers and cited in support of this suspicion his observation of lung cancer in several individuals who had suffered previously attacks of occupational lead poisoning. A similar suspicion was subsequently advanced in regard to the causation of a brain tumor in a lead worker by PORTAL. Referring to the known myelotoxic action of lead, BOYLAND *et al.* recently suggested that lead might cause leukemia in individuals upon prolonged exposure. This proposition deserves consideration, since polycythemia has been observed occasionally to be present in lead workers as the result of a stimulating action of lead on the proliferative activity of the bone marrow. Finally, MILLAR recently voiced his suspicion as to the existence of causal connections between the relative frequency of gastrointestinal cancers and exposure to environmental lead on the basis of his geochemical studies in England.

Although epidemiological investigations conducted by JECKLIN and by DINGWALL-FORDYCE and LANE on worker groups exposed to lead have not provided any support to such suppositions, recent studies on rats exposed to lead sulfate and lead phosphate for experimental and environmental reasons have clearly demonstrated that lead is a carcinogen to the kidneys of rats (Zollinger; van Esch, van Genderen and Vink; Boyland, Dukes, Grover and Mitchley; Kilham, Low, Conti and Dallenbach; Dukes). These observations should be kept in mind whenever lead should assume again importance as a medicinal agent.

Conclusions

The appraisal of cancer hazards from the use of arsenicals and metals in drugs establishes the fact that proven risks to man have resulted from a medicinal use of arsenicals, particularly inorganic arsenicals and that greatly increased attention should be extended to a probable similar action of organic arsenicals. Among the medicinally used metals and metal compounds, those having established carcinogenic effects on man, i.e. chromium and nickel, but have as yet not displayed an established similar effect when employed in medicinal preparations, should be utilized in medical practice with distinct caution. Whenever possible and practical, they should be replaced by noncarcinogenic substitutes. A similar policy of caution and discrimination should be adopted for medicinal preparations containing cobalt, iron and selenium, whenever, they are to be administered over extended periods and with little or no medical supervision. The chances that the medical use of other metals, such as zinc, mercury, copper, tantalum, aluminum, silver, gold and lead, may bring excessive and specific cancer risks to patients appear to be very slight, if not non-existent.

In view of the obvious frequent failures to obtain cancer cures with the available therapeutic measures and the slim hope of developing in the foreseeable future reliable and generally effective carcinostatic chemicals, it behooves the medical profession to apply the information on the carcinogenic effects of some drugs in the diagnostic and therapeutic management of patients by avoiding the use of such medicinal preparations. This plea seems to be appropriate because of the distinct reluctance of some members of the medical profession to admit the carcinogenic potency of some materials recognized to be carcinogenic upon occupational exposure when contained in drugs (ultraviolet radiation, coal tar, arsenicals).

References

The list of references following this important article was originally much more comprehensive. Considering the possibility for the readers to find the majority of references to the standard contributions, firstly published by Dr. W. C. Hueper, we felt obliged to suggest to him to reduce his bibliography. We gratefully appreciate his readiness to this end.

R. Truhaut

General

Hueper, W. C., *Occupational tumors and allied diseases*, p. 897. Springfield (Ill.): C. C. Thomas 1942.
— *Occupational and environmental cancers of the respiratory system*, p. 226. New York: Springer 1966.
Hueper, W. C., and Conway, W. D., *Chemical carcinogenesis and cancers*, p. 592. Springfield (Ill.): C. C. Thomas 1965.

Arsenic

Arhelger, S. W., and Kremen, A. J., Arsenical epitheliomas of medicinal origin. *Surgery* 30, 977—986 (1951).
Belote, G. H., The association of carcinoma of the tongue and syphilis, as determined by positive serologic tests. *J. Amer. med. Ass.* 94, 1985—1986 (1930).
Biltz, G., Beobachtung zur Frage des Psoriasiskarzinoms. *Derm. Wschr.* 128, 667—67 (1953).

BOUTWELL, R. K., A carcinogenicity evaluation of potassium arsenite and arsanilic acid. *Agric. and Food Chem.* **11**, 381—385 (1963).

BOWEN, A. L., LEWIS, T. L. T., and EDWARDS, W. R., Acute arsenical poisoning due to acetarsol pessaries. *Brit. med. J.* **1961** I, 1282—1283.

DÖLLE, W., and MARTIN, G. A., Hepatic cirrhosis after neosalvarsan treatment. *Acta hepatosplenol. (Stuttg.)* **8**, 227—233 (1961).

DÖRKEN, H., Einige Daten bei 290 Frauen mit Lungenkrebs. I. Über Lues als Vorkrankheit. *Oncologia (Basel)* **16**, 325—338 (1963).

EBERT, M. H., Die histologischen Veränderungen nach einmaliger Salvarsanapplikation in der Haut. *Arch. Derm. Syph. (Berl.)* **158**, 365 (1929).

EPSTEIN, F., Toxicity of carbasone. *J. Amer. med. Ass.* **106**, 769—772 (1936).

GRAHAM, J. H., and HELWIG, F. B., Bowen's diseases and its relationship to systemic cancer. *Arch. Derm.* **80**, 133—159 (1959); **83**, 738—758 (1961).

— MAZZANTI, G. R., and HELWIG, E. B., Chemistry of Bowen's disease: relationship to arsenic. *J. invest. Derm.* **37**, 317—330 (1961).

GROSSE, H., Lues und Krebs. *Hautarzt* **8**, 258—261 (1957).

HARBITZ, H., Development of tumor (fibrosarcoma) after injection of salvarsan. *Lancet* **1927** I, 70.

HELLER, J., Weitere Mitteilungen über schwere Arsenmelanosen und Hyperkeratosen nach kombinierter Neosalvarsan- und Salicylquecksilberbehandlung. *Arch. Derm. Syph. (Berl.)* **130**, 309—310 (1921).

HUEPER, W. C., Effects of neoarsphenamine on spontaneous breast tumours of mice. *Amer. J. Cancer* **17**, 106—115 (1933).

HUTCHINSON, J., Salvarsan and arsenic cancer. *Brit. med. J.* **1911** I, 976.

LACASSAGNE, A., BUU-HOI, N. P., ROYER, R., and RUDALI, G., Sur le pouvoir oncogène de certains dérivés organiques de l'arsenic. *C.R. Soc. Biol. (Paris)* **145**, 1451—1453 (1951).

MINKOWITZ, S., Multiple carcinomata following ingestion of medicinal arsenic. *Ann. intern. med.* **60**, 296—299 (1964).

NEUBAUER, O., Arsenical cancer: a review. *Brit. J. Cancer* **1**, 192—244 (1947).

NEUMANN, E., and SCHWANK, R., Multiple keratoses and carcinomas due to arsenic. *Acta Univ. Carol. Med. (Praha).* Suppl. **10**, 219—226 (1960).

PETERKA, E. S., LYNCH, FR., and GOLTZ, R. W., An association between Bowen's disease and internal cancer. *Arch. Derm.* **84**, 623—629 (1961).

PHILIP, C., Arsenkeratose nach Salvarsaninjektion. *Münch. med. Wschr.* **62**, 1248 (1915).

PUTNAM, FR. L., Psoriasis: Arsenical keratoses; superficial epitheliomatosis. *Arch. Derm. Syph (Chic)* **51**, 221 (1945).

ROBSON, A. O., and JELLIFFE, A. M., Medicinal arsenic poisoning and lung cancer. *Brit. med. J.* **1963** I, 207—209.

ROJEL, J., The interaction between uterine cancer and syphilis. *Acta path. microbiol. scand.*, Suppl. **97**, 82 (1953).

ROSAHN, P. D., The occurrence of malignant disease in syphilitic individuals. *Amer. J. Syph.* **38**, 413—421 (1954).

ROSSET, M., Arsenical keratoses associated with carcinomas of the internal organs. *Canad. med. Ass. J.* **78**, 416—419 (1958).

ROTHMAN, S., and FELSHER, Z., Leukoderma following arsenical dermatitis (malignant melanoma). *Arch. Derm. Syph. (Chic.)* **52**, 64 (1945).

SCHMENZNER, G., u. WALTHER, H., Multiple Basaliome auf Psoriasis vulgaris nach längerer Arsenbehandlung. *Zbl. Haut- u. Geschl.-Kr.* **28**, 204—209 (1960).

SCOTT, A., A retention of arsenic in the late cutaneous complications of its administration. *Brit. J. Derm.* **70**, 195—200 (1958)

SOMMERS, S. C., and McMANUS, R. G., Multiple arsenical cancers of the skin and internal organs. *Cancer (Philad)* **6**, 347—359 (1953).

UNNA, P. J., MEMMESHEIMER, JR. A., u. HERZBERG, J. J., Das Carcinom bei Psoriasis vulgaris-post hoc oder proper hoc? *Arch. klin. exp. Med.* **217**, 321—339 (1963).

WILLIAMSON, A. W. R., Arsenical skin cancer and lung cancer. *Guy's Hosp. Rep.* **109**, 42—45 (1960).

Chromium

BASCOM, J., PHILIPP, L. D., HAGLIN, J. J., and REILEY, R. R., The use of hip protheses in fresh fractures. *J. Amer. med. Ass.* **169**, 1863—1866 (1959).

BLÜMLEIN, H., Bösartige Tumoren nach Steckschußverletzungen. *Arch. Ohr.-, Nas.- u. Kehlk.-Heilk.* **171**, 239—244 (1958).

COLBERT, R. M., Removal of benign larynx tumor with potassium bichromate. *Arch. Otolaryng.* **8**, 715—716 (1928).

FRANK, H., and GREY, S. J., The determination of plasma volume in man with radioactive chromic chloride. *J. clin. Invest.* **32**, 991—999 (1953).

FRANKLIN, M., Chromic acid poisoning due to use of drug for gonorrheal cervicitis. *Clin. Obstet. Gynec.* **29**, 199—207 (1927).

KIRKLAND, T. S., Chromic acid in aural suppuration. *Med. J. Aust.* **1**, 684 (1930).

KRAINTZ, L., and TALMADGE, R. V., Distribution of radioactivity following intravenous administration of trivalent chromium-51 in the rat and rabbit. *Proc. Soc. exp. Biol. (N.Y.)* **81**, 490—492 (1952).

LOEWENTHAL, L. J. A., Reaction in green tattoos. *Arch. Derm.* **82**, 235—236 (1960).

LUBINUS, H., Ungewöhnliche Knochentumoren nach Küntschernagelung. *Zbl. Chir.* **75**, 1375—1360 (1950).

McDOUGALL, A., Malignant tumour at site of bone plating. *J. Bone Jt Surg.* **38**, 709—713 (1956).

PETGES, G., Chromic acid ointment in therapy of verruca. *Médecine* **13**, 778—782 (1932).

TÄGE, K. H., Testing of metals in orthopedic surgery. *Chirurg* **33**, 129—135 (1962).

TIETZ, N. W. HIRSCH, E. F., and NEYMAN, B., Spectrographic study of trace elements in cancerous and noncancerous human tissues. *J. Amer. med. Ass.* **165**, 2187—2192 (1957).

STRUPPLER, V., Sarkome nach Knochennagelung. *Mschr. Unfallheilk.* **62**, 121—127 (1959).

ZAROU, D. M., LICHTMAN, H. C., and HELLMAN, L. M., The transmission of chromium-51 tagged maternal erythrocytes from mother to fetus. *Amer. J. Obstet. Gynec.* **88**, 565—567 (1964).

Nickel

LAIN, E. S., Electrogalvanic lesions of the oral cavity produced by metallic dentures. *J. Amer. med. Ass.* **100**, 717—718 (1933).

—, and CAUGHRON, G. S., Electrogalvanic phenomena of the oral cavity caused by dissimilar metallic restorations. *J. Amer. dent. Ass.* **23**, 1641 (1936).

MACDONALD, W. J., Chemical and electrogalvanic burns of the tongue. *New Engl. J. Med.* **211**, 585 (1934).

MELCZER, N., u. KISS, J., Beiträge zur Entstehungsweise der Leukoplakia oris. *Z. Krebsforsch.* **61**, 673—675 (1957).

MITCHELL, D. F., SHANKWALKER, G. B., and SHAZER, S., Determining the tumorigenicity of dental materials. *J. dent. Res.* **39**, 1023—1028 (1960).

REINHARD, M. C., and SOLOMON, H. A., Electrical currents from dental metals as an etiologic factor in oral cancer. *Amer. J. Cancer* **22**, 606—609 (1934).

Cobalt

CASTELLI, D., and VARETTO, L., Erythropoietic action of cobalt glutamate. *Gazz. med. ital.* **111**, 253—260 (1952).

GAIRDNER, D., MARKS, J., and ROSCOE, J. D., Goitrogenic hazard of cobalt. *Lancet* **1947 II**, 256—258.

GLASS, G. B. J., LEE, D. H., SKEGGS, H. R., and STANLEY, J. L., Hydroxycobalamin. *J. Amer. med. Ass.* **183**, 425—429 (1963).

GROSS, R. T., KRISS, J. P., and SPAET, T. H., Haematopoietic and goitrogenic effects of cobaltous chloride in patients with sickle cell anemia. *Amer. J. Dis. Child.* **88**, 503—504 (1954).

HEATH, J. C., and DANIEL, M. R., The production of malignant tumours by cobalt in the rat: intrathoracic tumours. *Brit. J. Cancer* **16**, 474—478 (1962).

JAIMET, C. H., and THODE, H. G., Thyroid function studies on children receiving cobalt therapy. *J. Amer. med. Ass.* **158**, 1353—1355 (1955).

KLIPSTEIN, F. A., Iron and vitamin B_{12} deficiency following subtotal gastrectomy. Report of a patient developing polycythemia vera following treatment. *Ann. intern. Med.* **57**, 133—139 (1962).

KRISS, J. P., CARNES, W. H., and GROSS, R. T., Hypothyroidism and thyroid hyperplasia in patients treated with cobalt. *J. Amer. med. Ass.* **157**, 117—121 (1955).

WEAVER, J. C., KOSTAINSEK, V. M., and RICHARDS, D. N., Cobalt tumor of the thyroid gland. *Calif. Med.* **85**, 110—113 (1956).

Iron

BAKER, S. B. DE C., GOLBERG, L., MARTIN L. E., and SMITH, J. P., Tissue changes following injection of iron-dextran complex. *J. Path. Bact.* **82**, 453—470 (1961).

FIELDING, J., Sarcoma induction by iron-carbohydrate complexes. *Brit. med. J.* **1962 I**, 1800—1803.

GOLBERG, L., Die Wirkung von Eiseninjektionen im Tierversuch. *Arzneimittel-Forsch.* **13**, 939—945 (1963).

HADDOW, A., and HORNING, E. S., On the carcinogenicity of an iron-dextran complex. *J. nat. Cancer Inst.* **24**, 109—146 (1960).

—, and ROE, F. J., Induction of sarcomata in rabbits. *Brit. med. J.* **1964 I**, 1593—1594.

KUNZ, J., SHABAD, L., HENZE, K., u. DAVID, H., Experimentelle Untersuchungen zur cancerogenen Wirkung von Eisendextran (Ursoferran). *Acta biol. med. germ.* **10**, 602—614 (1963).

LUNDIN, P. M., The carcinogenic action of complex iron preparations. *Brit. J. Cancer* **15**, 838—847 (1961).

RICHMOND, H. G., Induction of sarcoma in the rat iron-dextran complex. *Brit. med. J.* **1959** I, 947—949.

SAMUELS, L. D., Leukemoid reaction to parenteral iron-dextran complex. *J. Amer. med. Ass.* **182**, 1334—1335 (1962).

ZOLLINGER, H. U., Weichteiltumoren bei Ratten nach sehr massiven Eiseninjektionen. *Schweiz med. Wschr.* **92**, 130—134 (1962).

Selenium

BERESTON, E. S., Use of selenium sulfide shampoo in seborrhoic dermatitis. *J. Amer. med. Ass.* **156**, 1246—1247 (1954).

COHEN, L. B., Use of selenium sulfide ointment in Blepharitis marginalis. *Amer. J. Ophthal.* **38**, 560—562 (1954).

Council of Pharmacy and Chemistry: Use of selenium sulfide for various seborrhoic conditions. *J. Amer. med. Ass.* **160**, 51 (1956).

FITZHUGH, O. G., NELSON, A. A., and BLISS, C. I., The chronic oral toxicity of selenium. *J. Pharmacol. exp. Ther.* **80**, 289—299 (1954).

GROVER, R. W., Diffuse hair loss associated with selenium (selsun) sulfide shampoo. *J. Amer. med. Ass.* **160**, 1397—1398 (1956).

GRUENWALD, P., Malformations caused by necrosis in the embryo. Illustrated by the effect of selenium compounds on chick embryos. *Amer. J. Path.* **34**, 77—103 (1958).

McCONNELL, K. P., Passage of selenium through mammary glands of the white rat and its distribution of selenium in the milk with proteins after subcutaneous injection of sodium selenate. *J. biol. Chem.* **173**, 653—657 (1948).

ORENREICH, N., Selenium disulfide shampoo. *Arch. Derm.* **90**, 76—82 (1964).

SEIFTER, J., EHRICH, W. E., HUDYMA, G., and MUELLER, G., Thyroid adenomas in rats receiving selenium. *Science* **103**, 762 (1946).

TSCHERKES, L. A., VOLGAREV, M. N., and APTEKAN, S. G., Selenium-induced tumours. *Acta Un. int. Cancr.* **19**, 632—633 (1963).

Zinc

ACKERMAN, L. V., and EBERHARD, T. P., The treatment of tumors with escharotics. *J. Miss. med. Ass.* **40**, 163—167 (1943).

CARLETON, R. L., FRIEDMAN, N. B., and BOMZE, E. J., Experimental teratomas of the testis. *Cancer (Philad.)* **6**, 464—473 (1953).

GUTHRIE, J., Observations on the zinc induced testicular teratomas of fowl. *Brit. J. Cancer* **18**, 130—142 (1964).

HARDING, H. E., Some enquiries into the toxicology of zinc stearate. *Brit. J. industr. Med.* **15**, 130—132 (1958).

MOHS, F. E., Chemosurgery: A microscopically controlled method of cancer excision. *Arch. Surg.* **42**, 279—288 (1941).

RIVIÉRE, M. R., CHOUROULINKOV, I., et GUÉRIN, M., Production de tumeurs par injections intratesticulaires de chlorure de zinc chez le rat. *Bull. Ass. franç. Cancer* **47**, 55—87 (1960).

STOCKS, P., and DAVIES, R. I., Zinc and copper content of soils associated with the incidence of cancer of the stomach and other organs. *Brit. J. Cancer* **18**, 14—25 (1964).

SZILVAY, G. DE, Carcinogenic effects of zinc in drinking water. *Minerva med.* **55**, 1504—1505 (1964).

Copper

FALIN, L. I., u. ANISSIMOWA, W. W., Zur Pathologie der experimentellen teratoiden Geschwülste der Geschlechtsdrüsen. *Z. Krebsforsch.* **50**, 339—351 (1940).

ISAKA, H., On the experimental testicular tumor produced with copper sulphate locally injected in the rat. *Gann* **42**, 351—352 (1951).

Aluminium

BROWN, E. W., and WINKLE, W. VAN, Present status of aluminium in the therapy and prophylaxis of silicosis. *J. Amer. med. Ass.* **140**, 1024—1029 (1949).

CAMPBELL, I. R., CASS, J. S., CHOLAK, J., and KEHOE, R. A., Aluminum in the environment of man. *Arch. industr. Health* **15**, 359—448 (1957).

Council on Pharmacy and Chemistry: Aluminum hydroxide preparations. *J. Amer. med. Ass.* **117**, 1356—1359 (1941).

MEIKLEJPHN, A., The successful prevention of silicosis among china biscuit workers in the North Staffordshire potteries. *Brit. J. industr. Med.* **20**, 255—275 (1963).

SWENSSON, A., NORDENFELT, O., FORSSMAN, S., LUNDGREN, K. D., and OHMAN, H., Aluminum dust pneumoconiosis. A clinical study. *Arch. Gewerbepath. Gewerbehyg.* **19**, 131—148 (1962).

Tantalum

FULCHER, O. H., Tantalum as a metallic implant to repair cranial defects. *J. Amer. med. Ass.* **121**, 931—933 (1943).

OPPENHEIMER, B. S., OPPENHEIMER, E. T., DANISHEFSKY, I., and STOUT, A. P., Carcinogenic effect of metals in rodents. *Cancer Res.* **16**, 439—441 (1956).

Scholer, H. C., Repair of hernias with tantalum gauze. *J. Amer. med. Ass.* **152**, 775 (1953).

Silver and Gold

Irgang, S., Keratoderma and melanoderma accompanying therapy with a gold compound. *Arch. Derm. Syph. (Chic.)* **34**, 624—625 (1936).

Nothdurft, H., Die experimentelle Erzeugung von Sarkomen bei Ratten und Mäusen durch Implantation von Rundscheiben von Gold, Silber, Platin und Elfenbein. *Naturwissenschaften* **42**, 75—76 (1955).

Schmähl, D., u. Steinhoff, D., Versuche zur Krebserzeugung mit kolloidalen Silber- und Goldlösungen an Ratten. *Z. Krebsforsch.* **63**, 586—591 (1955).

Mercury

Druckrey, H., Hamperl, H., u. Schmähl, D., Cancerogene Wirkung von metallischem Quecksilber nach intraperitonealer Gabe bei Ratten. *Z. Krebsforsch.* **61**, 511—519 (1957).

Lead

Boyland, E., Dukes, C. E., Grover, P. L., and Mitchley, B. V. V., The induction of renal tumours by feeding lead acetate to rats. *Brit. J. Cancer* **16**, 283—288 (1962).

Esch, G. J. van, Genderen, H. van, and Vink, H. H., The induction of renal tumours by feeding of basic lead acetate to rats. *Brit. J. Cancer* **16**, 289—297 (1962).

Dukes, C. E., Clues to causes of cancer of the kidney. *Lancet* **1961** II, 1157.

Kilham, L., Low, R. J., Conti, S. F., and Dallenbach, F. D., Intranuclear inclusions and neoplasms of the kidneys of wild rats. *J. nat. Cancer Inst.* **29**, 863—885 (1962).

Millar, I. B., Gastro-intestinal cancer and geochemistry in North Montgomeryshire. *Brit. J. Cancer* **15**, 175—184 (1961).

On Potential Carcinogenecity of the Iron Macromolecular Complexes

F. J. C. Roe

Reader in Experimental Pathology, Chester Beatty Research Institute, University of London, and Associate Pathologist, Royal Marsden Hospital, London, Great Britain

Introduction

SAUNDERS (1958) provides a brief review of the history of iron in medical treatment. Oxides and carbonates of iron have found a place in therapy from ancient times. Their use is mentioned in the *Ebers Papyrus*, and Dioscorides, Galen, Celsus and Aetius advocated iron therapy in the treatment of splenic enlargement and menorrhagia. In 1661 SYDENHAM described the striking benefit of iron therapy in the treatment of chlorosis. LIEBIG, in 1843, gave the first clear description of the role of haemolgobin, and FORTES and THIVOLLE, in 1925, first demonstrated that plasma-iron is different from haemoglobin. These and related findings demonstrated beyond argument that iron is an essential ingredient of the human diet.

FIGUEROA'S (1958) view that "The great majority of patients suffering from iron deficiency can be treated with oral iron" is probably widely acceptable, especially if the word "iron" is interpreted as "bivalent organic iron" (UNDRITZ, 1958). The valid indications for parenteral iron therapy in the very few patients who require it include, according to FIGUEROA (1958): —

1. Where there is a failure to absorb adequate amounts of oral iron.

2. Where a patient cannot tolerate orally administered iron, or is unwilling or cannot be relied upon to continue oral iron therapy.

3. Where it is necessary to replace iron stores in cases of severe, predictable and frequent blood loss not amenable to medical or surgical correction.

4. Cases of iron-deficiency anaemia that have failed to respond to prolonged adequate oral iron therapy.

Of these indications the first is rare, except in patients with idiopathic steatorrhoea, or who have undergone extensive surgical removal of the small intestine, and the second is the most common. Referring to the use of parenteral iron therapy during the third trimester of pregnancy, FIGUEROA (1958) comments that it is debatable whether the small or moderate increase in haemoglobin more readily achievable by the parenteral administration than by the oral administration of iron is justified.

Iron macromolecular complexes suitable for parenteral administration.

1. Saccharated iron-oxide (Ferrivenin, Proferrin, Colliron, Neo-Ferrum, Iviron). — For intravenous injection only.

2. Iron-dextrin (Dextriferron, Astrafer). — For intravenous injection only.

3. Iron-dextran complex (Imferon). — For intramuscular or intravenous injection.

4. Iron-sorbitol-citric-acid complex (Jectofer). — For intramuscular injection only.

5. Iron-polyisomaltose (Ferrum Hausmann). — For intramuscular injection only.

If given in adequate and equivalent amounts these preparations are more or less equally effective in the treatment of iron-deficiency anaemia (FIGUEROA, 1958) This is at first sight surprising since there are marked differences in the degree of retention of iron at the injection site (FIELDING, 1962): iron-dextrin and iron-dextran are both retained locally to a far greater extent than iron-sorbitol-citric-acid complex. However, these differences refer to conditions in which animals are overloaded with iron. In the absence of overloading the somewhat more rapid clearance of the iron-sorbitol complex is, from the point of view of rapidity of haematological response, apparently offset by the more rapid excretion of its iron-content by the kidneys (LINDVALL and ANDERSSON, 1961).

General toxicity, other than carcinogenicity, of parenteral iron preparations.

The toxic effects, other than carcinogenicity, of saccharated iron oxide are discussed by NISSIM (1954) and BROWN and MOORE (1956). The material is strongly alkaline and hypertonic and gives rise to marked local inflammation if injected extravascularly. Both immediate and delayed systemic toxic effects are also frequent; the former are thought

to be due to individual hypersensitivity to impurities in the preparation, and the latter to the intravascular precipitation of the compound. The incidence of reactions has varied with the technique of administration from less than 0.2% to over 50% of injections. Intravenous iron-dextrin also gives rise to a range of toxic reactions, especially in patients simultaneously receiving oral iron (BLAZER and DEL RIEGO, 1962). From the point of view of the incidence and severity of such toxic reactions the introduction of iron-dextran for intramuscular use was a big step forward (SCOTT and GOVAN, 1954). Intramuscular injection of iron-sorbitol-citric acid complex (Jectofer) undoubtedly carries more risk of toxic response than does similar treatment with iron-dextran (SCOTT, 1962), and the simultaneous administration of iron orally seems to enhance this risk. Iron-polyisomaltose is similar to iron-dextran both chemically and in its relative lack of toxicity (MEREU and TONZ, 1961).

HADDOW and HORNING (1960) described the failure of hair to regrow after clipping over the site of injection of iron-dextran, and BAKER, GOLBERG, MARTIN and SMITH (1961) and FIELDING (1962) reported the development of alopecia, brown staining and loss of tissue elasticity at the site of injection of iron-dextran, but not of iron-sorbitol-citric-acid complex. BERESFORD, GOLBERG and SMITH (1957) reported acute inflammation and degeneration followed by rapid and complete regeneration following the intramuscular injection of iron-polysaccharide complexes of the iron-dextrin/iron-dextran type. ROE and HADDOW (1965) found that acute tenderness and swelling at the injection site was more marked in rats injected with iron-sorbitol-citric acid complex than with iron-dextran.

Induction of neoplasms at site of intra-muscular or subcutaneous injection of iron preparations

Reports of the induction of sarcomas and histocytomas at the site of sub-cutaneous intramuscular injection of various iron-carbohydrate complexes is summarised in Table I. The repeated injection of relatively large doses of

(1961) obtained a low yield of tumours in both rats and mice following repeated injections of iron-polyisomaltose (Ferrum Hausmann). MEREU and TONZ (1961) referred to negative results in animal tests for carcinogenicity of this product but gave no details.

In most of the experimental studies control animals have been injected with

Table I. *Carcinogenicity of various iron preparations administered by subcutaneous or intramuscular injection*

Preparation	No. of tests for Carcino-genicity	No. of tests in which positive results obtained	Species	References
Saccharated iron-oxide	3	2	Mouse	RICHMOND (1959); HADDOW and HORNING (1960); HADDOW, DUKES and MITCHLEY (1961)
Iron-dextrin	3	3	Rat Mouse	LUNDIN (1961); FIELDING (1962)
Iron-dextran	19	17	Rat Mouse Hamster Rabbit	RICHMOND (1959); HADDOW and HORNING (1960); GOLBERG, MARTIN and SMITH (1960); LUNDIN (1961); FIELDING (1962); KUNZ, SHAHAB, HENZE and HEINZE (1963); HADDOW ROE and MITCHLEY (1964); HADDOW and ROE (1964); ROE, HADDOW, DUKES and MITCHLEY (1964); ROE and HADDOW (1965)
Iron sorbitol citric acid complex	3	1*	Rat Mouse	LUNDIN (1961); FIELDING (1962); ROE and HADDOW (1965)
Iron polyisomaltose	2	2	Rat Mouse	HADDOW, DUKES and MITCHLEY (1961)

* Solitary benign fibroma among 20 rats.

saccharated iron-oxide, iron-dextrin or iron-dextran may induce such tumours in laboratory rodents: in many tests for carcinogenicity sarcomas have been in-duced in upwards of 50 per cent of animals injected with these substances. Iron-sorbitol-citric-acid complex (Jec-tofer), on the other hand, has given an essentially negative result in 3 fairly stringent tests (LUNDIN, 1961; FIEL-DING, 1962 and ROE and HADDOW, 1965). HADDOW, DUKES and MITCHLEY

the corresponding carbohydrate moiety of iron-carbohydrate complex under test. Almost without exception entirely negative results have been obtained in such control groups. A problem here is that the carbohydrate by itself has a much smaller molecular size (ca. 2,500) than the iron-macromolecular complex which it forms with iron (ca. 180,000 — see ERIKSSON, 1961). HUEPER (1959), however, tested 11 different dextrans ranging in molecular weight from

37,000 to several million in rats, mice and rabbits: injection-site sarcomas were induced by none of these materials.

Sarcoma-induction in relation to amount injected at one site

Roe, Haddow, Dukes and Mitchley (1964) compared the effect of giving 24 weekly injections of 0.5 ml iron-dextran into one, two, four or six subcutaneous sites in comparable groups of

seen in animals injected in 4 or 6 sites tended to be more benign than that seen in animals injected in only 1 or 2 sites. A further interesting observation was that multiple tumours were frequently seen at individual injection sites.

Carcinogenicity in relation to iron-overloading

Golberg, Martin and Smith (1960) studied the effects of overloading animals

Table II. *Incidence and time of induction of rapidly growing tumours (RGT) at the injection site*

No. of rats	Injection sites per rat	RGT	Time of appearance of first RGT	Average time of appearance of RGT
24	1	14	329	501
24	2	6	460	667
24	4	9	449	706
24	6	3	522	674
32	0	0	—	—

Table III. *Risk of tumour developing at injection site*

Injection sites per rat	Dose of iron-dextran per site	Sites examined at autopsy	Sites with malignant tumours	(per cent)	Sites with benign or malignant tumours	(per cent)
1	12 ml.	22	14	(63.6)	14	(63.6)
2	6 ml.	46	9	(19.6)	11	(23.9)
4	4 ml.	96	20	(20.8)	29	(30.2)
6	2 ml.	138	12	(8.7)	17	(12.3)

rats. A spectrum of local tumours was induced, including benign fibromas, small, slowly growing sarcomas and rapidly growing sarcomas. Table II shows that the incidence of rapidly growing tumours fell and the average latent interval before they appeared rose as the number of injection-sites used increased. Table III demonstrates that, although the risk of tumour development at any one site fell as the number of injection-sites increased, the risk that the animal would develop a tumour at one of its injection-sites actually increased! However, the type of tumour

with iron. Their results indicated that the escape of iron from the site of injection was much slower in iron-overloaded animals than in normal animals. In addition, biochemical changes in the liver, serum and region of injection were observed in the former but not in the latter. Finally they asserted that local tumour induction only occurs in iron-overloaded animals. They saw, for example, no sarcomas in response to weekly intramuscular injections of 0.02ml iron-dextran in mice and only one sarcoma in 50 mice injected once weekly with 0.1 ml. However, in the latter case

survival was poor. More recently HAD-
DOW and ROE (1964) reported a high
incidence of sarcomas in mice receiving
0.05 ml iron-dextran weekly (total dose
2.35 mls) and one out of 20 rats given
90 weekly injections of 0.01 mls developed a sarcoma (Table IV, V). In a
current experiment sarcomas have appeared in response to only 2 injections,
each of 0.75 ml iron-dextran (see Table VI).

Clearly the risk of tumour induction recedes as the size of the local
dose is reduced, but particularly in the
light of the results just referred to it is
by no means certain that the degree of
general overloading with iron is of
any significance.

The relationship of dose to body size

HADDOW and HORNING (1960) and
ROE (1961) have argued cogently that

Table IV. *Carcinogenic response to different doses of iron-dextran (imferon) injected subcutaneously in CB ♂ rats (Wistar)*

No. of doses (Imferon)	Size of each dose (ml.)	Total dose (ml.)	Injection site sarcomas	No. of rats injected	Minimum induction time (days)
30	1.0	30	20	30*	145
20	0.5	10	8	20	426
64	0.05	3.2	2	20	478
90	0.01	0.9	1	20	736

* A further 8 rats had local histiocytomas.

Table V. *Carcinogenic response to different doses of iron-dextran (Imferon) injected subcutaneously in CB ♂ mice (Stock)*

No. of doses (Imferon)	Size of each dose (ml.)	Total dose (ml.)	Injection site sarcomas	No. of rats injected	Minimum induction time (days)
30	0.3	9.0	14	30	182
47	0.05	2.35	12	30	168
87	0.01	0.87	0	20	—

Table VI. *Effect of dose in induction of sarcomas at the site of injection of iron-dextran*

Group	No. of S.C. injections of 0.75 ml. iron-dextran into R. flank	Total dose of iron-dextran	No. of rats in group	Position 16 months after start of experiment		
				Survivors	Injection site sarcomas*	Time of appearance of sarcomas (months)
A	16	12 ml.	16	3	5	12, 14, 14, 14, 16
B	8	6 ml.	32	17	2	9, 15
C	4	3 ml.	64	29	0**	
D	2	1.5 ml.	128	71	3	13, 14, 14
E	0	0	64	33	0	

* All histologically confirmed.
** One benign fibroma.

the induction of sarcomas at the site of injection is a "local" phenomenon. Therefore, it is the actual size of the dose and not its size relative to whole body size which matters. The size of individual cells in man is of the same order as in experimental animals and a particular volume of injected material will come into contact with approximately the same number of cells in all species. Thus the ratio of dose to body weight is only of importance if it can be shown that the local induction of sarcomas by the injected material is dependent on a general dose-dependent effect on the body as a whole. So far this has not been demonstrated.

Evidence for carcinogenicity other than locally at the site of injection

HUEPER (1957, 1959) examined a wide variety of macromolecular substances for carcinogenicity, administering them intravenously, subcutaneously (by injection or implantation), or intraperitoneally to rats, mice or rabbits. Only one of 30 substances examined, silastic rubber (a silicone polymer), gave unequivocal evidence of tumour induction at the site of subcutaneous implantation. On the other hand, many of the test substances appeared to increase the incidence of tumours of the reticulo-endothelial system. These findings of HUEPER and the observations of HADDOW, DUKES and MITCHLEY (1961) that simple iron salts, such as ferric citrate, ferric salicylate, ferrous sulphate, ferrous lactate or ferrous gluconate, do not induce injection-site sarcomas, suggest that the local carcinogenicity of iron-macromolecular complexes is attributable neither to the carbohydrate alone, nor to the iron alone, but to the complexes themselves. On the other hand, the fact that a variety of macromolecules seem able to induce cancer of the reti-

culo-endothelial system, suggests that there may be a hazard of *distant carcinogenesis*, (i.e. the induction of tumours at sites distant from the point of injection) following the parenteral administration of iron-carbohydrate complexes also.

Most of the tests of iron-carbohydrate complexes for carcinogenicity have been designed specifically to study the induction of tumours locally at the site of injection. For such purposes a control group containing the same number of animals as the test group is appropriate. Much larger control groups are likely to be necessary for studying the effect of treatment on the incidence of tumours of *all* sites and tissues of the body. HADDOW and HORNING (1960) observed a number of unusual tumours in their iron-dextran treated animals, including a bronchogenic carcinoma in a rat. HADDOW (1963), from a survey of his many experiments with iron-dextran, regarded the yield of tumours at sites remote from the injection-site as "unquestionably significant". But LUNDIN (1961) commented on the absence of liver tumours in his iron-dextran treated animals, despite the large deposits of iron in the organ, and ROE and LANCASTER (1964) felt that more information was necessary before such a conclusion could be reached. ROE, HADDOW, DUKES and MITCHLEY (1964) recorded the occurrence of various types of tumour in both iron-dextran treated rats and in untreated control groups. More recently, ROE and HADDOW (1965) observed more 'distant' tumours of various types in rats injected repeatedly with iron-sorbitol-citric-acid than with iron-dextran in similar dosage. LANGVAD (1964) reported an experiment in which 50 male and 50 female mice of the St/El A strain were injected repeatedly with iron-dextran, each animal receiving a total of 2 mls of the substance. Seven per cent of the males and 58% of the females developed tumours. The corresponding rates for untreated controls were 0% and 20%, respectively. LANGVAD (1964) suggested that oncogenic viruses used in other experiments in the same laboratory at the time might, through contamination, have been wholly or partly responsible for the differences recorded. However, even if it were shown that iron-dextran acts as no more than a co-factor in the induction of tumours of distant sites, its use is hardly to be regarded as being without potential carcinogenic hazard for man.

Obviously the problem cannot be resolved until the results of careful studies on much larger groups of animals are available.

Evidence of carcinogenic effect of iron macromolecular complexes in man

To date there has, to our knowledge, been no fully acceptable report of the occurrence of sarcoma at the site of injection of iron-macromolecular complexes in man. CROWLEY and STILL (1960) reported the occurrence of a metastasis in the buttock at the site of previous iron-dextran injections in a case of cancer of the cervix uteri. ROBINSON, BELL and STURDY (1960) reported a case in which an undifferentiated soft-tissue sarcoma arose at the site of injection of iron dextran into the region of the deltoid muscle $3^1/_4$ years previously. Excess iron was present at the tumour site, though it was not proved to be iron-dextran. It was thought unlikely that the tumour was a metastasis, but the possibility could not be excluded. GOLBERG (1960) subsequently quoted the opinion of Professor R. A. WILLIS that the lesion observed by ROBINSON and his colleagues was not a neoplasm. Where there is a difference in opinion

between pathologists on the histopathological nature of a lesion, it is logical to take into account the macroscopic appearances and clinical details. The case history provided by ROBINSON and his colleagues is more in keeping with neoplasia than with any alternative diagnosis.

In any event, as pointed out by many authors, the induction of sarcomas in man by injected iron complexes, if it occurs at all, is likely to take many years. It is still less than 20 years since use of this type of iron preparation became widespread, so that there remains the possibility that the minimum induction period for man has not yet been exhausted.

If the main carcinogenic effect in man is a local one, then it is likely that it will be observed sooner rather than later, since localised soft-tissue sarcomas are relatively uncommon. If, however, the main danger is a slightly increased risk of cancer of many different sites, then nothing short of a major long-term prospective epidemiological survey is likely to reveal the hazard.

BAKER, GOLBERG, MARTIN and SMITH (1961) were interested in establishing the carcinogenic safety of iron-dextran for man. With this intention, they compared the local tissue response to injection in different species. Rabbits and dogs showed less residual iron at the injection-site, and a greater hepatic uptake of iron than mice and rats. Nevertheless, HADDOW, ROE and MITCHLEY (1964) encountered two cases of local sarcoma in 6 rabbits injected with iron-dextran. Most of the specimens obtained by BAKER *et al* (1961) from iron-dextran injection-sites in man showed no evidence of fibrosis, but in 2 cases fibrosis and the heavy accumulation of siderophages were seen. These are precisely the changes which precede tumour formation in experimental animals.

Is iron, per se, carcinogenic?

There is no evidence that iron as such is carcinogenic, though it is doubtful whether it has been deliberately tested for carcinogenicity to an adequate extent. There have been no reports of an excessive incidence of cancer in animals deliberately overloaded with simple iron compounds, and with possibly one exception, referred to above (see Langvad, 1964), the carcinogenic effect of iron-macromolecular complexes appears to be limited to the site of its injection into the body. Overloading with iron leads to its excessive storage in the liver, i.e. 'haemochromatosis'. In this condition the iron is stored as an organic complex, for which Golberg and Smith (1960) suggested the name "haptosiderin". These workers also suggested that where haemochromatosis arises spontaneously, it does so as an expression of an inborn error of metabolism involving the overproduction of haptosiderin. In induced haemochromatosis, on the other hand, the excess of haptosiderin is secondary to overloading with iron. Cirrhosis tends to accompany both spontaneous and induced haemochromatosis, but according to Golberg and Smith adequate protein and vitamin E in the diet delay or prevent its occurrence. Although in general there is undoubtedly an association between cirrhosis and liver cancer, in the particular case of the cirrhosis which accompanies haemochromatosis the association is very weak (Sheldon, 1935; Willis, 1953). Foulds and Stewart (1956) and Hueper (1956) both observed a high incidence of bronchial carcinoma in haematite miners, and concluded that sidero-silicosis predisposed to neoplasia. Doll (1958) did not regard the evidence for the association as conclusive, but Campbell (1940) reported a higher incidence of adenomatous lung tumours in mice exposed to mixtures of silica and iron oxide than in untreated controls.

The mechanism of carcinogenesis by iron macromolecular complexes

There has been much speculation with regard to the mechanism of carcinogenesis by macromolecular materials in general and by iron-carbohydrate complexes in particular. As pointed out above, the induction of local tumours cannot be attributed solely either to the iron or to the carbohydrate moiety of the various molecules. Carcinogenicity is somehow linked to the nature of the complex itself. In this connection it is of special interest that aluminium-dextran is also highly productive of local sarcomas on injection: Haddow, Dukes and Mitchley (1961) recorded the induction of 11 sarcomas in 40 mice given repeated subcutaneous injections of this complex. Preparations of chromium-dextran, copper-dextran and bismuth-dextran, on the other hand, were more or less inactive. The macromolecular compounds studied by Hueper (1959) were largely ineffective in the induction of local tumours. Hence macromolecularity itself is not a sufficient explanation of carcinogenicity.

Haddow and Horning (1960) suggested that blockage of the reticuloendothelial system with, perhaps, interference with immune processes might be implicated. Fielding (1962) saw evidence of lymphatic blockage after the injection of iron-dextran or iron-dextrin, but not after injection of iron-sorbitol-citric-acid. Richmond (1959) suggested that the carbohydrate complex might enable the passage of iron across intracellular membranes normally impervious to it. He subsequently (RICHMOND, 1962) showed that iron-dextran gives rise to cytological changes indicative of intracellular oxidation. He thought that the changes were not dissimilar from some of the effects of ionising radiation, and suggested that they could explain the carcinogenicity of iron-dextran. TURNER (1964) reported that the response of fowl fibrocytes grown *in vitro*, to iron-dextran, resembled that to known carcinogens. HADDOW and HORNING (1960) reviewed the literature concerning the interference with iron metabolism by carcinogenic agents, but came to no real conclusion with regard to the likely mechanism of action of iron-complexes.

It is, perhaps, tempting to regard carcinogenesis by iron-carbohydrate complexes as being related to carcinogenesis by other metals, e.g. arsenic, beryllium, cadmium, chromium, cobalt lead and nickel (see ROE and LANCASTER, 1964). However, on present evidence it would certainly be unwise to presume that this is so. In the cases of all the other metals the evidence strongly suggests that the metal itself is implicated. But in the case of iron, the only acceptable evidence of carcinogenicity relates to iron-carbohydrate complexes and, possibly, combinations of iron with silica. Aluminium alone behaves in a similar fashion.

ROE and LANCASTER (1964) suggested that the induction of cancer by the subcutaneous injection of chemically unreactive materials such as the iron macromolecular complexes may be more akin to the "Oppenheimer effect" than to chemical carcinogenesis. On the other hand, HUEPER (1959) contended that chemical mechanisms have not been excluded in the case of sarcoma induction by the implantation of plastic materials. Moreover, as ROE and LANCASTER (1964) themselves pointed out, by no me-

ans all chemically unreactive substances, even those which remain permanently at the injection-site, induce sarcomas.

The consideration of the mechanism of carcinogenesis by iron-carbohydrate complexes should, perhaps, begin with a description of the changes which precede the appearance of tumours. On this subject there is general agreement that the first change is the uptake of the injected material by histiocytes (siderophages). In these cells the iron is thereafter stored as newly formed ferritin (MUIR and GOLBERG, 1961). Siderophages are also found in the local lymph nodes, and other cells of the reticulo-endothelial system, generally, take up and store the iron as ferritin. However, the movement of iron away from the injection site, certainly in animals overloaded with iron, is slow (BAKER, GOLBERG, MARTIN and SMITH, 1961) and both siderophages and extracellular iron-containing material persists locally until tumour development ensues. The development of a mass of siderophages clearly depends on the proliferation of histiocytes and in some instances this proliferation leads to the formation of a histiocytic neoplasm (histiocytoma) in which many of the cells are not laden with iron. After a period of some months, depending on the species, proliferation of histiocytes gives place to fibroblastic activity. It is not certain whether fibroblasts are derived from siderophages or merely stimulated to divide by the presence of the siderophages. The onset of fibroplasia is appreciable, clinically, in that the injection site becomes firm and thickened. Such areas of thickening remain unchanged or enlarge slowly over a period of several months. Suddenly, usually it seems from one edge of the thickened lesion, a rapidly growing nodule appears. The growth of this lesion is progressive and necessitates the sacrifice of the animal within a matter of days or weeks from the time it first became palpable.

The stage of fibroblastic proliferation appears to be an essential preliminary in the induction of sarcomas. This is true not only of their induction by iron-macromolecular complexes but by all agents, including implanted sponges, plastic films, and metal objects. In our experience chemically unreactive substances which do not induce sarcomas at the site of their subcutaneous or intramuscular injection, also do not stimulate fibroblastic proliferation. This still leaves open the question of whether the induction of tumours by iron-carbohydrate complexes is chemical or physical in nature. Cadmium-precipitated ferritin was shown to be carcinogenic by Haddow, Roe, Dukes and Mitchley (1964), but a similar carcinogenic effect by cadmium itself was also demonstrated. It is not yet known whether cadmium-free ferritin is able to induce sarcomas if injected subcutaneously. If it can be shown that iron complexes induce tumours at sites remote from their injection, then an essentially chemical mechanism will seem more likely. At present, in our opinion, a physical mechanism similar to that which operates in the case of the 'Oppenheimer effect', seems most plausible.

Conclusion

From the point of view of future policy the mechanism of carcinogenesis by subcutaneously or intramuscularly administered macromolecular iron complexes is of academic interest only. In the case of their intravenous administration, however, it is highly relevant. At present there is no clear-cut evidence of carcinogenic hazard from intravenously administered iron-carbohydrate complexes, nor is there adequate evidence of their safety in this respect. Long-term experiments on a large scale in several species are urgently needed to investigate this problem. In the meantime, the possibility of carcinogenic response should be borne in mind by those proposing to administer iron parenterally. The reasons for preferring parenteral administration to the oral route are few (Figueroa, 1958). When administration by this route is justified, the apparently greater carcinogenic risk of some preparations, as compared with others, should be taken into account along with evidence of other types of toxicity in choosing the most suitable preparation. Overloading with iron should be avoided. The size of individual injections should be small and multiple injections should be distributed through several sites and not given all into the same site. Because the latent interval for sarcoma induction in man is likely to be more than 15 or 20 years there need, on present evidence, be little hesitation in administering iron complexes by subcutaneous or intramuscular injection into patients whose life expectancy is shorter than this. Much more caution should be exercised in the case of younger patients. In particular, it is most doubtful whether the administration of iron by the parenteral route to pregnant women, more or less as a routine measure, is at all justified.

References

Baker, S. B. de C., Golberg, L., Martin, L. E., and Smith, J. P., Tissue changes following injection of iron-dextran complex. *J. Path. Bact.* **82**, 453—470 (1961).

Beresford, C. R., Golberg, L., and Smith, J. P., Local effects and mechanism of absorption of iron preparations administered intramuscularly. *Brit. J. Pharmacol.* **12**, 107—114 (1957).

BROWN, E. B., and MOORE, C. V., Parenterally administered iron in the treatment of hypochronic anaemia. *Prog. Hemat.* 1, 22—46 (1956).

CAMPBELL, J. A., Effects of precipitated silica and iron oxide on the incidence of primary lung tumors in mice. *Brit. med. J.* 1940 II, 275—280.

CROWLEY, J. D., and STILL, W. J. S., Metastatic carcinoma at the site of injection of iron-dextran complex. *Brit. med. J.* 1960 I, 1411—1412.

DOLL, R., *Present knownledge of the causation of carcinoma of the lung.* Chapter in: Carcinoma of the lung, ed. by J. R. BIGNALL, p. 53—55. Edinburgh and London: Livingstone 1958.

ERIKSSON, F. R. cit. by SVARD, P. O., and LINDVALL, S., Mechanism of absorption of two intramuscular iron preparations. *J. Pharm. Pharmacol.* 13, 650—653 (1961).

FAULDS, J. S., and STEWART, M. J., Carcinoma of the lung in haematite miners. *J. Path. Bact.* 72, 353—366 (1956).

FIELDING, J., Sarcoma induction by iron-carbohydrate complexes. *Brit. med. J.* 1962 I, 1800—1803.

FIGUEROA, W. G., *Parenteral treatment of iron deficiency.* Chapter in: Iron metabolism, ed. by F. GROSS, p. 426—440. Berlin-Göttingen-Heidelberg: Springer 1964.

GOLBERG, L., Hazards of iron-dextran. *Brit. med. J.* 1960 II, 1598—1599.

— MARTIN, L. E., and SMITH, J. P., Iron overloading phenomena in animals. *Toxicol. appl. Pharmacol.* 2, 683—707 (1960).

— , and SMITH, J. P., Iron overloading and hepatic vulnerability. *Amer. J. Path.* 36, 125—149 (1960).

HADDOW, A., Advances in knowledge of the carcinogenic process ,1958—1962. *Acta Un. int. Cancr.* 19, 453—457 (1963)

— DUKES, C. E., and MITCHLEY, B. C. V., Carcinogenicity of iron preparations and metal carbohydrate complexes. *Ann. Rep. Brit. Emp. Cancer Campaign* 39, 74—76 (1961).

—, and HORNING, E. S., On the carcinogenicity of an iron-dextran complex. *J. nat. Cancer Inst.* 24, 109—147 (1960).

—, and ROE, F. J. C., Iron-dextran and sarcomata. *Brit. med. J.* 1964 II, 119—121.

— — DUKES, C. E., and MITCHLEY, B. C. V., Cadmium neoplasia: Sarcomata at the site of injection of cadmium sulphate in rats and mice. *Brit. J. Cancer* 18, 667—673 (1964).

— —, and MITCHLEY, B. C. V., Induction of sarcomata in rabbits by intramuscular injection of iron-dextran ("Imferon"). *Brit. med. J.* 1964 I, 1593—1594.

HUEPER, W. C., A quest into the environmental causes of lung cancer. Public Health Monograph No 36, U.S. Public Health Service Publication No 452 (1956).

— Experimental carcinogenic studies in macromolecular chemicals: I: Neoplastic reactions in rats and mice after parenteral introduction of polyvinyl pyrrolidones. *Cancer (Philad.)* 10, 8—18 (1957).

— Carcinogenic studies on water-soluble and insoluble macromolecules. *Arch. Path.* 67, 589—617 (1959).

KUNZ, J., SHAHAB, L., HENZE, K., and HEINZ, D., Experimentelle Untersuchungen zur cancerogenen Wirkung von Eisendextran (Ursoferran). *Acta biol. med. germ.* 10, 602—614 (1963).

LANGVAD, E., "Imferon", carcinogen or co-carcinogen? Internal factors determining the course of oncogenic virus infection? Report from Fibiger Laboratory, Copenhagen, at Symposium in Stockholm, April, 1964.

LINDVALL, S., and ANDERSSON, N. S. E., Studies on a new intramuscular haematinic, iron-sorbitol. *Brit. J. Pharmacol.* 17, 358—371 (1961).

LUNDIN, P. M., The carcinogenic action of complex iron preparations. *Brit. J. Cancer* 15, 838—847 (1961).

MEREU, T., u. TÖNZ, O., Die Eisenmangelanämie des Kindes und ihre Behandlung mit Eisenpolyisomaltosat. *Dtsch. med. Wschr.* 86, 1259—1266 (1961).

MUIR, A. R., and GOLBERG, L., Observations on subcutaneous macrophages, phagocytosis of iron-dextran and ferritin synthesis. *Quart. J. exp. Physiol.* 46, 289—298 (1961).

NISSIM, J. A., Toxic reactions after intravenous saccharated iron oxide in man. *Brit. med. J.* 1954 I, 352—356.

RICHMOND, H. G., Induction of sarcoma in the rat by iron-dextran complex. *Brit. med. J.* 1959 I, 947—949.

— The toxic effects of iron-dextran complex on mammalian cells in tissue culture. *Brit. J. Cancer* 15, 594—606 (1961).

ROBINSON, C. E. G., BELL, D. N., and STURDY, J. H.., Possible association of malignant neoplasm with iron-dextran injection: a case report. *Brit. med. J.* 1960 II, 648—650.

ROE, F. J. C., Cancer hazards in our environment. The use of animal experiments in their detection and evaluation. *N. S. med. Bull.* 40, 134—147 (1961).

— HADDOW, A., DUK s, C. E., and MITCHLEY, B. C. V., Iron-dextran carcinogenesis in rats:

Effect of distributing injected material between one, two, four, or six sites. *Brit. J. Cancer* **18**, 801—808 (1964).

ROE, F. J. C., and LANCASTER, M. C., Natural, metallic and other substances as carcinogens. *Brit. med. Bull.* **20**, 127—133 (1964).

SAUNDERS, J. B. DE C. M., *Iron and the development of medicine.* Chapter in: Iron in clinical medicine ed. by WALLERSTEIN, R. O., and METTIER, S. R., p. 1—4. Berkeley and Los Angeles: University California Press 1958.

SCOTT, J. M., Toxicity of iron sorbitol citrate. *Brit. med. J.* **1962** II, 480—481.

SCOTT, J. M., and GOVAN, A. D. T., Anaemia of pregnancy treated with intramuscular iron. *Brit. med. J.* **1954** II, 1257—1259.

SHELDON, J. H., *Haemochromatosis.* London: Oxford University Press 1935.

TURNER, C. J., Morphological effect of iron-dextran on fowl fibrocytes *in vitro. Brit. J. Cancer* **17**, 731—737 (1963).

UNDRITZ, E., *Oral treatment of iron deficiency.* Chapter in: Iron metabolism, ed. by F. GROSS, p. 406—425. Berlin-Göttingen-Heidelberg: Springer 1964.

WILLIS, R. A., *Pathology of tumours*, p. 434. London: Butterworth & Co. 1953.

Discussion of papers by Drs. Hueper and Roe

Berenblum: It might be that the right animal for revealing the carcinogenic potentiality of arsenic has not yet been used. Alternatively, arsenic may be a co-carcinogen. I suggest that arsenic should be tested to see if it enhances the activity of known carcinogenic agents.

Boyland: The ferret may be a suitable animal to reveal carcinogenicity of arsenic.

Saffiotti: I support Prof. BERENBLUM's suggestion to investigate the effects of arsenic combined with treatments with general carcinogens. Some combined tests, such as those of Dr. HUEPER and some in our laboratory have failed so far to reveal activity. However, the right combination might be rare. Dr. ROE mentioned our finding that benzo[a]pyrene, in combination with iron oxide produces carcinogenic effects in the lungs. I wish to emphasise that our results do not indicate any carcinogenic effects of iron oxide *per se.* In our experimental conditions, it only acts as a carrier of the carcinogen into the lungs and the soluble carcinogen is then eluted out from it. Most tumours do not arise at the site of iron deposition, but from the mucosa of the larger bronchi. We also tested cobalt oxide, which was shown by GILMAN to be carcinogenic by intramuscular injection in mice and rats. We introduced cobalt oxide in the lungs of hamsters by repeated intratracheal injections and we found that it induced a sort of cystic dilatation of the bronchioles; some areas around these lesions appear frankly neoplastic. Our histological study of the lesions, however, is not complete.

Doll: I agree with Dr. HUEPER that inorganic arsenic can cause cancers of the skin and lung, but the evidence that it can cause other types of cancer is weak, and there is not, in my opinion, any clear evidence that organic arsenicals can cause any form of cancer. The DANISH data showed that cancer of the cervix was commoner in women who had positive W.R.s than in others, but this was entirely accounted for by the greater proportion of prostitutes in the former. Among prostitutes the incidence of cervix cancer was the same, irrespective of whether they had had a positive W.R. in the past or not. Whether arsenic can act by itself, or whether it requires the presence of some other factor is unknown.

I agree also that some groups of men who have worked as nickel refiners have had a grossly increased incidence of cancer of the lung and nose. I doubt, however, whether the causative factor is exposure to nickel carbonyl. The greatest excess among the WELSH workers was in those men who worked with the crude ore and the same diseases are appearing in Canada where the crude ore is now being refined. In Wales there has been no hazard to men who started employment after about 1924, although the presence of a risk was not suspected until 1927. The main hazard may be due to compounds of nickel such as nickel arsenide or nickel sulphide, rather than to the pure metal.

It may be relevant to Dr. HUEPER's suggestion about cobalt that a recent study has shown a slight excess of leukaemia in patients under treatment for pernicious anaemia.

Rudali: For my part I am a little sceptical about the dangers for man from chromium and nickel. Dr. HUEPER's experiments involving the injection of rats with powdered metals are obviously not open to objection. On the other hand I think that in the case of the chromium or nickel protheses which remain in the human body there is very little diffusion of carcinogenically active materials.

Finally I should like to aks Dr. HUEPER if he has any personal experience with cadmium in the light of Dr. ROE's demonstration of the production of testicular tumours by cadmium salts.

Higginson: There are arsenical compounds which are carcinogenic in man but apparently not in animals and the iron compounds which are carcinogenic in animals but apparently not in man. It seems that the difficulties of extrapolation from animal experiments to man are indeed great.

Druckrey: One important question is: — are human beings more susceptible than animals?

Frazer: The studies reported by Dr. ROE are of considerable scientific interest. However, I should like to make a general point with regard to evaluation of toxic risks in man, with which the Symposium is concerned. If experience of use in man is available, there seems to be little point in doing further animal experiments to establish safety, since there will always be an element of doubt about their extrapolation to man. Admittedly, cancer is a long-term effect and it is not easy to unravel the tangled skein of cause and effect in this field. Nevertheless, a great many people have had parenteral iron preparations over the last 20 years. Is it not in these patients that we must seek the answer to this question? I have used parenteral iron preparations for many years in patients with upper intestinal enteropathies and we have certainly not seen any local ill effects, nor any other evidence of carcinogenic action. However, the problem clearly calls for detailed and controlled study.

Baker: In considering the relative carcinogenicity of various compounds has the total amount of iron injected been taken into consideration? It is impossible to give large amounts of most iron compounds because of local toxicity with ulceration.

Dr. ROE has argued that the injection is a local phenomenon and therefore it is the actual amount at one site that is important and not the dose in relation to body weight. This is a matter of comparative anatomy. In man and the larger animals the injected material spreads along the intramuscular septa which are capable of dispersing quite large volumes of fluid. In small animals, where the muscle fibres are very much larger, relative to the body size, the septa and fascial spaces are virtually absent. After a therapeutic injection in man, the dose is spread over a volume of tissue far greater than the total volume of a rat.

In relation to dose it is instructive to look at the histological picture. After a small dose of iron-dextran the iron is rapidly phagocytosed and within 48 hours it is all within macrophages in the form of haemosiderin, a physiological form of iron. If, however, large amounts of iron are given into the same site, then phagocytosis is slower. At these injection sites, the macrophages become overloaded with iron and die, the liberated iron is rephagocytosed and so one gets a continuous proliferation and death of macrophages.

It is dangerous to compare carcinogenesis due to iron-dextran and aluminium-dextran, the two reactions could hardly be more different. Iron-dextran is avidly picked up, whereas the aluminium-dextran remains as a depot in the tissues for weeks. Iron causes massive fibrosis, aluminium seems, if anything, to inhibit fibrosis; the depot is eventually walled off by a thin fibrous capsule.

Shabad: I agree with the suggestion made by Dr. ROE that the mechanism of the carcinogenic action of the iron-dextran is similar to that of plastic films.

Poel: What does Dr. ROE mean by "The Oppenheimer effect"?

Truhaut: In connection with Dr. HUEPER's report, may I point out that SCHMÄHL and STEINHOFF (1960) obtained spindle cell sarcoma at the site of injection after repeated subcutaneous administration of colloidal silver to rats. Comparatively negative results were obtained with colloidal gold. Also I should like to point out that cobalt benzenesulfonate is given sometimes by intramuscular route, as a peripheral vasodilatator and spasmolytic. HEATH has shown that the intramuscular injection of pure cobalt metal powder induces malignant tumours at the injection site in rats.

A propos of Dr. ROE's report, it seems to me interesting that tannins have a great affinity for iron ions leading to the formation of insoluble compounds. This might be considered as a mechanism of carcinogenic action of tannins.

Reference

SCHMÄHL, D., and STEINHOFF, D., Versuche zur Krebserzeugung mit kolloidalen Silber- und Goldlösungen an Ratten. *Z. Krebsforsch.* **63**, 586 (1960).

Hueper: In connection with possible co-carcinogenic action of arsenic mentioned by BERENBLUM I should like to point out that arsenic cancers in man are formed at sites where arsenic is retained. Their development is thus identical with that of other metal cancers and polymer cancers. These also become manifest at sites where after introduction these materials are retained, or where in the case of macromolecular colloidal solutions they are injected repeatedly, so as to produce a prolonged effect. Under such circumstances, both water soluble and insoluble carbon and silicon polymers have proved to be carcinogenic.

In reply to Professor TRUHAUT, I have no experience of colloidal suspensions, and none with cobalt injected parenterally.

To Dr. RUDALI I reply that cancer is easily produced in animals (rats) with pure nickel, and I am convinced that nickel does the job. I have not done experiments with cadmium.

In connection with Dr. HIGGINSON's point, I don't consider iron as a carcinogen.

Finally, I should like to remind Dr. DOLL that SUNDERMAN et al. (1959) induced carcinoma of various histological types in the lungs of rats surviving for two years or more after exposure to nickel carbonyl by inhalation.

Reference

SUNDERMAN, F. W., DONNELLY, A. J., WEST, B., and KINCAID, J. F., Nickel poisoning. IX Carcinogenesis in rats exposed to nickel carbonyl. *Arch. industr. Health* **20**, 36 (1959).

Roe: I agree with Professor FRAZER that data obtained from epidemiological studies on the hundreds of thousands of people treated with iron-dextran would, in many ways, be more helpful than further data from animal studies. Nevertheless, it is more difficult to obtain these epidemiological data than one might expect. We at one time approached the College of General Practitioners in Britain to see if they would initiate a study, but no reply was forthcoming. Personally, I am more worried about the pos-

sible carcinogenic effects of intravenously administered iron complexes than about the possibility of sarcoma-induction by local injections. In the latter case a cause and effect relation is likely to become apparent, sooner or later, even if no deliberate study is made. But if the intravenous injection of materials slightly increases the incidence of cancer at a number of different sites, only a very detailed and carefully controlled study on large numbers of individuals will bring this to light.

In answer to Dr. RUDALI, I would point out that the carcinogenic effect of cadmium on the testis appears to be an indirect one. Atrophy of the testes follows immediately after exposure to cadmium above a certain threshold level. According to GOULD and his colleagues in Florida, atrophy is due to selective damage to the testicular artery and to the pampiniform plexus of veins. The development, much later, of Leydig-cell tumours is secondary to testicular atrophy.

Dr. POEL has asked what do I mean by "The Oppenheimer Effect". I mean the induction of cancer by the implantation of chemically unreactive materials, where the physical shape and state of the implanted material plays a determining role in cancer induction. An example from our own laboratory is appropriate. Two groups of rats were implanted with pieces of polyvinyl sponge of the same size but of different shape: $33 \times 33 \times 2$ mm or $20 \times 20 \times 5$ mm. A high incidence of sarcomas was seen in the second group and a negligible incidence in the first.

Dr. BAKER has pointed out that the local reaction to aluminium-dextran is quite different from that to iron-dextran, although both induce sarcomas at the injection site. I cannot argue from personal experience in this matter, but am grateful to him for pointing this out.

Risques cancérogènes des Traceurs radioactifs utilisés pour le Diagnostic

M. Tubiana

Institut Gustave Roussy-Villejuif (Seine)

et N. C. Parmentier

Département de la Protection Sanitaire, Commissariat à l'Energie Atomique, Fontenay-aux-Roses (Seine)

Toute évaluation du risque cancérogène associé à l'utilisation chez l'homme de corps radioactifs, dans un but diagnostic ou thérapeutique, se heurte à des difficultés immenses, semblables d'ailleurs à celles soulevées par l'analyse des risques du radiodiagnostic: d'une part, les données humaines se rapportent à des doses beaucoup plus élevées que celles utilisées en pratique courante et l'extrapolation à des doses plus faibles est incertaine en l'absence de théories satisfaisantes sur le mécanisme de la radiocancérogénese, d'autre part, les expériences animales ont généralement été effectuées sur des rongeurs de petite taille et de courte durée de vie, leur utilisation pour prévoir les risques humains, est donc aléatoire, d'autant plus qu'il ne se dégage encore aucune vue d'ensemble cohérente.

I. L'iode Radioactif et la Thyroïde

L'iode 131 est de loin l'isotope le plus utilisé en clinique. En raison de son importance pratique, c'est donc le cas de l'irradiation thyroidïenne que nous considérerons d'abord en détail.

Les sources d'information sont multiples mais concernent essentiellement l'irradiation externe de la thyroïde.

1. De nombreux auteurs ont signalé dans les antécédents d'une proportion non négligeable de malades atteints de cancers de la thyroïde l'existence d'une irradiation cervicale, en particulier chez les sujets jeunes. Duffy et Fitzgerald signalèrent ainsi dès 1950 que sur 28 cancers de la thyroïde atteignant des enfants ou de jeunes adultes, 10 avaient été irradiés pour hypertrophie thymique. Plusieurs travaux ont, depuis, rapporté des faits semblables. Une étude générale de Winship (1961) portant sur 562 cas de cancers de la thyroïde de l'enfant, retrouve des antécédents d'irradiation chez 37% d'entre eux. Saenger (1963) dans une analyse d'observations précédemment publiées, trouve sur 255 cas, 45% d'antécédents d'irradiation. Le tableau suivant résume ces résultats.

En France, les proportions sont moindres puisque sur 16 cas d'enfants présentant des cancers de la thyroïde, nous n'avons retrouvé que 3 cas d'irradiation antérieure. Ceci est sans doute dû à ce que les irradiations thymiques n'ont pas été aussi fréquemment effectuées que dans d'autres pays (Coliez 1956).

Chez l'adulte, la proportion d'antécédents d'irradiation est beaucoup plus

Tableau I

Auteurs	Nombre de malades enfants atteints de cancer	% de malades irradiés	Periode de latence (années)	Dose estimée
Winship, Rosvoll, 1960	Total 562 directement questionnés 277	37% 80%	3—6—14	180—6000
Revue de Saenger et coll.	255	45%	3—24	100—2700

faible, puisque sur une série de 156 malades, nous n'avons trouvé que 3 cas, qui d'ailleurs avaient été irradiés avant l'âge de 20 ans (Coliez, 1956). Sur 638 cas de cancer de la thyroïde, colligés au Japon par Takahashi, 29 soit 4,5% avaient eu leur thyroïde irradiée, alors que dans le groupe témoin de 1535 sujets, 9 seulement ont des antécédents d'irradiation thyroidienne.

rissons et enfants irradiés pour hypertrophie thymique, on observait un nombre de cancers de la thyroïde beaucoup plus élevé que chez un groupe témoin. Une analyse récente du devenir de ce groupe (Pifer, 1963) a confirmé ce fait. Cependant, cette enquête, comme les autres enquêtes du même type, s'expose à une critique fondamentale, car le groupe étudié diffère de la population témoin

Tableau II

Auteurs	Nombre de malades adultes ayant un cancer	Nombre d'irradiés
Takahashi et coll. (1964)	638	29
Coliez, Tubiana* (1956)	156	3

* Les 3 cas ont d'ailleurs été irradiés avant l'âge de 20 ans

Plusieurs dizaines de cas de cancers de la thyroïde présentant des antécédents d'irradiation ont été rapportés dans la littérature; cependant, si ces observations individuelles permettent d'affirmer le rôle cancérogène possible d'une irradiation et d'estimer le temps de latence, elles ne permettent pas d'évaluer la fréquence de cette éventualité.

2. C'est pourquoi, une autre série de travaux s'est attachée, en suivant le devenir d'un groupe de sujets irradiés, à dénombrer la fréquence avec laquelle survient chez eux, un cancer de la thyroïde. La première de ces enquêtes (Simpson, 1955) avait montré que parmi des nour

non seulement parce qu'il a été irradié, mais aussi parce qu'existait initialement une hypertrophie thymique, des infections rhino-pharyngées ou d'autres états pathologiques ayant justifié une irradiation. Bien que ceci soit peu vraisemblable, on ne peut pas totalement exclure la possibilité d'une fréquence plus grande des cancers de la thyroïde chez de tels sujets. Dans l'enquête de Conti, les nouveaux-nés avaient eu le thymus irradié systématiquement à titre prophylactique. Aucun cancer n'a été observé dans ce groupe, mais le champ d'irradiation était peut-être suffisamment petit pour que la thyroïde n'ait pas été irradiée.

En réunissant, ce qui est de pratique discutable, l'ensemble de ces enquêtes, on obtient un groupe de 7561 sujets irradiés dans l'enfance et suivis jusqu'à la fin de l'adolescence, parmi lesquels 21 cas de cancers de la thyroïde ont été observés, alors qu'aucun n'a été observé chez les sujets témoins parmi lesquels, en théorie, aurait dû survenir 0,3 cas de cancer thyroïdien. La fréquence des cancers chez les sujets dont la thyroïde a reçu, au cours des premiers mois ou années de la vie, une dose de quelques centaines de rads, paraît donc de près de cent fois augmentée. Ces résultats ne peuvent cependant pas être acceptés sans précaution, car les sujets irradiés présentaient des troubles pathologiques qui les prédisposaient peut-être au cancer de la thyroïde. Mais, le fait que la fréquence soit liée aux modalités d'irradiation (PIFER, 1964) constitue un argument supplémentaire en faveur d'une relation entre l'irradiation et le cancer.

Soulignons de plus qu'HANFORD, sur un groupe de 162 sujets (adolescents ou adultes jeunes) irradiés pour adénopathie cervicale tuberculeuse avec des doses de l'ordre de 300 à 1500 rads, observe 7 cancers de la thyroïde, ce qui représente une forte augmentation de la fréquence.

Les enquêtes effectuées sur le devenir de sujets irradiés à un âge plus avancé, donnent des résultats moins nets. QUIMBY et WERNER ont colligé seulement 3 cas de cancer de la thyroïde, survenus après irradiation thyroïdienne, à des doses de l'ordre de 3000 rads, pour hyperthyroïdie. Comme entre 1920 et 1940 cette technique a été utilisée pour plusieurs milliers de malades, cette irradiation n'a pu être que peu cancérogène.

DELAWTER et WINSHIP n'observent aucun cas de cancer de la thyroïde dans un groupe de 222 sujets dont la région thyroïdienne avait été irradiée après l'âge de 19 ans et qui avaient été en moyenne suivis pendant 22,5 ans. Cependant, la fréquence des cancers thyroïdiens chez les sujets irradiés à Hiroshima et Nagasaki paraît augmentée; SOCOLOW rapporte 19 cas de cancers thyroïdiens sur 14.970 sujets irradiés (par des doses évaluées entre 35 et 2600 rads) alors qu'il n'y a que 2 cas sur 4992 sujets témoins non exposés; ZELDIS trouve que la fréquence des cancers de la thyroïde varie en raison inverse de la distance à l'hypocentre et est environ triplée chez les sujets irradiés à moins de 1400 m de l'hypocentre.

Au total donc, il semble que chez l'enfant, quelques centaines de rads provoquent une nette augmentation de la fréquence des cancers thyroïdiens. Des cancers ont été observés après une irradiation effectuée à l'âge adulte, mais généralement après des doses plus fortes.

3. BEACH et DOLPHIN en analysant les cas précédents, ont essayé d'établir une relation entre la dose et la fréquence du cancer. Les 192 cas étudiés sont compatibles avec une augmentation de la fréquence d'environ 1,7% par 500 rads. Ce résultat ne peut être accepté qu'avec prudence. Dans ces observations, la période de latence moyenne entre l'irradiation et la découverte du cancer était de 11 ans; cette durée ne paraît pas être influencée par l'âge, le sexe ou la dose.

4. Si l'on admettait que cette relation reste valable pour des doses plus faibles et pour des irradiations effectuées avec de l'iode 131, on arriverait à une fréquence d'environ 0,15% après administration d'iode radioactif pour examen, puisque dans ces cas la dose reçue par la thyroïde est de l'ordre de 50 rads; ceci représenterait déjà une augmentation notable de la fréquence des cancers. En fait, une telle évaluation est très hasardeuse.

a) Il n'y a pratiquement aucun argument en faveur de l'extrapolation linéaire jusqu'à des doses très faibles. L'effet cancérogène de faibles doses de radiations inférieures à 100 rads, n'a pu être observé pour aucun tissu et dans aucun cas chez l'homme ou l'animal, l'existence d'une relation linéaire entre la dose et la fréquence ne peut être considérée comme certaine. Cette extrapolation ne serait justifiée que s'il existait une théorie satisfaisante de la radiocancérogenèse, selon laquelle un cancer pourrait être provoqué par une lésion unique, par exemple une mutation maligne (mutation génique ou lésion chromosomique). Il serait alors concevable qu'il n'existe pas de seuil, que toute irradiation, si faible soit-elle, comporte un risque cancérogène, et que la relation entre la dose et l'effet puisse être linéaire.

Ceci est loin d'être prouvé et selon la plupart des analyses récentes, l'association de plusieurs facteurs ou plusieurs mutations (au minimum 2) paraît nécessaire pour rendre compte des faits observés (Upton, Mole, Lamerton). Si tel était le cas, la fréquence des cancers devrait croître plus rapidement que la dose (comme le carré ou le cube de la dose) et une extrapolation linéaire fournirait une estimation par excès.

b) Rien ne prouve que les faits observés après irradiation par rayons X soient valables après irradiation interne par isotopes. Il y a en effet au moins deux différences importantes: le débit et la distribution de la dose.

La fréquence des mutations varie avec le débit et paraît 3 à 5 fois plus basse pour des débits faibles. L'effet leucémogénétique après irradiation de la souris passe, pour une même dose de 1000 rads, de 39% pour un débit de 81 R/h à 5% pour un débit de 1,3 R/h (Mole). Or les débits de dose, après ingestion diagnostique d'iode 131, sont très

bas, de l'ordre de 0,1 rad/heure. Pour des doses thérapeutiques, ils restent relativement modérés, très inférieurs en tout cas à ceux utilisés en radiothérapie.

L'hétérogénéité de la dose a des conséquences plus difficiles à prévoir. Théoriquement, on pourrait concevoir aussi bien un accroissement des risques, du fait des fortes doses reçues par certaines cellules, qu'une diminution du risque, puisque certaines cellules sont peu irradiées. Quelques travaux expérimentaux ont comparé les effets d'une irradiation par RX ou iode 131. Chez le rat, Abbatt et Doniach ont constaté que 30 μ Ci qui délivrent à la thyroïde une dose estimée entre 10.000 et 15.000 rads, inhibent la réponse de la thyroïde à une substanco goitrigène, de façon équivalent à 1000 rads de RX. Au point de vue cancérogène, Doniach (1956) observe le même rapport des doses. Cette différence d'un facteur 10 entre les effets de deux types d'irradiation ne peut pas être uniquement attribuée aux variations de débit; le mode de répartition de la dose à l'échelle cellulaire doit donc jouer un rôle important.

Ces constatations expérimentales s'accordent avec les faits cliniques. Bien que plusieurs dizaines de milliers d'hyperthyroïdiens aient été traités depuis 20 ans par l'iode 131 (on peut estimer qu'en moyenne les thyroïdes traitées ont reçu 10.000 rads), un seul cas de cancer est rapporté dans la littérature (Sheline), encore s'agit-il d'un sujet qui avait été traité alors qu'il était enfant. L'ensemble est d'ailleurs intéressant au point de vue relation entre l'âge et la susceptibilité de la thyroïde à l'effet des radiations; sur les 18 sujets hyperthyroïdiens qui au moment du traitement avaient moins de 20 ans et pour lesquels le recul moyen est de 11 ans, il observe un cas de cancer thyroïdien et 5 tumeurs bénignes thyroïdiennes. Il observe deux tumeurs bénignes sur les 52 cas traités entre 20 et 30 ans et aucune sur les 186 sujets traités après 30 ans.

Il est certes trop tôt pour dire que le traitement de l'hyperthyroïdie par l'iode 131 ne comporte pas de risque cancérogène, puisque pour JELLIFFE, le délai d'apparition est de l'ordre de 25 ans, mais chaque année qui passe montre que ce risque est peut-être moindre qu'on ne l'avait redouté.

5. Les travaux expérimentaux éclairent certains aspects de l'induction par les radiations de tumeurs thyroïdiennes. La fréquence des tumeurs thyroïdiennes est beaucoup plus grande si la thyroïde après avoir été irradiée est soumise à une stimulation prolongée par la TSH, telle celle déterminée par l'administration de goitrigène (DONIACH, 1958) ou un régime pauvre en iode. Ceci est d'ailleurs analogue à ce qui avait été observé pour certains cancérogènes chimiques, tels l'acétylamino.2.fluorène (BIELSCHOWSKY, 1955). On peut rapprocher ce fait de la grande susceptibilité de la la thyroïde de l'enfant. Le poids de la thyroïde passe de 1,5 g. chez le nourrisson à 30 g. chez l'adulte, soit une multiplication par un facteur 20, voisine de celle observée chez l'animal après traitement par goitrigène; dans les deux cas, les mitoses fréquentes et la stimulation du tissu paraissent permettre l'extériorisation d'une lésion provoquée par les radiations. Le processus semble correspondre à un mécanisme en deux phases. GOLDBERG, 1964 a montré qu'après administration d'une dose très faible d'iode 131 (un microcurie) qui délivre à la glande quelques centaines de rads, la stimulation de la glande par thyroïdectomie subtotale fait apparaître des tumeurs malignes, mais la fréquence de ces tumeurs est très diminuée par l'administration systématique d'extraits thyroïdiens mettant au repos l'hypophyse et la

thyroïde. Cependant, même chez des animaux traités par extraits, un cancer de la thyroïde a été observé après ingestion d'un microcurie; ce qui montre que la lésion déterminée par l'irradiation a donc une petite chance de se manifester, même en l'absence de stimulation. Inversement, d'ailleurs, des cancers ont été observés chez des animaux non irradiés mais recevant un régime carencé en iode ou après thyroïdectomie partielle, et dont la thyroïde est alors sous l'action d'une stimulation excessive. La stimulation par TSH et l'irradiation représentent donc deux facteurs cancérogènes dont l'association accroît considérablement l'activité.

En conclusion, le risque cancérogène de l'iode 131 utilisé à titre diagnostique ou même thérapeutique, paraît très faible chez des sujets de plus 30 ans. Il n'est pas négligeable, quoique difficile à évaluer, chez des sujets jeunes carencés en iode ou goitreux, dont la thyroïde est soumise à une stimulation par TSH endogène. Quelques conclusions pratiques se dégagent tout naturellement de ces faits :

a) quand un examen à l'iode radioactif comporte un risque même faible, (enfants, goîtreux, etc. . . . .) il faut avant de le prescrire, mettre en balance la valeur des renseignements qu'il peut apporter et ses risques. Il serait absurde de renoncer à des renseignements cliniquement utiles, en raison de craintes plus ou moins fondées; à l'inverse, il serait imprudent d'irradier sans raison valable.

b) Il faut autant que possible réduire la quantité d'iode radioactif utilisée pour effectuer ces examens. 20 µCi d'iode 131 suffisent pour effectuer des scintigraphies thyroïdiennes et des études des composés iodés plasmatiques, moins de 5 µCi suffisent pour une mesure de la fixation. La dose peut être encore diminuée en utilisant des moyens techniques plus sensibles soit des radioiodes à vie courte, tel l'iode 132, soit des radioiodes n'émettant pas de particules beta, tel l'iode 125.

c) A moins de contre-indication chirurgicale, il parait prudent de ne pas traiter d'hyperthyroïdies par l'iode radioactif chez des enfants ou des adultes jeunes. Au-delà de 35 ans, le risque de cancérogénèse parait faible et peut être considéré comme un risque acceptable.

d) Il ne faut jamais laisser un sujet dont la thyroïde a été irradiée, en état d'insuffisance thyroïdienne, même discrète. Il est donc prudent dans ce cas, de mettre la thyroïde au repos grâce à un régime riche en iode ou des extraits thyroïdiens.

II. La Leucémogénèse et les Isotopes

Nous considérerons brièvement le cas des autres cancers et des autres isotopes.

Toute irradiation totale de l'organisme fait courir un risque de leucémogénèse et chez l'animal on a constaté que le ^{32}P peut provoquer des leucémies (Holmberg); chez l'homme, depuis la première observation de leucémie apparue chez un malade traité par l'iode radioactif pour cancer de la thyroïde (Delarue, 1955) de nombreux autres cas ont été signalés: ceci n'est pas surprenant en raison des doses élevées utilisées dans ce cas, mais aucune étude d'ensemble n'a été effectuée sur ce sujet pour tenter d'établir une relation entre la dose et l'effet. Environ 20 cas de leucémies ont été signalés chez les hyperthyroïdiens traités par l'iode radioactif, mais comme la leucémie n'est pas une maladie rare et que le nombre de malades ayant reçu ce traitement est élevé, ceci peut n'être qu'une coïncidence. C'est ce que semble établir l'enquête de E. Pochin (1960) selon laquelle la fréquence des leucémies

n'est pas plus grande dans ce groupe de malades. Cependant, la proportion plus élevée de leucémies aiguës et de cas chez les hommes (Wald, Werner) montre que cette enquête mérite d'être poursuivie.

Chez les polyglobuliques traités par le phosphore radioactif on observe de nombreuses leucémies (Wald), mais il s'agit d'une hémopathie dont la transformation spontanée en leucémie n'est pas exceptionnelle, ce qui enlève beaucoup de valeur à ces constatations et rend impossible toute étude quantitative.

III. Les Cancers Osseux

De nombreux travaux expérimentaux ont montré l'augmentation de la fréquence de cancers osseux chez les animaux traités par phosphore ou strontium radioactifs. Chez la souris, la fréquence semble varier comme le carré de la quantité d'isotope administrée (2). A quantité totale égale, la fréquence dépend du débit de dose et de la façon dont l'irradiation est répartie dans le temps.

Chez l'homme, les seules données quantitatives proviennent de l'étude de sujets ayant reçu des injections thérapeutiques de radium ou victimes d'une intoxication professionnelle. Hasterlik par exemple trouve que parmi 40 sujets dont l'organisme contenait plus de 1 μCi de Ra, 14 avaient des néoplasies et sur 63 dont l'organisme contenait entre 0,1 et 1 μCi, 3 seulement. Ces chiffres correspondent à un risque d'environ 33 cas de cancer par million d'habitants, par an et par microcurie dans le premier groupe, de 22 dans le second.

IV. Cancers Provoqués par le Thorostrast et Cancers du Foie

Le Bioxyde de Thorium colloïdal ou thorostrat a été largement utilisé comme produit de contraste en radio-diagnostic, bien que dès 1933 OBERLING ait démontré son pouvoir cancérogène. Il paraît avoir déterminé l'apparition de nombreux cancers (LACASSAGNE, BATZENSCHLAGER). BLOMBERG, sur 908 malades ayant reçu du Thorostrast, trouve 6 cas de cancer hépatique. DAHLGREEN analysant 68 cas de cancers après thorostrast trouve que le délai d'apparition est en moyenne de 17 ans. Une cinquantaine de cancers primitifs du foie ont été provoqués par le thorotrast (LACASSAGNE, 1964) dans des pays où ce cancer est exceptionnel. Soulignons de plus qu'en dehors du cancer du foie le thorotrast par son produit de filiation le radium 228 est capable de provoquer des cancers osseux. Les doses délivrées au foie sont extrêmement difficiles à calculer, d'une part, à cause de la fixation élective dans le systéme reticulo-endothelial à la périphérie sous la capsule du foie et de la rate, d'autre part, à cause du Ra 228, dont l'élimination hors de la rate et du foie est mal connue et dont les produits de filiation ont un métabolisme particulier. En posant des hypothèses simplifiées, OBERHAUSEN en Allemagne, MARINELLI aux E.U. et GROSSIORD en France l'évaluent entre 1200 et 1500 rads. Enfin, il faut souligner que dans le cas du thorotrast, au problème de radiotoxicité, s'ajoute la toxicité chimique du produit, lié à la masse de thorotrast injectée, environ 10 g et au stabilisant ajouté, en particulier la dextrine dont certaines structures sont elles-mêmes cancérogènes. De ces cancers hépatiques, peuvent être rapprochés les cancers provoqués par l'or radioactif. Mais l'irradiation provoquée par cet émetteur est beaucoup plus homogène. C'est ainsi que HAREL *et coll.* observent chez le rat, après injections intra-péritonéales d'or colloïdal radioactif, des cancers du foie et que UPTON (1956) chez la souris, après in-

jection intraveineuse d'or colloïdal, provoque des hépatomes. Ceci ne fait que souligner la nécessité de réserver les traitements par colloïdes radioactifs à des malades présentant des tumeurs malignes.

V. Risques des Précurseurs Marqués de l'ADN

Bien que la thymidine tritiée et les autres précurseurs marqués de l'ADN ne soient pas utilisés de façon courante chez l'homme, leur intérêt pour suivre la cinétique des populations de cellules, amènera sans doute un nombre croissant d'auteurs à y recourir, c'est pourquoi il est nécessaire en terminant, d'envisager brièvement leurs risques.

La thymidine tritiée incorporée à l'ADN des chromosomes, provoque chez la souris des mutations (BATEMAN).

La dose reçue par la cellule est dans ce cas, sans signification puisqu'étant donné le faible parcours des particules, seul un très faible volume est irradié. Néanmoins sur des bases dosimétriques (AMELGOT) on a pu montrer que l'effet est vraisemblablement lié, non à la transmutation comme dans le cas du ^{32}P, mais à l'ionisation.

Chez la souris 1 μCi/g de thymidine tritiée ou 0,2 μCi/g de thymidine marquée au ^{14}C, semblent avoir un effet faiblement cancérogène (BASERGA); Ce sont des quantités relativement faibles, de l'ordre de grandeur de celle utilisée in vivo pour les études de cinétique de population. Ceci montre qu'il faut être très prudent avant d'autoriser l'utilisation de ces substances chez l'homme et qu'il serait préférable de restreindre leur emploi aux malades ne présentant qu'une faible espérance de vie.

Conclusion

Les observations effectuées chez l'homme montrent que les rayonnements émis par les isotopes radioactifs dans l'organisme peuvent avoir une action cancérogène analogue à celle des rayons X; malheureusement les données sont trop fragmentaires pour permettre une évaluation des risques.

La plupart des cas de cancers observés sont consécutifs à des irradiations transcutanées de quelques centaines ou milliers de rads. Pour cette gamme de dose, les observations sont compatibles avec une relation linéaire entre la dose et l'effet. Dans les cas de tumeurs dues à une irradiation post-natale, l'accroissement de la fréquence des leucémies parait être d'environ 1 cas par rad par an et par million d'habitants [1]. C'est à une fréquence du même ordre que l'on arrive pour les cancers du corps thyroïde, si l'on admet que la période pendant laquelle le cancer risque de survenir est d'une vingtaine d'années [2]. Elle est plus difficile à évaluer mais serait du même ordre en ce qui concerne les tumeurs des os, après ingestion de radio-éléments (2).

Cependant, il est, en l'état actuel de nos connaissances, très hasardeux d'utiliser ces données pour évaluer le risque lié à l'administration d'isotopes radio-actifs. La dose délivrée lors d'irradiations internes par isotopes a un débit plus faible et une répartition plus hétérogène. Elle est, pour ces raisons, vraisemblablement moins efficace au moins pour la majeure partie des tissus.

De plus, l'utilisation des données recueillies après des doses moyennes ou élevées, pour prévoir l'effet de doses faibles de l'ordre d'une dizaine de rads est très incertaine et nécessite des hypothèses sur la relation entre la dose et l'effet. Or les mécanismes de la radio-cancérogénèse sont mal connus et complexes : à côté de lésions cellulaires direc-

tes, portant notamment sur le matériel génétique de la cellule, le rôle de la stimulation de la croissance tissulaire, des perturbations endocriniennes et des mécanismes d'immunité, peuvent être importants. Les expériences animales montrent que les relations peuvent être différentes selon les tissus considérés, le mode d'irradiation et l'intervalle des doses considérées. Dans aucun cas une relation linéaire n'a pu être démontrée sur un vaste intervalle de dose. L'avantage des extrapolations linéaires est de fournir une indication de la limite supérieure du risque, ce qui est souhaitable dans le domaine de la protection, mais leur précision est illusoire et il serait dangereux de se servir de telles évaluations pour discuter l'utilité d'examens ou de traitements utiles à la santé.

Avant de parvenir à un modèle cohérent de la radiocarcinogénèse, ce qui serait indispensable pour extrapoler de façon valable, de nombreuses expériences animales complémentaires seront nécessaires. Elles seront nécessairement longues et coûteuses, car elles doivent porter sur de vastes lots d'animaux irradiés à doses faibles. Parallèlement, les études épidémiologiques doivent être poursuivies, car elles seules sont susceptibles de fournir des indications pour l'homme et d'analyser le risque dans les différents sous-groupes d'une population en fonction notamment de l'âge et de l'état de santé. Ce n'est qu'à cette double condition que l'on peut espérer dans l'avenir parvenir à des évaluations plus précises. En attendant, il faut être prudent, ne recourir à une méthode isotopique pour le diagnostic que lorsque les méthodes classiques ne peuvent pas fournir de renseignements équivalents et toujours essayer de réduire la dose délivrée aux malades, afin d'obtenir le maximum d'informations pour le minimum de rads.

Bibliographie

[1] Rapport du Comité Scientifique des Nations Unies pour l'Etude des effets des Radiations ionisantes, *Suppl.* **16** (2/5216) 1962.

[2] Rapport du Comité Scientifique des Nations Unies pour l'Etude des effets des Radiations ionisantes, *Suppl.* **14** (2/5814) 1964.

ABBATT, J. D., DONIACH, I., HOWARD, P., FLANDERS, J. H., and LOGOTHEPOULOS, Comparison of the inhibition of goitrigenesis in the rat produced by X Rays and radioactive iodine. *Brit. J. Radiol.* **30**, 86 (1957).

ANDRE, L., Cancers thyroidiens apres irradiation. Rapport au Colloque sur les tumeurs de la thyroïde. Marseille 1964. Bâle: Karger, Edit. 1966.

APELGOT, S., et DUQUESNE, M., Energie dissipée par le tritium dans des microorganismes. *Int. J. Radiat. Biol.* **7**, 65 (1963).

BASERGA, R., LISCO, H., and KISIELSKI, W., Further observations on the induction of tumors in mice with radioactive thymidine. *Proc. Soc. exp. Biol. (N.Y.)* **110**, 687 (1962).

BATEMAN, A. J., and CHANDLEY, A. C., Mutations induced in the mouse with tritiated thymidine. *Nature (Lond.)* **193**, 705 (1962).

BATZENSCHLAGER, A., DORNER, M. et WEILL-BOUSSON, La pathologie tumorale du thorotrast chez l'homme. *Oncologia (Basel)* **16**, 28 (1963).

BEACH, S. A., and DOLPHIN, G. W., A study of the relationship between X rays dose delivered to the thyroïds on children and the subsequent development of malignant tumours. *Phys. in Med. Biol.* **6**, 583 (1962).

BENSTEDT, J. P., BLACKETT, N. M., and LAMERTON, L. F., Histological and dosimetric considerations of bone tumour production with radioactive phosphorus. *Brit. J. Radiol.* **34**, 160 (1961).

BLOMBERG, R., LARSSON, L. E., and LINDELL, B., Late effects of thorotrast in cerebral angiography. *Acta radiol. (Stockh.)* **1**, 996 (1963).

COLIEZ, R., TUBIANA, M., DUTREIX, J., et LAUGIER, A., La place de l'iode radioactif dans le diagnostic et le traitement du cancer de la thyroïde. Résultats de l'étude de 168 cas. *Bull. Ass. franç. Cancer* **43**, 218 (1956).

CONTI, E. A., PATTON, G. D., CONTI, J. E., and HEMPELMANN, L. H., Present health of children given X-ray treatment to the anterior mediastinum in infancy. *Radiology* **74**, 386—391 (1960).

DAHLGREN, S., Thorotrast tumours. *Acta pathol. microbiol. scand.* **53**, 147 (1961).

DELAWTER, D. S., and WINSHIP, T., Follow up of adults treated with RX for thyroïd disease. *Cancer* **16**, 1028 (1963).

DELARUE, J., TUBIANA, M., et DUTREIX, J., Cancer de la thyroïde traité par l'iode radioactif. Terminaison par une leucémie aigue. *Bull. Ass. franç. Cancer* **40**, 263 (1953).

DONIACH, I., Comparison of the carcinogenetic effect of X-radiation with radioactive iodine on the rat's thyroïd. *Brit. J. Cancer* **11**, 67 (1956).

— Experimental induction of tumours of the thyroïd by radiation. *Brit. med. Bull.* **14**, 181 (1958).

DUFFY, B. J. jr., and FITZGERALD, P. K. J., Thyroïd cancer in childhood and adolescence. A report on 28 cases. *Cancer* **3**, 1018 (1950).

FINKEL, M. P., BERGSTRAND, P. J., and BISKIS, B. O., The latent period, incidence and growth of 90 Sr induced osteosarcoma in mice. *Radiology* **77**, 269 (1961).

GOLDBERG, R. C., NICHOLS, C. W., LINDSAY, S., and CHAIKOFF, I. K. C., Induction of neoplasm in the thyroïd gland of the rat by subtotal thyroïdectomy and by injection of one microcurie of I $_{131}$. *Cancer Res.* **24**, 35 (1964).

GROSSIORD, A., ROUCAYROL, B., DUPERRAT, P. F., CECCALDI, L., et MEEUS BITH, Adénocancer du foie avec cirrhose 21 ans après une artériographie au thorotrast. *Sem. Hôp. Paris.* **32**, 1728 (1956).

HANFORD, J. M., QUIMBY, E. H., and FRANTZ, V., Cancer arising many years after radiation therapy, incidence after irradiation of benign lesions in neck. *J. Amer. med. Ass.* **181**, 404 (1962).

HAREL, J., GUERIN, M., TUBIANA, M. et ABBATUCCI, J., Production de tumeurs malignes (hépatomes et autres) par injection intrapéritonéale d'or radioactif chez le rat blanc. *Bull. Ass. franç. Cancer* **43**, 423 (1956).

HASTERLIK, R. J., FINKEL, A. J., and MILLER, C. E., The cancer hazards of industrial and accidental exposures to radioactive isotopes. *Ann. N.Y. Acad. Sci.* **114**, 832 (1964).

HOLMBERG, E. A. D., PASQUALINI, C. D., ARINI, E., PAVLOVSKY, A., and LABASE, S. L., Leukemogenic effect of radioactive phosphorus in mice. *Cancer Res.* **24**, 1745 (1964).

JELLIFFE, A. M., and JONES, K. M., Thyroïd cancer after irradiation in adult life. *Clin. Radiol.* **11**, 162 (1960).

Lacassagne, A., De l'abus de l'utilisation des radioéléments pour le diagnostic médical. *Condition de Vie et Santé* **2**, 120 (1957).

— Des tumeurs du foie provoquées par les radiations. *Rev. franç. Etud. clin. biol.* **9**, 269 (1964).

Lamerton, L. F., Radiation carcinogenesis. *Brit. med. Bull.* **20**, 2, 134 (1964).

Latourette, H. B., and Hodges, F. J., Incidence of neoplasia after irradiation of thymic region. *Amer. J. Roentgenol.* **82**, 667 (1959).

Lindsay, S., and Chaikoff, E. L., The effects of irradiation on the thyroïd gland. *Cancer Res.* **24**, 1099 (1964).

Mole, R. H., Patterns of response to whole body irradiation: effect of dose, intensity, exposure time on duration of life and tumour production. *Brit. J. Radiol.* **32**, 497 (1959).

— Bone tumour production in mice by strontium 90. *Brit. J. Cancer* **17**, 524 (1963).

Oberling, C., et Guerin, M., Action du thorotrast sur le sarcome de Jensen du rat blanc. *Bull. Ass. franç. Cancer* **22**, 469 (1933).

Pifer, J. W., and Hempelman, L. H., Radiation induced thyroïd carcinoma. *Ann. N.Y. Acad. Sci.* **114**, 2, 838 (1964).

— Toyooka, R. W., Murray, W. R., Ames, W. R., and Hempelmann, L. H., Neoplasms in children treated with X-rays for thymic enlargement. I. Neoplasms and mortality. *J. nat. Cancer Inst.* **31**, 1333 (1963).

Pochin, E., Leukaemia following radioiodine in treatment of thyrotoxicosis. *Brit. med. J.* **1960** II, 1545.

Quimby, E. H., and Werner, S. C., Late radiation effects in roentgen therapy for hyperthyroïdism. Their possible bearing on the use of radioactive iodine. *J. Amer. med. Ass.* **140**, 1046 (1949).

Roussy, G., et Guerin, M., Le cancer expérimental du foie provoqué par le dioxyde de Thorium. *Presse méd.* **61**, 761 (1941).

Saenger, E. L., Seltzer, R. A., Sterling, T. D., and Kereiakes, J. G., Carcinogenic effects of I_{131} compared with X-irradiation. *Hlth Phys.* **9**, 1371 (1963).

— Silberman, E. N., Sterling, T. D., and Turner, M. E., Neoplasia following therapeutic irradiation for benign conditions in childhood. *Radiology* **74**, 889 (1960).

Sheline, G. E., Lindsay, S., Mac Cormack, K. R., and Galante, M., Thyroïd nodules occuring late after treatment of thyroïtoxicosis with radioiodine. *J. clin. Endocr.* **22**, 8 (1962).

Simpson, C. L., Hempelmann, L. H., and Fuller, L. M., Neoplasia in children treated with X-rays in infancy for thymic enlargement. *Radiology* **64**, 840 (1955).

Takahashi, S., Kitabashi, T., and Wakabayashi, Cité dans [2].

Taylor, S., Induction of thyroid cancer in rat on low iodine diets. Current topics in Thyroid Research-*Proceedings. Fifth Int. Thyroïd conference. Rome 1965.*

Upton, A. C., The dose response relation in Radiation induced cancer. *Cancer Res.* **21**, 717 (1961).

Wald, N., Thomas, G. E., and Brown, G., Hematologic manifestation of radiation exposure in man. *Progr. Hemat.* **3**, 1 (1962).

Werner, S. C., Gittelsohn, A. M., and Brill, A. B., Leukemia following radioiodine therapy of hyperthyroïdism. *J. Amer. med. Ass.* **177**, 646 (1961).

Winship, T., and Rosvoll, R. V., Childhood thyroïd carcinoma. *Cancer* **14**, 734 (1961).

Zeldis, L. J., Jablon, S., and Ishida, M., Current status of studies of carcinogenesis in Hiroshima and Nagasaki. *Ann. N.Y. Acad. Sci.* **114**, 225 (1964).

Evaluation of Possible Carcinogenicity of Petroleum Products in Therapeutic Use

W. Lijinsky

Associate Professor of Oncology

U. Saffiotti

Associate Professor of Oncology

P. Shubik

Professor of Oncology

The Chicago Medical School, Institute for Medical Research,
Division of Oncology, Chicago, Ill.

Many industrial products in common medicinal and cosmetic use vary widely in chemical composition. While some samples are highly refined, others might be much less so. This is certainly true of a residual material from petroleum fractionation such as petrolatum, for which there are no criteria other than color, oil content and similar physical characteristics.

Mineral oil (the wax-free oil obtained from the lube distillate fraction of petroleum) is used mainly as a laxative and also has some cosmetic uses. For these purposes the mineral oil is highly refined and a control method for assurance of its purity has been developed by the Food and Drug Administration (Haenni *et al.*, 1962).

Petroleum waxes (the oil-free wax obtained from the lube distillate fraction of petroleum) are used medicinally for hardening ointments, in addition to their many uses in the food processing industry. Standard criteria for the control of their purity are also available (Howard, Haenni and Joe, 1965).

Petrolatums (derived from the high boiling residues of petroleum distillation, or from tank bottoms) are used directly as wound dressings in large quantities and also are the bases for the compounding of many ointments and cosmetics, in which an inert base is preferred. For these materials there are no criteria to control their safety and their composition conforms only to those standards, such as color and oil content, as are important commercially.

When confronted with the problem of assessing the possible carcinogenicity of these petroleum products, the following considerations should be kept in mind.

Some means of standardization of such materials is needed. This can be accomplished by a combination of uniform manufacturing procedure from a definable starting material and establishment of standard chemical analytical criteria. Obviously the composition of petroleum crudes varies very widely, particularly in their aromatic content. If the crudes from which materials for medicinal use are prepared are principally those of low initial aromatic content, the likelihood of the presence of carcinogens in the final products is reduced. This might also minimize the amount of refining necessary to meet quality standards set for medicinal use. Simpler chemical analytical methods can be devised for materials manufactured by more uniform procedures than is possible for materials derived by a variety of processes. This has been demonstrated in our study of petroleum waxes (SHUBIK et al., 1962) in which the only samples exceeding the standards set by the Food and Drug Administration were those prepared by an atypical method of manufacture.

Because of the very large number of samples of any one type of material produced, it is essential that an analytical control method be simple and rapid. It would be desirable to analyze every single sample of the products; this presents some practical difficulties but the closer we can approach this ideal the more assurance we have of the lack of hazards in the material.

The simplest analytical procedure for the control of possibly carcinogenic polynuclear hydrocarbons in petroleum products would be a spectrometric measurement of the material itself. This has been one of the criteria for purity of medicinal mineral oil in the U.S.A. (HAENNI and HALL, 1960). If the background absorbing material is too high, a suitable extract of the material can be made by solvent extraction and/or chromatography, which can then be examined spectrometrically (HAENNI et al., 1962; LIJINSKY et al., 1963a; HOWARD et al., 1965). The total absorbance limits are then set within certain wavelength ranges and they represent the maximum tolerated limits of concentrations of any or all polynuclear hydro-

carbons (obviously including all the noncarcinogenic ones).

The criteria set for quality of these materials should be such as to assure no carcinogenic hazard. This is more easily said than done. Regulations like the "Delaney clause" in U.S. Public Law 85—929 (1958) that set a zero tolerance level for carcinogens are more idealistic than practical. The limits are certainly dependent on the sensitivity of available analytical methods to identify carcinogens in a mixture, since levels below this sensitivity will remain undetected. These levels at the present moment are of the order of 1 part in a billion $(1:10^9)$ for compounds such as benzo(a)pyrene in petroleum wax and mineral oils. The methods that reach such sensitivity are very lengthy and therefore unsuitable as routine control procedures of industrial and commercial products.

For these reasons a compromise had to be reached and routine control analytical methods currently in use limit the maximum concentration of any known carcinogenic polynuclear hydrocarbon to 0.1 p.p.m. when the absorbance is due entirely to this one polynuclear compound; if several compounds are present, the effective limit is very much lower because the limit represents the combined absorbance of all compounds present.

It is conceivable that methods for excluding specific carcinogens at a concentration considerably lower than 0.1 p.p.m. will be developed based, for example, on gas chromatography. Some progress is being made in this direction (LIJINSKY et al., 1965a). These analytical methods are necessarily limited to the control of well defined known carcinogens for which reference standards are available. A further limitation is represented by the use of less highly refined petroleum products, such as petrolatums, for which it is difficult to establish chemical control procedures because of their high content of background absorbing material. In these, it is possible that some compounds which have not yet been identified are yet carcinogenic. The only way of detecting the presence of such compounds is by biological testing.

Biological testing of these petroleum products themselves is a lengthy and expensive procedure. It is nevertheless a minimum requirement for the evaluation of their safety for human use.

We have conducted one such large scale testing program on petroleum waxes (SHUBIK et al., 1962). It included a preliminary physico-chemical screening of 209 samples of waxes, of which 32 representative samples were submitted to chemical analysis. Of these, five samples were selected as a representative cross-section of the materials and used for detailed biological testing. Each sample was tested by three routes of administration on three species of animals, subdivided by sex, namely by feeding to rats (100 rats per group fed for 2 years with 10% levels of wax in the diet); by skin painting on mice and rabbits (90 mice per group painted with 15% solutions of wax in benzene 3 times per week for their lifespan; 8 rabbits per group treated in the same way for their lifespan up to 4 years); by subcutaneous implantation of wax disks in mice (100 mice per group implanted with a wax disk 20 mm in diameter and 2 mm thick). In addition, two waxes were fractionated by chromatography on magnesia/Celite and their concentrated aromatic fractions as well as their filtrates were also tested biologically.

The results of the tests, run together with appropriate solvent treated and untreated controls, showed no evidence of any carcinogenic effect in the feeding

and skin painting tests. The subcutaneous implantations of wax disks produced local fibrosarcomas comparable to those induced by similar implants of plastics and metals, but no distant tumorigenic effect. The incidence of sarcomas at the site of the implants could not be accounted for by any detectable chemical carcinogen but appeared related on the other hand to the physical nature of the implant, particularly the melting point of the wax; powdered wax implants were ineffective. It was concluded that the subcutaneous tests were indeed an inappropriate and unreliable testing procedure for the purpose of safety evaluation of such materials to be used by the oral route.

No hazard was detected with any of the feeding or skin painting studies, nor did any evidence of hazards result from chemical analyses. Based on the negative biological findings, a fairly rapid chemical procedure for controlling the quality of waxes for human use was developed (HOWARD et al., 1965) by the Food and Drug Administration. This was designed so as to approve essentially all of the waxes tested and yet minimize the possible trace amount of carcinogens that could be present in any future sample of wax. Following completion of the wax program, we undertook investigations of other petroleum products.

A number of mineral oil samples were analyzed (LIJINSKY et al., 1963b) and found to contain only minute quantities of polynuclear compounds. No known hydrocarbons were identified at a concentration of 1 part per billion, a level at which such compounds were identified in commercial solvents (LIJINSKY and RAHA, 1961). Biological testing of the mineral oils did not warrant a high priority.

On the other hand more extensive work on the petrolatums was indicated.

In the course of these studies on petrolatum we became aware of several new aspects of the problem of the evaluation of carcinogenic hazards in petroleum products.

Chemical analysis of several samples of petrolatum from different manufacturers by methods sensitive to 1 part per billion of individual polynuclear hydrocarbons showed the absence of any known carcinogen at this concentration (Lijinsky et al., 1963b). However, in several samples, the total concentration of the problem, the other sample in the same experimental conditions also gave negative results (Table I).

It was realized that such a test was not entirely adequate for this material, which, in human use, is applied often undiluted and for very long periods of time. Therefore, a procedure was devised in which the likely carcinogens were concentrated into a small portion, the effective dose of which could be much higher than that obtainable applying the original material. Forty kilograms

Table I. *Skin tumor induction with an amber petrolatum*

Treatment	Sex	Initial number of mice	Survivors at weeks 30 50 70	Total number of Tumor bearing mice	Tumors	Carcinomas	Regressions	Average latent period for all tumors (in weeks)
Petrolatum (15% in isooctane)[a]	♀	30	30 27 19	2	2	—	1	71
	♂	30	25 22 13	2	3[b]	—	2	60

[a] Applied twice weekly to the dorsal skin of Swiss mice, 3 drops (approximately 60 microliters) per application.
[b] One papilloma under chin.

centration of noncarcinogenic polynuclear compounds was an order of magnitude higher than in any petroleum wax examined. In spite of the failure to detect any known carcinogens in the petrolatums, it was decided to test biologically two samples representative of the least degree of refining, recognizing the possibility that there exists in such material hitherto unidentified compounds with carcinogenic properties.

The two samples of petrolatum were tested by skin application on groups of 30 male and 30 female Swiss mice as 15% solutions in iso-octane. Survival of the mice was good and no significant tumor incidence was found after lifetime treatment. Results of the test of one sample are reported elsewhere (Lijinsky et al., 1965b). The testing of of one petrolatum sample were chromatographed in iso-octane on silica gel columns and the aliphatic material washed into the filtrate with iso-octane. The adsorbed aromatic material was eluted with benzene and the residual oil after evaporation of the solvent comprised 1.2% of the petrolatum. The crude aromatic concentrate was fractionated by partition between cyclohexane and nitromethane, the latter being a selective solvent for polynuclear compounds. After distillation of the nitromethane the pale yellow oily residue amounted to 0.15% of the original sample. Portions of the aromatic concentrate and the cyclohexane and nitromethane subfractions were diluted with iso-octane to a volume corresponding to a 50 fold higher concentration than that of the component in the original petrolatum sample. The three aromatic fractions were biologically tested by skin painting on groups of 30 male and 30 female Swiss mice; twice weekly treatments were continued throughout the life of the animals (LIJINSKY et al., 1965b).

material extracted by nitromethane was undertaken in an effort to establish the nature of the carcinogen or carcinogens present. The results of this further work are reported here. The major identified polynuclear constituent of this fraction was pyrene (or alkyl derivatives of

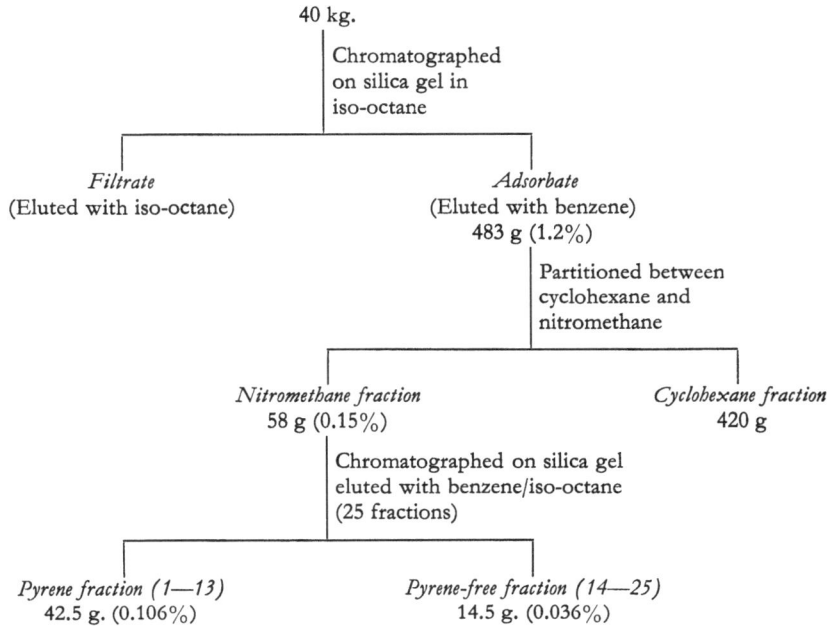

Fig. 1. Fractionation of amber petrolatum

The fractionation scheme used is shown in Fig. 1. The results of the biological tests of the petrolatum and its fractions (LIJINSKY et al., 1965b) show that there is no doubt that the aromatic extract of the petrolatum and its two subfractions are carcinogenic to mouse skin. These results can be compared with similar tests of an aromatic extract of a microcrystalline wax; in this case not a single tumor was induced (SHUBIK et al., 1962).

Since no known carcinogen was identified by analysis of the petrolatum sample and yet biological tests showed carcinogenic activity of the aromatic extract, further fractionation of the

pyrene) and the fractionation consisted of a division into material adsorbed less strongly or as strongly as pyrene, and that adsorbed more strongly than pyrene, as determined by spectrometric examination of the fractions. This separation was achieved by chromatography on silica gel, using mixtures of iso-octane and benzene containing increasing proportions of benzene as elutants. Twenty-five 250 ml fractions were collected and all of those showing absorption spectra of pyrene were pooled (pyrene fraction). All of the subsequent fractions were also pooled (pyrene-free fraction). Approximately three-quarters of the material was in the pyrene fraction. After evaporation of the solvents both fractions were diluted with iso-octane to an equivalent of 50 times their concentration in the petrolatum and tested biologically by skin application in Swiss mice. These tests are not yet complete. The animals are in the 80th week of treatment and the results so far are shown in Table II.

It appears that the carcinogenic activity is concentrated mainly in the

sent in this carcinogenic fraction of petrolatum have not been established, but is seems likely that they are alkyl derivatives of benzanthrene, benzophenanthrene or chrysene. It is hoped that further fractionation of this mixture, combined with biological testing and chemical analysis will reveal the identity of the carcinogen or carcinogens present.

The results of our studies indicate that, in dealing with this type of material,

Table II. *Skin tumor induction with subfractions of aromatic component of amber petrolatum*

Treatment[a]	Sex	Mice	Number[b] of			Average latent period for all tumors (in weeks)
			Tumor bearing animals	Tumors	Carcinomas	
Pyrene fraction[c]	♂	20	6	9	1	54
	♀	20	0	0	0	—
Pyrene-free fraction[c]	♂	20	1	1	1	47
	♀	20	6	11	6	69

a Applied twice weekly to the dorsal skin of Swiss mice, one drop (approximately 20 microliters) per application.

b Observed so far up to the 80th week of treatment.

c The material from 40 kg of petrolatum was diluted to 800 ml. with iso-octane.

pyrene-free fraction and is associated with compounds more strongly adsorbed than pyrene. Elemental analysis showed that this pyrene-free fraction, which was suspected to contain heteropolynuclear compounds, in fact contained only carbon and hydrogen. This fraction and the pyrene fraction were examined by mass spectrometry using a high resolution instrument (Associated Electrical Industries MS 9). Ions with masses of 234 and 236 were prominent, which can be due to polynuclear compounds with a maximum of four fused rings. Peak matching with ions from a hydrocarbon of known molecular weight showed that the compounds present were indeed hydrocarbons and contained no oyxgen, nitrogen or sulfur atoms. The structures of the compounds pre-

prepared from a source (such as petroleum) likely to contain carcinogens and not subsequently highly refined, it is dangerous to draw negative conclusions about their possible carcinogenic effect simply from chemical analysis. Biological testing of the materials and extracts of them are a necessity. Although such testing is expensive and time-consuming, it can not be dispensed with until such materials are standardized and more is known about the chemical composition of their aromatic components.

The following conclusions can be drawn.

Some means of standardization of petroleum products for medicinal and cosmetic use is needed. This can be achieved by a combination of uniform manufacturing procedure from definable starting materials and establishment of standard chemical analytical criteria.

An essential prerequisite of any chemical method of standardization of such materials is suitable biological testing for carcinogenic activity. This testing can be of the material itself or of a suitably prepared extract, depending on the number of animals to be employed, the feasible dose of material and other considerations. Having established that the material is either carcinogenic or noncarcinogenic, a basis may be established for the formulation of appropriate chemical criteria of safety.

The number of chemical carcinogens in the environment might be much larger than was supposed. Large groups of such compounds, hitherto unsuspected of carcinogenic activity, might await discovery. The current emphasis on detection of such well known carcinogens as benzo(a)pyrene might be misplaced, since they might well be a much less significant factor than the unidentified carcinogens which occur. It is known, for example, that the carcinogenic activity of coal tar, creosote and tobacco tar can not be accounted for by their measured content of known carcinogens (BERENBLUM and SCHOENTAL, 1947; LIJINSKY et al., 1957; WYNDER and HOFFMANN, 1959). The activity unaccounted for might well be due to such unknown compounds as have been shown to occur in our sample of petrolatum.

Acknowledgment

Dr. LIJINSKY and Dr. SAFFIOTTI are supported by Research Career Development Awards, respectively No. K3-CA-25, 041 and No. K3-CA-25, 027, and the experimental work by research grant No. CA-05170, all from the National Cancer Institute, National Institutes of Health, U.S. Public Health Service.

References

BERENBLUM, I., and SCHOENTAL, R., Carcinogenic constituents of coal tar. *Brit. J. Cancer* **1**, 157—165 (1947).

HAENNI, E. O., and HALL, M. A., Tentative ultraviolet absorption limits for mineral oils. *J. Ass. Offic. Agr. Chemists* **43**, 92—95 (1960).

—, JOE, F. L., HOWARD, J. W., and LEIBEL, R. L., A more sensitive and selective ultraviolet absorption criterion for mineral oil. *J. Ass. Offic. Agr. Chemists* **45**, 59—66 (1962).

HOWARD, J. W., HAENNI, E. O., and JOE, F. L., An ultraviolet absorption criterion for total polynuclear aromatic hydrocarbon content of petroleum waxes in food additive use. *J. Ass. Offic. Agr. Chemists* **48**, 304—315 (1965).

LIJINSKY, W., DOMSKY, I., MASON, G., RAMAHI, H. Y., and SAFAVI, T., The chromatographic determination of trace amounts of polynuclear hydrocarbons in petrolatum, mineral oil and coal tar. *Analyt. Chem.* **35**, 952—956 (1963b).

— —, and RAHA, C. R., A short method of testing petroleum waxes for the presence of polycyclic aromatic hydrocarbons. *J. Ass. Offic. Agr. Chemists* **46**, 725—731 (1963a).

LIJINSKY, W., DOMSKY, I., and WARD, J., A procedure for the detection of carcinogenic polynuclear hydrocarbons in petroleum waxes using electron capture. *J. Gas Chromatog.* **3**, 152—154 (1965a).

—, and RAHA, C. R., Polycyclic aromatic hydrocarbons in commercial solvents. *Toxicol. appl. Pharmacol.* **3**, 469—473 (1961).

—, SAFFIOTTI, U., and SHUBIK, P., A study of the chemical constitution and carcinogenic action of creosote oil. *J. Nat. Cancer Inst.* **18**, 687—692 (1957).

— — —, Skin tumorigenesis by an extract of amber petrolatum. *Toxicol. appl. Pharmacol.* **18**, 113—117 (1965b).

SHUBIK, P., SAFFIOTTI, U., LIJINSKY, W., PIETRA, G., RAPPAPORT, H., TOTH, B., RAHA, C. R., TOMATIS, L., FELDMAN, R., and RAMAHI, H., Studies on the toxicity of petroleum waxes. *Toxicol. appl. Pharmacol.* **4**, Suppl. 1—62 (1962).

WYNDER, E. L., and HOFFMANN, D., A study of tobacco carcinogenesis. VII. The role of higher polycyclic hydrocarbons. *Cancer (Philad.)* **12**, 1079—1086 (1959).

Discussion of Papers by Professor Tubiana and Doctor Parmentier and by Professors Lijinsky, Saffiotti and Shubik

Truhaut: Dr. SAFFIOTTI has drawn attention to the variation in composition of many pharmaceutical preparations. I feel that the possibility of intoxication from impurities should receive much more attention, standards of purity should be rigorous and analytical methods for verifying purity should be developed.

With regard to the report by Madame Parmentier, I should like to emphasise that the risk of carcinogenicity from radio-active tracers may be potentiated by other drugs; an example of this is the potentiation of the carcinogenicity of radio-active iodine by thiourea. Nevertheless, this particular combination of agents is frequently used in human medicine.

Boyland: It may be relevant that mineral oils from the Middle East differ from those from America in that they contain more sulphur.

Taylor: I feel that Madame Parmentier has taken too conservative a position with regard to hyperthyroidism. After all there is a risk from surgical treatment of this condition. One should balance the small risk of carcinoma against the usefulness of drug treatment.

Hueper: I know of a case where mineral oil produced by catalytic cracking was bought by a drug company for medicinal purposes.

The different behaviour of hard and soft paraffin waxes may be a dose phenomenon unrelated to the surface properties of the two waxes. I studied the case of a woman with bilateral paraffinomas of the breast. The paraffin wax had separated into soft and hard fractions and the former had caused phagocytosis and removed to the regional lymph nodes. Only the hard wax remained at the implantation site.

Rudali: I am much more suspicious than Madame Parmentier with regard to the long-term hazards from X-irradiation. Our experience with the effects of ionizing irradiation on animals indicates wide variation in susceptibility. The same is probably true in man. Therefore we should take into account heredity predisposition to the induction of cancer by irradiation.

Sometimes in the laboratory doses which one would expect to be safe produce cancer. In one of our experiments we saw bilateral ovarian tumours 2 years after ten exposures of female mice to 5 r.

Napalkov: I would like to associate myself with the comments of Professor TRUHAUT on the potential dangers of combined exposure to radio-iodine and anti-thyroid compounds. Incidentally, some anti-thyroid compounds have been shown to induce liver tumours in animals, and this effect is not necessarily mediated via the pituitary.

Réponse du Docteur Parmentier: Les problèmes soulevés par M. Le Professeur TRUHAUT et M. le Docteur NAPALKOV se rejoignent. Il est en effet possible que l'association irradiation et antithyroïdiens de synthèse augmente la fréquence des cancers thyroïdiens, comme le suggère l'expérimentation animale. Mais, ce problème doit être lié à la quantité d'antithyroïdiens administrée: en effet, si la dose est trop élevée, la sécrétion thyroïdienne est déprimée et la sécrétion TSH augmentée et nous trouvons dans le cas cité dans notre conférence. Par contre, il est très probable que, si les antithyroïdiens sont administrés en quantité juste nécessaire pour traiter l'hyperthyroïdie, le risque de cancérisation par l'association ne doit pas être plus élevé que le risque couru lors de l'administration isolée d'iode 131.

Je répondrais également simultanément à M. TAYLOR et M. RUDALI, bien que leur attitude devant les risques soient tout à fait opposées. L'iode 131 est utilisé en thérapeutique depuis 1948. Nous disposons donc d'un recul de 17 à 18 ans, encore assez court, nécessitant donc de rester encore prudent, de réserver ce traitement à l'adulte et de bien peser les risques vis à vis des bénéfices ou des risques encourus par d'autres thérapeutiques. Il faut de plus bien séparer l'utilisation de l'I_{131} en thérapeutique et en diagnostic, les doses et les débits de dose étant très différents puisque pour un test à l'I_{131}, les quantités d'activité nécessaires varient entre 5 μCi et 20 μCi. Le rejet total d'une telle technique serait donc absurde même si la dose ne donnant aucun effet est la dose nulle, comme le dit M. RUDALI. Il faut là encore raisonner en terme de probabilité et bien peser les avantages et les dangers: pour conclure, je rappellerai la dernière phase de notre rapport: «Il faut essayer d'obtenir le maximum d'informations pour le minimum de rads» sans pratiquer une attitude d'abstention complète.

Je répondrai enfin à M. SHABAD. Il est certain que les radioéléments ont ouvert un vaste champ d'exploration et ont le gros intérêt de permettre des recherches quantitatives. Mais le rôle de l'état physico-chimique du radioélément, utilisé, comme le prouve la fâcheuse expérience de thorotrast est loin d'être négligeable. Et certains isotopes peuvent associer un facteur de radiocarcinogénèse et un facteur de cancérisation physicochimique.

Saffiotti: In reply to Professor BOYLAND, I should like to point out that the materials we tested were American-derived. Regulations concerning the quality control of commercial petroleum products are necessary, but must be practical and enforceable. Such regulations have been established for mineral oil by the Food and Drug Administration. Similar regulatory controls should be developed in other countries.

A Propos de l'Activité oncogène de quelques hydrocarbures halogénés utilisés en thérapeutique

G. Rudali

Laboratoire de Génétique de l'Institut du Radium-Foundation Curie, Paris

La découverte de l'activité cancérigène des substances chimiques de synthèse au cours des 30 dernières années a permis de mettre en évidence cette propriété biologique chez environ mille composés. L'examen de l'activité de ces substances conduit à les diviser, assez arbitrairement, il est vrai, en deux groupes.

Dans le premier groupe on peut classer des composés comme le benzopyrène, les naphthylamines et leurs dérivés, l'aminofluorène, l'uréthane, etc... Ce sont des cancérigènes majeurs. Leur caractère essentiel est leur activité élevée, souvent après des temps de latence relativement courts et pour des espèces variées. Certains d'entre eux se trouvent en quantités abondantes dans notre biosphère comme composants ou comme impuretés des produits alimentaires, des déchets industriels ou ménagers, des engrais, des insecticides, des matières premières de la grande industrie, des substances médicamenteuses, etc...

Les substances qui constituent le deuxième groupe, celui des cancérigènes mineurs ont, en général, une activité limitée à une seule espèce. Souvent leur activité se limite à l'induction d'adénomes et atteint rarement le stade de la cancérisation proprement dite qui survient alors le plus souvent après des latences assez longues. Le risque de contamination pour l'espèce humaine par ces substances peut être considéré comme réduit ou nul. Soit qu'elles n'interviennent pas en quantité suffisantes ou à un rythme approprié dans le circuit métabolique de l'homme, soit qu'elles n'existent pas d'une façon générale dans la nature. C'est le cas des solutions concentrées de glucose [6], du styryl 430 [2], du mercure [3], de la neige carbonique [1], etc...

Il est probable que les dérivés halogénés de certains hydrocarbures aliphatiques, comme le tétrachlorure de carbone et le chloroforme seraient à ranger dans ce deuxième groupe. Il convient de faire observer, ne serait-ce qu'en raison de la vocation de ce symposium sur les médicaments que le danger de cancérisation de l'homme avec ces substances peut être considéré comme pratiquement nul, si l'on se place *stricto sensu* sur le plan des thérapeutes.

Aussi bien le tétrachlorure de carbone que le chloroforme sont des substances très volatiles ayant donc une action immédiate et fugace. Expérimentalement, elles se sont montrées cancérigènes pour le foie des souris. Cependant la production des tumeurs chez ces animaux nécessite de nombreuses administrations régulières pendant une longue période. Les administrations sporadiques ou à plus forte raison uniques sont sans effet apparent.

L'absorption de ces médicaments dans le passé, fut toujours rare, limitée dans le temps et, en raison même de leur toxicité aiguë étroitement surveillée. La dose cancérigène pour la souris semble se situer aux environs de 30 administrations de 1,5 cm³ par Kg. Chez l'espèce humaine les doses thérapeutiques sont de l'ordre de 0,05 cm³.

Je vous rappelle brièvement que le tétrachlorure de carbone fut longtemps recommandé comme antiseptique et comme parasiticide dans l'infestation

[11] ont également provoqué des hépatomes chez dessouris mâles de la lignée A.

Il nous a semblé intéressant de compléter ces travaux par une série d'expériences. Outre la tentative de produire des hépatomes chez les rats, animaux particulièrement sensibles aux hépatocancérigènes, comme l'amino-fluorène, le jaune de beurre ou la diéthylenitrosoamine, nous avons fait quelques expériences avec des substances halogénées simples, structuralement apparentées au tétrachlorure de carbone.

Tableau I. *Action du C Cl₄ sur le foie de rats. (2 gavages hebdomadaires de 0,5 cm³ d'une sol. à 50%)*

Régime	Nombre de rats	Cirrhoses	tumeurs	survie moy.
Normal	20	précoces 88⁰ j.	0	301
Carencé	10	tardives 147⁰ j	0	217

par les ankylostomes et les ascaris. Le chloroforme fut, pendant plusieurs décennies un des anesthésiques le plus en faveur chez les chirurgiens et les accoucheurs. Mais les narcoses en circuit fermé et les nouveaux anesthésiques ont permis de restreindere de plus en plus ses indications. Toutefois, il convient de ne pas perdre de vue que ces deux anciens médicaments continuent à être utilisés sur une très grande échelle dans l'industrie, où ces solvants ont de nombreuses applications.

L'action oncogène du tétrachlorure de carbone a été découverte par ED-WARDS en 1941 [4]. EDWARDS et ED-WARDS *et collab.* [5] ont montré que des gavages, administrés à des souris de quatre lignées différentes, avec 0,1 cm³ d'une solution huileuse à 40%, produisent chez ces animaux des tumeurs hépatocytiques en 60 à 90% des cas, selon l'origine génétique des animaux. Par la suite nous avons confirmé ces résultats, en collaboration avec MARIANI [8] chez des souris XVII / G. STOWELL *et collab.*

Expérience n° 1

Trente rats males du commerce (sans origine génétique connue) d'un poids moyen de 193 g reçurent deux fois par semaine un gavage de 0,5 cm³ d'une solution huileuse à 50% de tétrachlorure de carbone. Vingt parmi eux eurent un régime alimentaire normal, c'est-à-dire équilibré. Les dix autres furent nourris evec le régime carencé en protéines et an vitamines qui sert habituellement dans les expériences de cancérisation du foie des rats par le jaune de beurre. Les survies des animaux s'échelonnèrent entre 83 et 397 jours dans le lot nourri avec le régime équilibré et de 63 à 285 jours dans le groupe carencé (moyenne de 301 et 217 jours).

Le tableau I montre qu'aucun des rats de cette expérience n'a présenté des adénomes et à plus forte raison des hépatomes malins. En revanche dans les deux groupes on a observé des cirrhoses, survenant plus tôt chez les carencés que dans le groupe recevant le régime équilibré.

Expérience n° 2

Simultanément avec ces expériences sur des rats deux autres furent entreprises avec des souris XVII/G, initialement âgées de 90 jours environ. Dans l'une d'elles on avait pour but de rechercher l'action éventuelle de dilutions relativement faibles: 25% au lieu de 40%. Dans l'autre on s'est servi des doses habituelles. Le but de cette deuxième

aux. Ces huit tumeurs furent greffées, chacune sous la peau de quatre souris appartenant à la même lignée et âgées de 45 à 60 jours. Aucun de ces 32 animaux dont 23 vécurent au moins un an, n' a développé une tumeur à l'emplacement de la greffe. Au sacrifice, on n'a trouvé aucune trace du greffon.

Une autre série d'expériences avait pour but de rechercher si d'autres

Tableau II. *Oncongenèse hépatique de souris XVII/G gavées avec du CCl⁴*

Solution de de CCl^4	Nombre de souris après 250 jours	Date apparition de la 1º tum. en jours	Date moy. app. des tum. en jours	Nombre tum.	T. p. %
25%	18	525	525	1	5
40%	12	250	307	11	91

Tableau III. *Réactions hépatiques de souris recevant des gavages avec des hydrocarbures aliphatiques chlorés*

Substance	Nombre de souris initiales	Nombre de souris valables	Lésions hépat. aigües	Nombre de tumeurs hépat.	Suvies moy. en jours
CH—Cl^3	24	5	++++	3	297
CHCl=CCl^2	28	24	—	0	/

expérience était la production de tumeurs hépatiques avec le dessein d'en étudier la transmissibilité par greffe. Les gavages avec 0,1 cm³ administrés deux fois par semaine furent poursuivis pendant 6 mois (50 gavages par animal).

Comme cela ressort du tableau II, une seule tumeur, assez tardive fut observée dans le lot recevant la solution à 25%. Par contre, comme dans des expériences précédentes, la fréquence des hépatomes fut de 91% chez les souris recevant la solution à 40%. Dans le lot de 12 souris gavées avec cette dernière solution 11 ont présenté des tumeurs apparues entre le 250e et le 401e jours. Parmi ces 11 tumeurs, 8 furent découvertes *in vivo*, lors des examens hebdomadaires systématiques des anim-

dérivés halogénés des hydrocarbures aliphatiques simples pouvaient avoir une action oncogène pour le foie des souris.

En premier lieu nous avons étudié le trichloréthylène. Cette substance, en effet, est parfois utilisée en tant qu'analgésique obstétrical, mais, en outre, il est également un solvant organique largement employé dans l'industrie.

Expérience n° 3

Nous avons administré à des souris NLC divisées en deux lots soit du chloroforme, soit du trichloréthylène, tous deux en solution huileuse à 40%. Les doses hebdomadaires étaient de deux gavages à 0,1 cm³. Comme cela ressort du tableau III le trichloréthylène n'a provoqué aucune tumeur; le chloroforme, en revanche, s'est montré légèrement oncogène. Il est intéressant de faire observer, que dans nos expériences le trichloréthylène n'a montré aucune hépatotoxicité aigüe: ni stéatose, ni nécrose, ni prolifération endothéliale ne furent notées.

Expérience n° 4

Une dernière expérience a été consacrée à la possibilité de maintenir le pouvoir oncogène en faisant différentes

mes. Si le tétrachlorure de carbone et le chloroforme possèdent une incontestable activité oncogène pour le foie de la Souris, il est intéressant de noter que cette propriété de ces molécules ne s'exerce pas chez les rats. Même chez les souris, les tumeurs provoquées par des gavages avec le tétrachlorure de carbone, et ceci à des doses très élevées, ne semblent pas avoir une réelle malignité. Les tentatives de transplantation sous-cutanée de ces tumeurs ont échoué dans tous les cas. On peut donc se

Tableau IV. *Action de différents dérivés halogénés du méthane sur des souris*

Substance	Nombre de souris init.	Souris avec longues survies	Dilution	Toxicité aigüe p. foie
$CBr-Cl^3$	58	6	10%	$++++$
CBr^2-Cl^2	28	7	10%	$+++$
$CHBr-Cl^2$	58	10	40%	$---$
$CHBr^2-Cl$	28	9	40%	$---$
CBr^4	27	16	40%	$---$

substitutions chlorées et bromées dans la molécule du méthane. Cinq substances ont servi pour ces exp'riences. Ces substances furent comme dans les autres expériences administrées par voie de gavage en solution huileuse à des souris de trois lignées différentes: XVII/G, NLC ou RIII/f. La dose administrée était de 0,1 cm³ par gavage de la solution huileuse à 40%, pour trois de ces composés et à 10% pour deux autres, dont la toxicité aigüe fut telle que l'utilisation de dilution plus concentrée se révéla impossible (voir tableau IV).

Aucune de ces cinq substances, malgré dans certains cas des lésions hépatiques toxiques assez graves, n'a provoqué à long terme des cancers ou des adénomes. Le tableau IV indique les résultats de ces expériences.

Discussion

Les expériences qui viennent d'être présentées soulèvent plusieurs problè-

demander si le tétrachlorure de carbone doit être considéré comme un agent cancérigène, dans le sens complet du mot. Des expériences récentes de SCHMÄHL et collab. [9] semblent indiquer que le tétrachlorure se comporte comme un co-cancérigène pour la diéthyl-nitrosamine au cours d'expériences de cancérisation du foie de rats.

Il est probable que le tétrachlorure peut être considéré comme inactif en tant qu'agent cancérigène du foie pour l'espèce humaine. Malgré sa large utilisation comme solvant industriel depuis de nombreuses décennies, il ne semble pas que ce composé ait provoqué des cancers professionnels.

En ce qui concerne le mode d'action des deux hydrocarbures chlorés ayant provoqué des tumeurs chez les souris il est difficile de formuler des hypothèses précises à ce propos. Néanmoins, il ne semble pas qu'il existe une corrélation directe entre la toxicité générale de ces composés sur la cellule hépatique et la production tardive des hépatomes.

Nous avons au cours de nos expériences étudié une série de dérivés halogénés du méthane et de l'éthylène. Ces composés mono-, bi-, tri-, ou tétrahalogénés dont certains produisent les mêmes lésions hépatotoxiques aigües que le tétrachlorure de carbone n'ontpas provoqué des tumeurs dans nos expériences.

Parmi ces substances, deux nous semblent particulièrement intéressantes sur le plan théorique. Le trichloréthylène n'a montré aucune activité oncogène. Il s'en suit que le nombre d'atomes de chlore dans ces molécules n'est pas le seul critère qui prête à ces composés l'activité oncogène. L'absence d'activité du bromo-trichloro-méthane me semble un fait particulièrement digne d'intérêt. En effet, ce composé se distingue du chloroforme, oncogène pour le foie, par la substitution d'un atome d'hydrogène par un atome de brome. Il a donc suffi d'opérer cette substitution pour enlever à la molécule son activité. Tout se passe donc comme si la présence de l'atome d'hydrogène était nécessaire pour que ces molécules soient oncogènes.

Ceci suggère avant tout, que l'agent actif serait un métabolite de ces hydrocarbures.

MEYER (cité d'après V. OETTINGEN [7]) a suggéré jadis, afin d'expliquer l'action toxique en général du tétrachlorure de carbone, que ce composé devait se décomposer dans la cellule hépatique pour donner, d'une part de l'acide chlorhydrique et d'autre part du phosgène. On peut donc se demander si le pouvoir oncogène de ces molécules ne proviendrait pas de la formation de ce gaz toxique. De toute manière, si techniquement il était possible d'étudier l'action oncogène éventuelle de ce dernier composé, l'expérience devrait être tentée.

Résumé

1. L'administration de tétrachlorure de carbone à des souris provoque chez ces animaux des hépatomes ayant des caractères histologiques de malignité mais qui ne sont pas transmissibles par des greffes. Le tétrachlorure de carbone, administré par des gavages à des rats ne provoque pas de tumeurs hépatiques chez ces animaux.

2. Le trichloréthylène, le tétrabromure de carbone, le brome-dichloro-carbone, le dibromo-dichlorocarbone, le dibromo-chlorocarbone et le trichloro-bromocarbone se sont montrés inactifs en tant qu'agents oncogènes pour le foie des souris.

3. On discute l'éventualité que l'action oncogène serait due à un métabolite du tétrachlorure de carbone: le phosgène. On envisage la possibilité que ces hydrocarbures halogénés puissent être des co-cancérigènes pour d'autres agents chimiques, comme le diéthylenitrosoamine.

J'exprime toute ma reconnaissance au Professeur M. MAGAT, de la Faculté des Sciences de Paris, qui a mis à ma disposition les cinq substances bromées qui furent utilisées dans ces expériences. Je remercie également Madame le Docteur N. YOURKOVSKI et Madame H. CHALVET pour leur collaboration technique.

Bibliographie

[1] BERENBLUM, I., Further investigation on the induction of tumours with carbon dioxide snow *Brit. J. exp. Path.* **11**, 208—211 (1930).

[2] BROWNING, C. H., GULBRANSEN, R., and NIVEN, J. S F., Sarcoma production in mice by a single subcutaneous injection of a benzoylamino quinoline styryl

compound. *J. Path. Bact.* **42**, 155—159 (1936).

[3] DRUCKREY, H., HAMPERL, H., u. SCHMÄHL, D , Cancerogene Wirkung von metallischem Quecksilber nach intraperitonealer Gabe bei Ratten *Z. Krebsforsch.* **61**, 511—519 (1957).

[4] EDWARDS, J. E., Hepatomas in mice induced with carbontetrachlorid. *J. nat. Cancer Inst.* **2**, 197—199 (1941).

[5] — HESTON, W. E., and DALTON, A. J., Induction of the carbon tetrachlorid hepatoma in strain L mice. *J. nat. Cancer Inst.* **3**, 297—301 (1943).

[6] NISHIYAMA, Y., Über die Sarkombildung durch wiederholte Injektionen der hochkonzentrierten Glukoselösung bei den mit o-Amidoazotoluol gefütterten Ratten. *Gann* **29**, 1—9 (1935).

[7] OETTINGEN, W. F. VON, The halogenated hydrocarbons: their toxicity and potential dangers. *J. industr. Hyg.* **19**, 349—448 (1937).

[8] RUDALI, G., et MARIANI, P. L., Sur la production de tumeurs du foie chez la Souris XVII/G a l'aide du tetrachlorure de carbone. *C.R. Soc. Biol.* (Paris) **144**, 1626—1627 (1950).

[9] SCHMÄHL, D., THOMAS, C., SATTLER, W., u. SCHEID, G. F., Experimentelle Untersuchungen zur Syncarcinogenese. III. Mitt.: Versuche zur Krebserzeugung bei Ratten bei gleichzeitiger Gabe von Diäthylnitrosamin und Tetrachlorkohlenstoff bzw. Athylalkohol; zugleich ein experimenteller Beitrag zur Frage der „Alkoholzirrhose". *Z. Krebsforsch.* (sous presse) (1965).

[10] STOWELL, R. E., and LEE, C. S., Histochemical studies of mouse liver after single feeding of carbon tetrachloride. *Arch. Path.* **50**, 519—537 (1950).

[11] — — TSUBOI, K. K., and VILLASANA, A., Histochemical and microchemical changes in experimental cirrhoses and hepatoma formation in mice by carbon tetrachloride. *Cancer Res.* **11**, 345—354 (1951).

Discussion

Della Porta: The resistance of the rat to liver tumour-induction by CCl$_4$ is a remarkable example of a species difference in reactivity to carcinogens. On the other hand, a group of research workers in Italy have observed hepatomas in CCl$_4$-treated rats (COSTA et al., 1963). In an experiment of our own, Syrian golden hamsters given CCl$_4$ for 30 weeks developed a 100% incidence of liver cell carcinomas (DELLA PORTA et al., 1961). As for the difficulty in transplanting CCl$_4$-induced hepatomas, LEDUC and WILSON (1959) suggested that the length of the interval between the last administration of CCl$_4$ and the transplantation may be important.

References

COSTA, A., WEBER, G., BARTOLONI ST. OMER, F., e CAMPANA, G., La cancrocirrosi sperimentale da CCl$_4$ nel ratto. *Arch. De Vecchi Anat. pat.* **39**, 303 (1963).

DELLA PORTA, G., TERRACINI, B., and SHUBIK, P., Induction with carbon tetrachloride of liver cell carcinomas in hamsters. *J. nat. Cancer Inst.* **26**, 855 (1961).

LEDUC, E. H., and WILSON, J. W., Transplantation of carbon tetrachloride-induced hepatomas in mice. *J. nat. Cancer Inst.* **22**, 581 (1959).

Truhaut: It is important to be sure that chloroform used in tests on mice is preserved by the addition of 0.5 per cent ethanol or that it is really pure. Phosgene may be formed by the photochemical oxidation of chloroform. This reaction is inhibited by ethanol. Has Dr. RUDALI tested bromoform, iodoform or trichlorethylene?

Rudali: We have not tested bromoform or iodoform. Trichlorethylene gave negative results in large scale experiments.

Frazer: Chloroform water is 0.25% solution of chloroform in water; it is widely used as a flavouring agent and preservative. I do not agree that one can condemn the use of chloroform water on the basis of Dr. RUDALI's report. I would agree, however, that chloroform water might be studied, both with regard to the presence of impurities and possible toxicity.

Drugs with Lactone Groups as Potential Carcinogens

Frank Dickens

Courtauld Institute of Biochemistry, Middlesex Hospital Medical School, London, W. 1

One of the most valuable features in the extension of our knowledge of carcinogens to include new types is the possible application of such work to the development of protective measures. This is particularly true in the instance of new drugs, where a knowledge of those types of chemical structure which are likely to be associated with carcinogenic properties is most essential. This is for two reasons, first to enable those introducing such new drugs to recognize on chemical grounds their possible carcinogenic risk, and secondly to apply to such compounds especially thorough biological tests in order to exclude as far as possible the therapeutic introduction of new potential carcinogens.

The particular area of this subject with which our own work has been concerned refers to the carcinogenic lactones, lactams and related compounds. These studies have been made jointly with my colleague Dr. H. E. H. Jones. When this work began, in 1956, the only lactone known to be carcinogenic appears to have been β-propiolactone (Walpole *et al.*, 1954; Dickens and Jones, 1961).

Carcinogenic Action of β-Propiolactone and its Derivatives

β-Propiolactone has been used fairly extensively as a sterilizing agent, including its use as an aerosol for sterilizing rooms (Beears and Roha, 1960). Since according to these authors the LD_{50} is only about 0.5—0.6 mg/litre for 2 hr. exposure in animals, it is obvious that great care is necessary in such usage. This also applies to its use in sterilizing plasma (Hartman, Lo Grippo and Kelly, 1954), arterial or bone grafts (Rains *et al.*, 1956), or as a toxoiding agent in place of formalin (Orlans and Jones, 1958). Roe and Salaman (1958) have drawn attention to the possible carcinogenic hazard involved in such uses.

Chemically, β-propiolactone is highly reactive, due to the strained 4-membered ring. It is an alkylating carcinogen, undergoing rapid electrophilic reactions, e.g. with the sulphydryl (—SH) group forming a thioether. In the case of cysteine the compound formed is S-2-carboxyethyl-cysteine (Dickens and Jones, 1961), as proved by isolation of the crystalline product.

Table I shows that β-propiolactone is capable both of the induction of sarcoma when repeated doses are given subcutaneously, or of skin carcinoma when repeatedly painted on the skin of animals. Recently in this laboratory it has been found that repeated intratracheal administration by intubation is capable of inducing malignant lung tumours in rats (Jones and Waynforth, unpublished observations).

In addition to a course of repeated doses, in this series, the integrity of the lactone ring is necessary for carcino-

Table I. *Carcinogenicity of β-Lactones and some related compounds*

Animal	Route	Dose (usually twice weekly)	Cancer animals/ survivors	Earliest appearance (weeks)	Authors
β-Propiolactone					
Rat	S.C.	2 mg. in oil	9[1]/12	27	Walpole *et al.*, 1954
Mouse	Skin	2.5% in acetone	5/29	21—40	Roe and Glendenning, 1956
Mouse	Skin	2.5% in acetone	20/45	16	Searle, 1961
Rat	S.C.	1 mg. in oil	14/14	29	Dickens and Jones, 1961
Rat	S.C.	0.1 mg. in oil	4/4	25	Dickens and Jones, 1961
Rat	S.C.	2 mg. in water	2/4	31	Dickens and Jones, 1961
Mouse	S.C.	20 μg. in oil	7/20	43	Dickens and Jones, 1965
Rat	Intra-tracheal	0.3 mg. in oil	1[2]/3	72	Dickens, Jones and Waynforth, 1966
Mouse	Skin	0.25—5% in acetone	27/149	ca. 20	Palmes *et al.*, 1962
β-Hydroxypropionic acid					
Rat	S.C.	1 mg. in water	0/3	contd. for 106 wks.	Dickens and Jones, 1963a
α-Carboxy-β-phenylpropiolactone					
Rat	S.C.	2 mg. in oil	1/4	91	Dickens and Jones, 1961
αα-Diphenyl-β-propiolactone					
Rat	S.C.	1 mg. in oil	1/3	89	Dickens and Jones, 1961
ββ-Dimethyl-trimethylene oxide					
Rat	S.C.	1 mg. in oil	2/4	83	Dickens and Jones, 1963a

[1] The oil used by these authors also gave some local tumours, without added propiolactone
[2] A squamous-cell carcinoma of bronchiolar epithelium.

genicity: the hydrolysis product β-hydroxypropionic acid for example was found by us to be inactive in this respect (Dickens and Jones, 1963a).

The 4-Membered Lactam Ring: Penicillin and Related Antibiotics

The demonstration (Table I) that even fairly small repeated doses of the 4-membered β-lactones could induce malignant tumours led us to test in the same way penicillin and later 6-amino-penicillanic acid, in both of which a 4-membered lactam ring occurs. Our standard technique consisted in twice-weekly subcutaneous injections into rats of 2 mg substance in 0.5 ml arachis oil, given as nearly as possible at the

same injection site and continued for many weeks. At the same time, control animals received injections of the oil alone. Not a single local tumour arose in any of these control rats (Table II). [More recently we have used batches of mice, given amounts of 0.1 ml arachis oil containing 0.5 mg of the substance to be tested, but in the control mice given oil alone one mammary tumour and one sarcoma have arisen at or near the injection site. This finding is contrary to the supposedly hypersensitive nature of the subcutaneous tissues of the rat, vis-a-vis the mouse, for tests of carcinogenicity, on which particularly Clayson (1962) has written. Care was taken to use one large batch of oil throughout these experiments.]

When 2 mg doses of crystalline sodium penicillin G (sodium benzyl penicillin), containing 1670 I.U./mg, in 0.5 ml arachis oil were injected twice weekly into two batches of rats, tu-

and JONES, 1965) in the same way as penicillin G, which is the benzyl derivative of this compound. After twice weekly injections of 2 mg doses for 65 weeks into 6 rats, only one rat of the

Table II. *Penicillin and antibiotic lactones as tumorigenic agents after their repeated subcutaneous injection*

Animal	Period injected (weeks)	Dose (twice weekly)	Cancer animals/ survivors	Earliest appearance (weeks)	Reference
Penicillin G (sodium salt)					
Rat	46—52	2 mg. in oil	2/8	59	DICKENS and JONES, 1961
Rat	78	2 mg. in oil	5/11	78	DICKENS and JONES, 1963a
6-Amino-penicillanic acid					
Rat	65	2 mg. in oil	1/6	84	DICKENS and JONES, 1965
Penicillic acid					
Rat	64	1 mg. in oil	4/4	48	DICKENS and JONES, 1961
Rat	61	0.1 mg. in oil	1/4	94	DICKENS and JONES, 1963a
Rat	52	2 mg. in water	4/5	56	DICKENS and JONES, 1963a
Mouse	65	0.2 mg. in oil	6/19	38	DICKENS and JONES, 1965
Sarkomycin					
Rat	65	2 mg. in oil	1/5	42	DICKENS and JONES, 1965
Patulin (clavacin)					
Rat	—	2 mg. in oil	Toxic	—	DICKENS and JONES, 1961
Rat	61	0.2 mg. in oil	4/4	58	DICKENS and JONES, 1961
Rat	64	0.2 mg. in oil	2/4	62	DICKENS and JONES, 1961
Parasorbic acid					
Rat	32	2 mg. in oil	4/5	61	DICKENS and JONES, 1963a
Rat	32	0.2 mg. in oil	4/6	63	DICKENS and JONES, 1963a
Oil controls					
Rat	54—61	0.5 ml. arachis oil only	0/24	—	DICKENS and JONES, 1961, 1963, 1965
Mouse	65	0.1 ml. arachis	1[1]/19	69	DICKENS and JONES, 1965

[1] Also 1 mammary adenocarcinoma in a mouse. All other cancers listed were local sarcomas at injection site (rats and mice).

mours arose at the injection site (Table II). The total incidence of rats bearing local malignant tumours in the two experiments was 7 among 19 rats so injected (DICKENS and JONES, 1961, 1963a). These tumours were sarcomas or fibrosarcomas, and some of them could be successfully transplanted to other rats.

6-Amino penicillanic acid (6-APA) has recently been tested by us (DICKENS

6 survivors bore a local tumour in the 84th week of the experiment (Table II) and this proved to be histologically a sarcoma, though it failed to grow on attempted transplantation. The order of carcinogenicity of 6-APA is thus very low. It would be important to know if this also applies to the newer penicillins in which substituents other than the benzyl group are attached to the 6-amino group of 6-APA (Phenoxyethyl peni-

cillin or Broxil, α-aminophenyl penicillin or Ampicillin, etc.). In this connexion it is of interest that the enzyme penicillinase, which specifically opens up the β-lactam structure and no other (CHAIN, 1960), does not attack the β-lactam ring in these newer penicillinase-resistant derivatives of 6-APA. There are therefore biological differences in behaviour which may perhaps also prove important in relation to carcinogenesis in this series.

A study of the literature shows that although numerous tests by other workers of the effects of administration of penicillins have been reported (see HARTWELL, 1951; SHUBIK and HARTWELL, 1957), these tests were either by oral administration or alternatively were continued only for short periods. Since according to our studies, penicillin G is a weak and slow-acting tumorigenic agent, it is not surprising that these previous trials have not revealed any carcinogenic action of the penicillins.

The chemical structure of the penicillins (and other β-lactam antibiotics such as the cephalosporins, which have yet to be tested) is such that its carcinogenic activity is not at all surprising. Penicillin reacts like β-propiolactone with the SH group of cysteine and similar sulphydryl compounds, with the opening of the 4-membered ring and loss of antibiotic properties (for probable mechanism and kinetics of this reaction, see NAKKEN et al., 1960; DICKENS and COOKE, 1965).

Obviously the other β-lactam antibiotics urgently need to be tested in a similar manner.

Carcinogenic Action of other Antibiotic Substances

Professor BOYLAND is dealing with this subject at this meeting and I will therefore restrict my comments to our own work in this field.

Many αβ-unsaturated lactones are bacteriostatic in varying degree (for a review see HAYNES, 1948). These include simple 5 or 6 membered lactone rings like angelica lactone and parasorbic acid, as well as more complex lactone structures such as protoanemonin, patulin (clavacin) and penicillic acid.

In our tests (cf. Table II), subcutaneous malignant tumours were produced in rats by repeated subcutaneous injection of each of these substances, although β-angelica lactone was only very weakly (and α-angelica lactone not at all) carcinogenically active. But the more active antibiotics patulin and penicillic acid, as well as the methyl derivative of protoanemonin, were active carcinogens in the rat (DICKENS and JONES, 1961, 1963a) and mouse (DICKENS and JONES, 1965).

The delta lactone of 2-hexenoic acid (parasorbic acid) provided an example of a simple six-membered lactone ring which shares antibiotic and growth-inhibitory properties with marked carcinogenic activity (DICKENS and JONES, 1963a; see Table II).

The biological activity (as antibiotics or in other respects) of most of these compounds has been shown to be abolished by prior incubation with sulphydryl compounds such as cysteine or glutathione. They probably, but not certainly, owe their carcinogenic action to their ability to act as alkylating agents under physiological conditions (see DICKENS, 1964).

The carcinogenic activity of other bacteriostatic or fungistatic compounds (Table III) such as phenyl vinyl ketone (DICKENS and JONES, 1965) and more weakly, the tumour growth inhibitory antibiotic sarkomycin (DICKENS and JONES, 1965) also gives considerable support to the idea that there may be some feature which is shared in the

Table III. *Carcinogenesis and structure*

References to propiolactones are given in Table I. The other compounds have been described by DICKENS and JONES, 1961, 1963a, 1963b, 1965. Results with dehydroacetic acid are work of DICKENS, JONES and WAYNFORTH, 1966.

mechanism of carcinogenesis on the one hand and anti-microbial action on the other. The recent Japanese work on this aspect will no doubt be included in Professor BOYLAND's contribution to this meeting.

It should be mentioned here that parasorbic acid, which our work has shown to be actively carcinogenic in animals (Table III), has been used therapeutically in man. It has been used for many years by Laplanders as a 'Spring tonic', being the active constituent of berries of the Mountain Ash (*Sorbus aucuparia L.*) in which the hexenolactone occurs to the extent of several percent. It is supposedly beneficial for the liver and for overcoming biliary stasis (WIDEN, 1931). More recently an antihaemorrhagic effect has also been claimed (SHINOWARA *et al.*, 1941) Professor BOYLAND has reported (BOYLAND, 1964) that commercial extracts of these berries are regularly on sale at druggists in Germany. Obviously, our finding that the essential oil (Sorbinöl, the old German name for parasorbic acid, or $(+)$-δ-hexenolactone) of the Mountain Ash berry is carcinogenic in animals, is an indication to avoid the use of a drug possessing such vague therapeutic properties.

The naturally occurring antibiotic lactones, and synthetic analogues of a number of these compounds, have been tested by GIARMAN (1948, 1949) for their effects on the isolated heart. The active constituents of the cardiac glycosides (digitalis, strophanthin and squill) all contain an unsaturated gamma- or delta-lactone substituent on C-17 of the cyclopentano-perhydrophenanthrene nucleus, of which complex the lactone moiety with its double bond is essential for cardiac activity (HAYNES, 1948; GIARMAN, 1949).

Few of these cardiac glycosides have been systematically tested for carcino-genic activity, no doubt because of their toxicity, but some negative results have been reported by SMITH and GARDNER (1939) and DRUCKREY (1940) for strophanthidin, digitonin, digitoxin and digitoxigenin. Nevertheless, many of these compounds contain $\alpha\beta$-unsaturated lactone rings of the types found by us to be carcinogenic; their pharmacological action can be imitiated by SH poisons such as *o*-iodobenzoic acid and iodoacetamide, and addition of SH compounds such as cysteine can inhibit their cardiac activity. As a preliminary to testing for carcinogenicity the glycosides themselves, we are at present testing instead a number of the unsaturated lactones for which GIARMAN (1948, 1949) has reported marked cardiotoxic activity (vulpinic acid, pulvinic acid dilactone) as well as the less active ascorbic acids and hydroxymethyl furfural. GIARMAN reported also appreciable cardiac activity for several of the substances which we later showed to be carcinogenic (patulin, or clavacin, penicillin acid, parasorbic acid) as well as for β-angelica lactone (weakly carcinogenic in our tests) and α-angelica lactone (negative in our tests). The suggestion of some common feature in these widely differing pharmacological activities is therefore quite strong and requires further study.

Phenolic Lactones as Carcinogens

In relation to the lactonic carcinogens already described, the coumarin group may be briefly mentioned here. The facts that aflatoxin, produced by the growth on foodstuffs of the mould *Aspergillus flavus*, is a very active carcinogen (BARNES and BUTLER, 1964; DICKENS and JONES, 1963b, 1965), and that it contains the coumarin structure, is relevant to this discussion, although coumarin itself and coumalic acid failed to give tumours in our recent tests (Dickens and Jones, 1965), but tests of both substances were not clear-cut because of their toxicity. Dicoumarol (and the later related compounds) as an anticoagulant drug deserves special attention, and we are at present testing this substance for possible carcinogenic activity. Previous experiments (by feeding) have been inadequate as they extended only over 40 days or 3 months (Hueck, 1951).

Other substances in this class, used as drugs, include the vitamin P analogues (hisperidin, hisperidin methyl chalcone, etc.), the testing of which may be of importance as they are administered over prolonged periods with a view to decreasing the capillary fragility of the patient.

Conclusion

With all drugs there is probably some risk, and it is therefore always necessary to balance the risk against the benefit to the patient.

In general, a fairly long exposure to a potential carcinogen is a necessary factor in carcinogenesis, although there are some exceptions to this (e.g. nitrosamines, benzidine). In the case of the lactones and lactams, repeated applications have so far proved quite necessary for carcinogenesis. We have several examples of this with the present series of compounds.

Consequently, special attention ought to be directed to those potentially carcinogenic drugs which are customarily or sometimes administered over long periods.

No one has suggested that the use of penicillin should be abandoned because a minute percentage of those treated have suffered from severe allergies, or sometimes even fatal reactions. Similar considerations also probably apply to the drugs discussed in this paper. Nevertheless, what is important is that those producing and using drugs of these particular classes should be aware of the facts revealed by animal experiments, that certain types of chemical structure are likely to be associated in some degree with carcinogenic properties.

References

Barnes, J. M., and Butler, W. H., Carcinogenic activity of aflatoxin in rats. *Nature (Lond.)* **202**, 1016 (1964).

Beears, W. L., and Roha, M., Propiolactone as a sterilant. II. *U.S. Govt. Research Reports* **32**, 22 (1959); *P.B. Report* 139748, *Chem. Abstr.* **54**, 17791 (1960).

Boyland, E., Biochemical aspects of carcinogenesis with special reference to alkylating agents and some antibiotics. Proc. 7th Eurotox Meeting, Brussels, 3—6 June, 1964. *Food and Cosmetics Toxicology* **2**, 655 (1964).

Chain, E., Some new antibiotics. *New Scientist*, 29th September, 838 (1960).

Clayson, D. B., *Chemical carcinogenesis*. London: J. & A. Churchill 1962.

Dickens, F., Carcinogenic lactones and related substances. *Brit. med. Bull.* **20**, 96 (1964).

—, and Cooke, J., Rates of hydrolysis and interaction with cysteine of some carcinogenic lactones and related substances. *Brit. J. Cancer* **19**, 404 (1965).

Dickens, F., and Jones, H. E. H., Carcinogenic activity of a series of reactive lactones and related substances. *Brit. J. Cancer* **15**, 85 (1961).

— — Further studies on the carcinogenic and growth-inhibitory activity of lactones and related substances. *Brit. J. Cancer* **17**, 100 (1963a).

— — The carcinogenic action of aflatoxin after its subcutaneous injection in the rat. *Brit. J. Cancer* **17**, 691 (1963b).

— — Further studies on the carcinogenic activity of certain lactones and related substances in the rat and mouse. *Brit. J. Cancer* **19**, 392 (1965).

— —, and Waynforth, H. B., Oral, subcutaneous and intratracheal administration of carcinogenic lactones and related substances:

the intratracheal administration of cigarette tar in the rat. *Brit. J. Cancer* **20**, 134 (1966).

DRUCKREY, H., Über oestrogene und cancerogene Wirkung. *Z. Krebsforsch.* **50**, 27 (1940).

GIARMAN, N. J., Antibiotic lactones and synthetic analogs. I. Cardiotoxic effects on the isolated frog heart. *J. Pharmacol. exp. Ther.* **94**, 232 (1948).

— Antibiotic lactones and synthetic analogs. II. Cardiotonic effects on the isolated frog heart. *J. Pharmacol. exp. Ther.* **96**, 119 (1949).

HARTMAN, F. W., LO GRIPPO, G., and KELLY. A. R., Preparation and sterilization of blood plasma. *Amer. J. clin. Path.* **24**, 339 (1954).

HARTWELL, J. L., Survey of compounds tested for carcinogenic activity. U.S. Public Health Service 1951.

HAYNES, L. J., Physiologically active unsaturated lactones. *Quart. Rev. chem. Soc. London* **2**, 46 (1948).

HUECK, O., Histologische Untersuchungen an Versuchstier über die Wirkung hoher Dicumarol und Tromexandosen auf die Leber und andere Organe. *Naunyn-Schmiedelbergs Arch. exp. Path. Pharmak.* **212**, 302 (1951),

NAKKEN, K. F., ELDJARN, L., and PIHL, A., The mechanism of inactivation of penicillin by cysteine and other mercaptoamines. *Biochem. Pharmacol.* **3**, 89 (1960).

ORLANS, E. S., and JONES, V. E., Beta-propiolactone as a toxoiding agent. *Nature (Lond.)* **182**, 1216 (1958).

PALMES, E. D., ORRIS, L., and NELSON, N., Skin irritation and skin tumour production by beta propiolactone (BPL). *Amer. industr. Hyg. Ass. J.* **23**, 257 (1962).

RAINS, A. J. H., CRAWFORD, N., SHARPE, S. H., SHREWSBURY, J. F. D., and BARSON, G. J., Management of an artery-graft bank with special reference to sterilization by β-propiolactone. *Lancet* **1956 II**, 830.

ROE, F. J. C., and SALAMAN, M. H., Sterilization of arterial grafts. *Brit. med. J.* **1958 I**, 942.

SEARLE, C. E., Experiments on the carcinogenicity and reactivity of β-propiolactone. *Brit. J. Cancer* **15**, 804 (1961).

SHUBIK, P., and HARTWELL, J. L., Survey of compounds tested for carcinogenic activity, Suppl. I. U.S. Public Health Service 1957.

SHINOWARA, G. Y., DELOR, J., and MEANS, J. W., Clinical and laboratory investigations on the extract of the European Mountain Ash berry, with particular reference to its antihaemorrhagee activity. *J. Lab. clin. Med.* **27**, 897 (1941).

SMITH, P. K., and GARDNER, W. U., A note on the lack of carcinogenic action of some cardiac glucosides and saponins. *Yale J. Biol. Med.* **11**, 187 (1939).

WALPOLE, A. L., ROBERTS, D. C., ROSE, F. L., HENDRY, J. A., and HOMER, R. F., Cytotoxic agents: IV, The carcinogenic actions of some monofunctional ethyleneimine derivatives. *Brit. J. Pharmacol.* **9**, 306 (1954).

Discussion

Frazer: Is there a single authenticated case of a local tumour at the site of the penicillin injection amongst the millions of people who have benefited from the parenteral injection of penicillin in various forms?

Roe: In the letter which Dr. SALAMAN and I wrote to the British Medical Journal (see reference) our main concern was for technicians exposed to β-propiolactone in the course of sterilizing materials such as arterial grafts for surgical use. In one article on this subject, β-propiolactone was described as "relatively innocuous" and it was stated that "a concentrated solution may damage the skin and a mist is injurious to the eyes and respiratory tract". SALAMAN and I recommended stringent precautions in the handling of the substance. We were also concerned about the possibility that β-propiolactone itself, or its metabolic products, remaining in serum or arterial grafts sterilized by it, might exert a carcinogenic effect. Recently, LAWS and ZINNEMANN (1963) produced evidence providing some reassurance on this point.

References

LAWS, J. O., and ZINNEMANN, K., Tissue reaction to heterografts sterilised with beta-propiolactone. *J. Path. Bact.* **86**, 21—23 (1963).

ROE, F. J. C., and SALAMAN, M. H., Sterilization of arterial grafts. *Brit. med. J.* **1958 I**, 942.

Truhaut: At one time it was proposed to use β-propiolactone for disinfecting the air particularly in hospital wards. Considerable information with regard to this will be found in a number of the American Journal of Hospital Pharmacy published during 1961. Here seems to be a shining example of the importance which must be given to the toxicological assessment of a compound before its use is authorised, especially on a large scale.

Truhaut: Did you also use 4'-nitro-4-benzylpyridine for testing the alkylating reactivity of lactones?

Dickens: We have studied reactivity with sulphydryl groups, but not with this reagent.

Pyrrolizidine (Senecio) Alkaloids and other Natural Drugs as Potential Carcinogens

R. Schoental

Member of the Scientific Staff of the Medical Research Council
Toxicology Research Unit, Medical Research Council Laboratories,
Woodmansterne Road, Carshalton, Surrey, Great Britain

Introduction

It is gratifying to note that the existence of natural carcinogens is no more disregarded. After all man suffered and died of cancer long before the advent of synthetics. In the 20 minutes at my disposal I can do no more than to draw attention to a few points which came to my notice in the course of the last 15 years during which I have been interested in natural toxic products, especially those used as medicines by primitive and not so primitive peoples.

I am not going to recapitulate to you the results of studies which led to the recognition of pyrrolizidine alkaloids, aflatoxins, luteoskyrin and cycasin as very effective hepatocarcinogens. These have been reviewed (SCHOENTAL, 1963; KRAYBILL and SHIMKIN, 1964; WOGAN, 1965, and in the Proceedings of the Third Conference on the Toxicity of CYCADS, 1964, respectively). My intention is to discuss how most profitably to select priority problems for study in the field of natural toxic substances.

Though there exist very many herbals and books on medicinal botany from various countries (ASPREY and THORNTON, 1955; CHOPRA, 1933; CULPEPER; DALZIEL, 1937; DRAGENDORFF, 1898; DIOSCORIDES; WREN, 1956; KIRTIKAR et al., 1936; NADKARNI, 1927; STANER and BOUTIQUE, 1937; PERROTT, 1943/44; READ, 1936 etc.) these are not necessarily comprehensive, as many plants might be in use by country people which have not come to the knowledge of the compilers of such books. The search for toxic or carcino genic agents would best be served by basing the selection of the plant materials on observations of toxicity in livestock.

Many fungal (FORGACS and CARLL, 1962) and plant materials have been reported to be toxic to livestock (STEYN, 1934; HURST, 1942; WATT and BREYER-BRANDWIJK, 1962; KINGSBURY, 1964 etc.). Most of the toxic principles have either not yet been identified or not appropriately tested for chronic toxicity and carcinogenic action. Perusal of such books would be helpful, though the problems selected will no doubt depend on the individual cancer worker and his interests.

Social workers and anthropologists will have to disentangle whether, and which particular natural products are involved in human tumour cases. Our task is to recognise the existence, to isolate and to study the structures, and the mode of action of natural products which can induce tumours in animals. The finding in recent years that many substances of diverse chemical structures can cause the same type of tumour, had a salutary effect on our thinking about the mechanism of carcinogenesis which was previously based mainly on the structures of polycyclic compounds (compare SCHOENTAL, 1963, 1964).

The naturally occurring toxic substances (like the ones produced synthetically) can roughly be divided into 3 types, though often the distinction may only be a question of dosage.

1. Compounds which are *acutely* toxic; these either kill in the course of a few hours or days after their ingestion, or cause only transitory upset, followed by complete recovery. Most of the known alkaloids, cardiac glycosides and bacterial toxins are of this type. Their toxic properties have been recognised long ago, as the connection between cause and effect is easy to trace. Many of the acute effects due to such substances are studied by the classical pharmacological methods. It has not been adequately established whether all their effects are really reversible or whether chronic lesions can result from some of these toxic compounds.

2. Compounds which do not cause acute fatalities, though they may or may not induce some malaise or short illness, which wears off in time and appears to be followed by recovery. Yet, by some mechanisms, mostly unknown, the initial lesions progress insidiously and can result in chronic illness and death, a long time after such compounds have been ingested. Certain hepatotoxins, carcinogens and possibly agents causing demyelination or other neurological diseases belong to this type. The connection between the ingestion of the causative materials and the effects which only become apparent many months or years later might be very difficult, or impossible, to trace.

3. Compounds which are significantly more toxic to the foetus or to the very young than to the adult. When ingested by pregnant or lactating females, the latter may remain unscathed, yet the foetus *in utero* or the suckling young, may suffer the ill effects. Again, when the toxic action on the offspring is acute, cause and effect are easy to recognise, but when the toxin initiates delayed chronic lesions, the connection between the cause and effect is not so obvious, and might be difficult to trace. Certain teratogenic, lathyrogenic and carcinogenic compounds belong to this type.

In special circumstances it may be possible to recognise agents producing delayed chronic diseases if such disease occur with relatively high frequency in particular localities or in groups exposed to a common environmental factor. Many compounds responsible for certain diseases known to occur among workers in specific industries were traced, and such illness could be prevented or eliminated by taking appropriate protective measures (good ventilation, protective clothing, etc.) or by modifying the industrial procedures, as in the manufacture of dyes for which β-naphthylamine was used. From studies of industrial hazards much fundamental knowledge of great scientific importance has been gained, especially in the field of carcinogenic agents. A recent example is the recognition that mesothelioma of the lung can follow many years after exposure to certain types of asbestos (WAGNER, et al., 1960).

However, the tracing of aetiological factors of diseases which are encountered under primitive conditions of life, in the tropics and subtropics, is obviously much more difficult. Genetic and nutritional factors which are known to modify or predispose to the effects of various toxins, have often been suspected to be responsible for certain pathological conditions, until the real toxic agent has been eventually discovered.

Some of the pathological conditions encountered in communities living under 'natural' conditions, have been known to disappear with the advent of 'industrialised' way of life. Primary liver cancer can serve as an example. In U.S.A. its incidence is similar among the white and the Negro populations; but among some Negro communities in Africa (including Western Africa, from where the American Negroes came) it is often very high indeed (KENNAWAY, 1944; FINDLAY, 1950). The aetiology of many such conditions is still mostly unknown or uncertain, but they are likely to be related to 'natural' environmental factors. It would be of great importance, academic and practical, to identify the natural toxic factors, the conditions under which they operate and how the respective 'diseases' develop, before the spreading of a uniform way of life will make this impossible. The inquiry must cover all the materials, whether ingested as food, as medicine or charm, used for external application, inhalation etc. The toxic factors may be of animal, plant or microbial origin. The task is enormous and some judicious selection is essential. There is already enough evidence that certain tumours may be caused by natural products, as substances isolated from natural sources can reproduce similar conditions in experimental animals.

Pyrrolizidine (Senecio) Alkaloids

Pyrrolizidine (Senecio) alkaloids were among the first to be suggested, as possible 'natural' aetiological factors in the high incidence of liver diseases (kwashiorkor, liver cirrhosis and primary liver tumours) in the Tropics and Subtropics (SCHOENTAL, 1955). There exist more than 2000 species of Senecio, Crotalaria, Heliotropium and of other genera, among which certain species

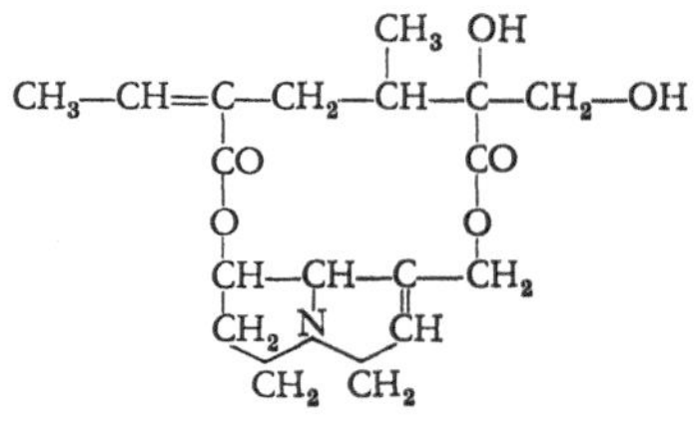

Fig. 1. The structure of retrorsine, a carcinogenic pyrrolizidine alkaloid

have been found to contain pyrrolizidine alkaloids. However, no more than 100—150 of these plant species have as yet been examined chemically for the presence of alkaloids, and even fewer have been tested for toxicity in animals. The available data are sufficient already to indicate the potential hazards in using plants of these genera before making sure that any particular batch of plants does not contain toxic alkaloids. Recently a number of Crotalaria species have been found to contain non-hepatotoxic alkaloids; however even these should still be re-tested, with the view of excluding a possibility that their long term ingestion may cause some other types of tumours.

Oesophageal lesions in horses, known as Chillagoe disease in Queensland, are believed to be due to the ingestion of *Crotalaria aridicola* (quoted by CULVENOR and SMITH, 1962). Oesophageal tumours have been found also in cattle in Kenya (PLOWRIGHT, 1955), and are likely to be caused by "natural" carcinogens, whether present in the ingested forage or formed in the course of its digestion and microbial fermentation. The recently described high incidence of oesophageal cancer among the Bantu in Transkei (BURELL, 1962) could conceivably be due to similar causes.

The study of the hepatotoxic pyrrolizidine alkaloids dislcosed that (1) a single dose (of the order of LD_{30-50}) may be able to induce chronic liver disease, including primary liver hepatoma, which becomes apparent a long time after the ingestion of the causative agent; (2) that the hepatotoxic agent can pass through the placenta and be excreted in the milk, when ingested by a pregnant or a lactating female, respectively (SCHOENTAL, 1959); (3) that the foetus and the very young are more sensitive to the action of the toxic pyrrolizidine alkaloids than are adults; and (4) that the adult male is more sensitive to these toxins than the adult female (compare: SCHOENTAL, 1963).

These characteristics apply not only to the toxic pyrrolizidine alkaloids but also to other "natural" (and synthetic) carcinogens, such as aflatoxins (ALLCROFT and LEWIS, 1963), cycasin (MICKELSON et al., 1964) etc. When the foetus or the young are affected by a carcinogenic agent, they may develop tumours quite young.

Cycasin

Of particular interest was the finding of carcinogenic properties of cycasin, the glycoside of methylazoxymethanol, present in nuts and leaves of the tree, *Cycas circinalis* L, which is widely distributed throughout the Tropics and Subtropics (LAQUEUR et al., 1963; LAQUEUR, 1964). The nuts are a source of starch, often used as food after appropriate preparation, including soaking in water (WHITING, 1963, 1964).

Aqueous emulsions of the fresh cycad nuts have been used as dressings of skin ulcers and wounds and appear to promote their healing (O'GARA et al., 1964). Other species of Cycadaceae include Encephalartos and Zamias; some are toxic and like *Macrozamia communis* may contain macrozamin (LANGLEY et al., 1951). The active principle of both, cycasin and macrozamin, is the unstable aglycone, methylazoxymethanol,

$$CH_3-\underset{\underset{O}{\downarrow}}{N}=N-CH_2OH.$$

The latter was obtained by hydrolysis of cycasin with emulsin, the β-glycosidase of almonds (KOBAYASHI and MATSUOMTO, 1965). This compound is active as a carcinogen by both, the oral and the intraperitoneal routes. Its more stable derivative, obtained by acetylation, is also active when injected intraperitoneally, while cycasin is effective only by the oral route and is not active in germ-free rats; evidently cycasin is hydrolysed by the intestinal flora, and only the aglycone is carcinogenic. Intraperitoneal injections of methylazoxymethanol induce tumours in the liver, kidneys and intestines (LAQUEUR and MATSUMOTO, 1966).

The chemical resemblance of this "natural" product to the synthetic carcinogen, dimethylnitrosamine, is striking. Both act probably *via* diazomethane, formed in the course of their metabolic degradation (MAGEE and SCHOENTAL, 1964). Recently cycasin has been shown to act as a methylating agent *in vitro* and to methylate phenol to anisole when heated with concentrated sulphuric acid (RIGGS, 1965).

A related glycoside, elaiomycin, has been isolated from *Streptomyces hepaticus* by HASKELL et al., (1954); this has antibiotic properties against *Mycobacterium tuberculosis* and causes liver cirrhosis in the guinea pig. It might cause liver tumours as well (WEISS, 1964).

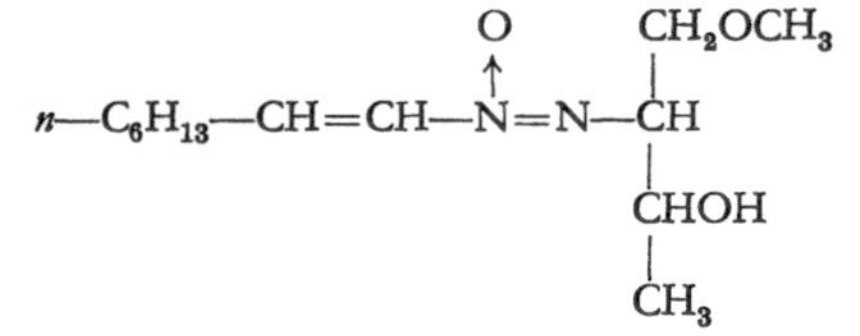

$$n-C_6H_{13}-CH{=}CH-\overset{\overset{O}{\uparrow}}{N}{=}N-\underset{\underset{\underset{\underset{CH_3}{|}}{CHOH}}{|}}{\overset{\overset{CH_2OCH_3}{|}}{CH}}$$

elaiomycin

The antibiotics, *hygroscopins*, isolated by Japanese workers, appear to have related structures (quoted by WEISS, 1964). In view of the possibility that cycasin can be identified in the form of its trimethylsilyl-derivative by gas chromatography, the search for this type of compounds not only among plants but also among micro-organisms should be facilitated (WEISS, 1964). The cycas toxin has been shown to affect many animal species, but whether it can be responsible for the neurological conditions observed in the Marianas and in some parts of Japan and New Guinea is not certain.

Alkylnitroso-compounds could also be formed from "natural" materials which are rich in nitrites or nitrates. As example can serve the case of the herring-meals which were prepared from herrings preserved with sodium nitrite. Some batches of such herring meals were hepatotoxic when fed to sheep. This species appears exceedingly sensitive to the hepatotoxic action of dimethyl-nitrosamine, which together with some other, not yet identified nitroso-compounds has been detected in the toxic herring-meals (SAKSHAUG et al., 1965).

Whether nitroso-derivatives of nicotine and of the other alkaloidal and amine constituents of tobacco play a part in the carcinogenic effects of cigarette-smoke is still uncertain (BOYLAND et al., 1964). The carcinogenic

alkylnitroso-compounds are believed to act through alkylation of certain cell constituents. It is conceivable that such alkylations could occur in the course of de-alkylation of alkoxy-groups or similar processes in which free alkyl radicals might be formed.

Fungal Metabolites

Several types of hepatotoxic and hepatocarcinogenic materials have been found among fungal metabolites; the study of this source of potential carcinogens, has been till recently, neglected. The present trend indicates that appropriate attention will now be devoted to these substances, a great many of which have already been chemically identified (MILLER, 1961), but not yet tested for carcinogenic activity. Aflatoxins from

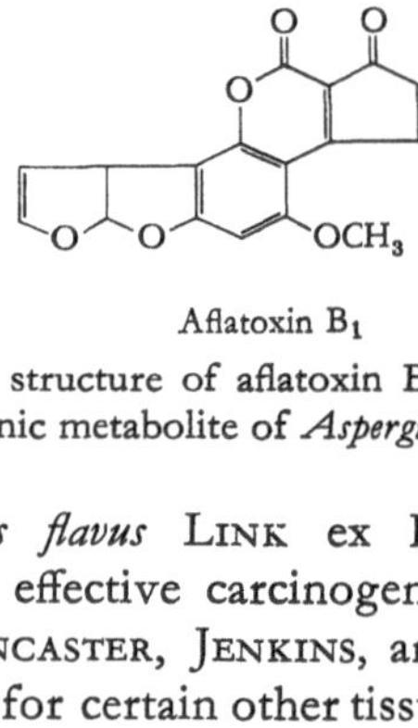

Aflatoxin B₁

Fig. 2. The structure of aflatoxin B_1, a potent carcinogenic metabolite of *Aspergillus flavus*

Aspergillus flavus LINK ex FRIES are extremely effective carcinogens for the liver (LANCASTER, JENKINS, and PHILP, 1961) and for certain other tissues of the rat (BARNES and BUTLER, 1964; DICKENS and JONES, 1963a, 1965). Ochratoxin A from *A. ochraceus* WILH has been reported to cause fatty livers (VAN DER MERWE, et al., 1965), luteoskyrin and a cyclic, chlorine containing peptide from *Penicillium islandicum* Sopp have been reported by Japanese workers to produce liver tumours. Grisefulvin present in *P. griseofulvum* and in several other Penicillium species, induced hepatomas in mice (WESTON-HURST and PAGET, 1963; DE MATTEIS et al., 1966). Actinomycins, L and S have been reported to induce sarcoma in mice when injected subcutaneously, actinomycin S being the more effective (KAWAMATA, et al., 1959). Among the many fungal species present in Nature (estimated as 40,000—250,000) there is little doubt that still some other metabolites will be found carcinogenic (compare KRAYBILL and SHIMKIN, 1964).

Lactones

The reported carcinogenic activity of β-propiolactone and of certain other simple α,β-unsaturated lactones (DICKENS and JONES, 1961, 1963b, 1965) suggests the need for further testing of this type of compounds, which are often encountered among natural products of plant or microbial origin (HAYNES, 1948). Some steroidal saponins and cardiac glycosides contain α,β-unsaturated lactone rings; many of such substances have been used as traditional drugs. Recently, cardiac glycosides with α,β-unsaturated lactone rings have been found to be cytotoxic in tissue culture (KUPCHAN, et al., 1964; KELLY, et al., 1965).

Oestrogens

The African male is reported to often suffer from gynaecomastia and high incidence of breast tumours (TROWELL, 1948). Excessive intake of oestrogens can cause tumours of the sex organs, as discovered first by LACASSAGNE (1932). Some plants contain substances which show oestrogenic activity when ingested. The best known example is genistein, the 5,7,4'-trihydroxy-iso-flavone, present in red clover, Trifolium subterraneum, Leguminosae, and in other Trifolium and Prunus species. Though the oestrogenic activity of genistein is very low (about 10^{-5} of the activity of oestrone), the amount of clover eaten by sheep was sufficient to cause great

losses in sheep breeding industry in Western Australia (BRADBURY and WHITE, 1954).

A more effective oral oestrogen, miroestrol, has been isolated from the root of Pueraria mirifica (Leguminosae), a plant growing in North Thailand, which has been traditionally used as a rejuvenating drug for old men and women, but not recommended for young people (CAIN, 1960). The root is known in Thailand as kwao keur, and in Burma as pankse. The presence of oestrone in date palm kernels described by BUTENANDT and JACOBI (1933) has been recently confirmed (HEFTMANN et al., 1965). Small quantity of oestriol has been isolated from willow catkins and flowers (SKARZYNSKI, 1933).

Organo-Selenium Compounds

Plants and microorganisms which contain organo-selenium compounds (SHRIFT, 1964) are of obvious interest in view of the reported carcinogenic action of selenium. Ingestion of the nut-like seeds of Lecythis ollaria (monkey-nut, coco de mono), a deciduous tree in Central and South America caused toxic effects in man and livestock. The seeds contain seleno-cystathionine,

$$HOOC—CH(NH_2)—CH_2—Se—$$
$$—CH_2—CH_2—CH(NH_2)COOH$$

a compound which occurs also in Astragalus species and Stanleya pinnata. Whether chronic lesions or tumours can result from the ingestion of these plant materials has not been established. The cytotoxic action of seleno-cystathionine in tissue culture suggests carcinogenic potentialities (ARONOV and KERDEL-VEGAS, 1965; KERDEL-VEGAS, et al., 1965).

Chronic selenium poisoning may be involved in a condition in sheep in

South Africa, known as geeldikkop, which is a photosensitisation syndrome with jaundice (BROWN, 1963). Geeldikkop was previously suspected to be caused by the ingestion of the plant, *Lippia rehmanni* Pears, which like *Lippia pretorensis* Pears and *Lantana camara* L contains triterpenoid acids. It is possible that both factors play a part in geeldikkop. It is of interest that angelic acid, the unsaturated, branched chain, five carbon acid, encountered among the hepatotoxic pyrrolizidine alkaloids, is present in some of these triterpenoids.

A great many plants have been reported to cause jaundice in livestock (KINGSBURY, 1964), and most of these have not yet been appropriately studied. Jaundice may be the result of various causes including parenchymal liver cell or bile duct damage by hepatotoxic agents.

Goitrogenic Organo-Sulphur Compounds

Among plants, especially the Cruciferae, many contain organo-sulphur compounds which are goitrogenic. When cows ingest such materials, they may excrete in the milk goitrogens; and these have been suspected as the cause of goitre in Australia (BACHELARD and TRIKOJUS, 1960). It would be interesting to know, whether the natural goitrogens can induce thyroid and liver tumours as is the case with e.g. thiourea. Plants of the Brassica species are used frequently as food, lactagogues etc. in many parts of the world.

Almost every drug, "natural" or synthetic is potentially toxic and its use involves taking a calculated risk. The latter has to be balanced against the beneficial effects expected in any particular case. The risk is greater in the case of herbs and crude products, which are difficult to standardise and the pharmacological properties of which may vary, not only from batch to batch, but also may change on keeping. In addition, many of the traditional herbal remedies appear to have no beneficial action, as is the case of the toxic pyrrolizidine alkaloids. The long term effects and carcinogenic potentialities of "natural" drugs have only been studied in very few cases, and much remains to be done in this field.

Until proved safe, drugs suspected of carcinogenic potentialities should obviously not be allowed to be indiscriminately sold for the use of women during pregnancy and lactation and of young children. Unfortunately, many drugs are used exactly for such cases, whether as emmenagogues, lactagogues, abortifacients etc., or for the numerous diseases of childhood.

Summary

The finding of effective carcinogens among "natural" materials of plant and microbial origin indicates the need for further study of natural products, known or suspected to be used as drugs etc., especially those used for the treatment of women during pregnancy and lactation and of young children.

The choice of materials for carcinogenic studies could profitably be guided by reports of toxicity to livestock, and by the known correlations between carcinogenic activity and cytotoxic, goitrogenic, growth inhibitory and oestrogenic action. In appropriate cases selection could be based on structures, as in the case of pyrrolizidine alkaloids, α,β-unsaturated lactones, etc.

The difficulties are discussed of connecting a chronic disease, such as cancer, with a causative agent, which might have been ingested a long time before the disease becomes apparent.

References

ALLCROFT, R., and LEWIS, G., Groundnut toxicity in cattle: Experimental poisoning of calves and a report on clinical effects in older cattle. *Vet. Rec.* **75**, 487—493 (1963).

ARONOW, L., and KERDEL-VEGAS, F., Selenocystathionine, a pharmacologically active factor in the seeds of *Lecythis ollaria*. *Nature (Lond.)* **205**, 1185—1186 (1965).

ASPREY, G. F., and THORNTON, P., Medicinal plants of Jamaica. *W. Indian med. J.* part I, **2**, 233—252 (1953); — part II, **3**, 17—41 (1954); — part III, **4**, 69—82 (1955); — part IV, **4**, 145—168 (1955).

BACHELARD, H. S., and TRIKOJUS, V. M., Plant thioglycosides and the problem of endemic goitre in Australia. *Nature (Lond.)* **185**, 80—82 (1960).

BARNES, J. M., and BUTLER, W. H., Carcinogenic activity of aflatoxin to rats. *Nature (Lond.)* **202**, 1016 (1964).

BOYLAND, E., ROE, F. J. C., GORROD, J. W., and MITCHLEY, B. C. V., The carcinogenicity of nitrosoanabasine; a possible constituent of tobacco smoke. *Brit. J. Cancer* **18**, 265—270 (1964).

BRADBURY, R. B., and WHITE, D. E., Estrogens and related substances in plants. *Vitam. and Horm.* **12**, 207—233 (1954).

BROWN, J. M. M., Biochemical lesions in the pathogenesis of geeldikkop *(Tribulosis ovis)* and enzootic icterus in sheep in South Africa. *Ann. N.Y. Acad. Sci.* **104**, 504—538 (1963).

BURRELL, R. J. W., Esophageal cancer among Bantu in the Transkei. *J. nat. Cancer Inst.* **28**, 495—514 (1962).

BUTENANDT, A., and JACOBI, H., The female sexual hormone. X. The preparation of a crystalline plant tokokinin (thelykinin) and its identification with the α-follicular hormone. *Hoppe-Seylers Z. physiol. Chem.* **218**, 104—112 (1933).

CAIN, J. C., Miroestrol, an oestrogen from the plant *Pueraria Mirifica*. *Nature (Lond.)* **188**, 774—777 (1960).

CHOPRA, R. N., *Indigenous drugs of India*. Calcutta: The Arts Press 1933.

CULPEPER'S *Complete herbal*. (ed. C. F. LLOYD). London: Herbert Joseph Ltd. 1947.

CULVENOR, C. C. J., and SMITH, L. W., Alkaloids of *Crotalaria trifoliastrum* Willd and *C. aridicola* Domin. 1. Methyl ethers of supinidine and retronecine. *Aust. J. Chem.* **15**, 121—129 (1962).

DALZIEL, J. M., *The useful plants of West Tropical Africa*. London: Crown Agents 1937.

DICKENS, F., and JONES, H. E. H., Carcinogenic activity of a series of reactive lactones and related substances. *Brit. J. Cancer* **15**, 85—100 (1961).

— — The carcinogenic action of aflatoxin after its subcutaneous injection in the rat. *Brit. J. Cancer* **17**, 691—698 (1963a).

— — Further studies on the carcinogenic and growth inhibitory activity of lactones and related substances. *Brit. J. Cancer* **17**, 100—108 (1963b).

— — Further studies on the carcinogenic action of certain lactones and related substances in the rat and mouse. *Brit. J. Cancer* **19**, 392—403 (1965).

DIOSCORIDES, *Greek herbal* (GUNTER, R. T., ed.). London: Oxford University Press 1934.

DRAGENDORFF, G., *Die Heilpflanzen der verschiedenen Völker und Zeiten*. Stuttgart: Ferdinand Enke 1898.

FINDLAY, G. M., Observations on primary liver carcinoma in West African soldiers. *J. roy. micr. Soc.* **70**, 166—172 (1950).

FORGACS, J., and CARLL, W. T., Mycotoxicoses. *Advanc. vet. Sci.* **7**, 274—382 (1962).

HASKELL, T. H., RYDER, A., and BARTZ, Q. R., Elaiomycin, a new tuberculostatic antibiotic. *Antibiot. and Chemother.* **4**, 141—144 (1954).

HAYNES, L. J., Physiologically active unsaturated lactones. *Quart. Rev. chem. Soc. of London* **2**, 46—72 (1948).

HEFTMANN, E., Ko SHUI-TZE, and BENNETT, R. D., Identification of estrone in date seeds by thin-layer chromatography. *Naturwissenschaften* **52**, 431—432 (1965).

HURST, E., *The poison plants of New South Wales*. Sydney: N.S.W. 1943.

KAWAMATA, J., NAKABAYASHI, N, KAWAI, A., FUJITA, H., IMANISHI, M., and IKEGAMI, R., Carcinogenic effect of actinomycin. *Biken's J.* **2**, 105—112 (1959).

KELLY, R. B., DANIELS, E. G., and SPAULDING, L. B., Cytotoxicity of cardiac principles. *J. med. Chem.* **8**, 547—548 (1965).

KENNAWAY, E. L., Cancer of the liver in the Negro in Africa and in America. *Cancer Res.* **4**, 571—577 (1944).

KERDEL-VEGAS, F., WAGNER, F., RUSSELL, P. B., GRANT, N. H., ALBURN, H. E., CLARK, D. E., and MILLER, J. A., Structure of the pharmacologically active factor in the seeds of *Lecythis ollaria*. *Nature (Lond.)* **205**, 1186—1187 (1965).

KINGSBURY, J. M., *Poisonous plants of the United States and Canada*. Englewood Cliffs, N.J.: Prentice-Hall 1964.

Kirtikar, K. R., Basu, B. D., and An, I. C. S., *Indian medicinal plants,* 2nd ed. Allahabad 1936.

Kobayashi, A., and Matsumoto, H., Studies on methylazoxymethanol, the aglycone of cycasin. Isolation, biological and chemical properties. *Arch. Biochem.* **110**, 373—380 (1965).

Kraybill, H. F., and Shimkin, M. B., Carcinogenesis related to foods contamination by processing and fungal metabolites. *Advanc. Cancer Res.* **8**, 191—248 (1964).

Kupchan, S. M., Hemingway, R. J., and Doskotch, R. W., Tumor inhibitors IV Apocannoside and cymarin, the cytotoxic principles of *Apocynum cannabinum* L. *J. med. Chem.* **7**, 803—804 (1964).

Lacassagne, A., Apparition de cancers de la mamelle chez la souris mâle, soumise à des injections de folliculine. *C. R. Acad. Sci. (Paris)* **195**, 630—632 (1932).

Langley, B. W., Lythgoe, B., and Riggs, N. V., Macrozamin, part. II. The aliphatic azoxy structure of the aglycone part. *J. chem. Soc.* 2309—2316 (1951).

Laqueur, G. L., Carcinogenic effects of cycad meal and cycasin (methyl-azoxymethanol glycoside) in rats and effects of cycasin in germ-free rats. *Fed. Proc.* **23**, 1386—1387 (1964).

—, and Matsumoto, H., Neoplasms in female Fischer rats following intraperitoneal injection of methylazoxymethanol. *J. nat. Cancer Inst.* **37**, 217—232 (1966).

— Mickelsen, O., Whiting, M. G., and Kurland, L. T., Carcinogenic properties of nuts from *Cycas Circinalis* L. indigenous to guam. *J. nat. Cancer Inst.* **31**, 919—933 (1963).

Lancaster, M. C., Jenkins, F. P., and Philp, J. McL., Toxicity associated with certain samples of groundnuts. *Nature (Lond.)* **192**, 1095—1096 (1961).

Magee, P. N., and Schoental, R., Carcinogenesis by nitroso-compounds. *Brit. med. Bull.* **20**, 102—106 (1964).

Matteis, F. de, Donnelly, A. J., and Runge, W. J., The effect of prolonged administration of griseofulvin in mice with reference to sex differences. *Cancer Res.* **26**, 721—726 (1966).

Merwe, K. J. van der, Steyn, P. S., Fourie, L., Scott, B. de, and Theron, J. J., Ochratoxin A, a toxic metabolite produced by *Aspergillus ochraceus* Wilh. *Nature (Lond.)* **205**, 1112—1113 (1965).

Mickelsen, O., Campbell, E., Yang, M., Mugera, G., and Whitehair, C. K., Studies with cycad. *Fed. Proc.* **23**, 1363—1365 (1964).

Miller, M. W., *The Pfizer handbook of microbial metabolites.* London: McGraw-Hill Book Co. Inc. 1961.

Nadkarni, K. M., *Indian materia medica.* Bombay: Nadkarni 1927.

O'Gara, R. W., Brown, J. M., and Whiting, M. G., Induction of hepatic and renal tumours by the topical application of aqueous extract of cycad nut to artificial skin ulcers in mice. *Fed. Proc.* **23**, 1383 (1964).

Perrott, E., *Matières premières du règne végétal.* Paris: Masson & Cie. 1943/44.

Plowright, W., Malignant neoplasia of the oesophagus and rumen of cattle in Kenya. *J. comp. Path.* **65**, 108—12 (1955).

Proceedings of the Third Conference on the Toxicity of Cycads. *Fed. Proc.* **23**, 1337—1388 (1964).

Read, B. E., *Chinese medicinal plants,* 3rd ed. Peking 1936.

Riggs, N. V., Decomposition and carcinogenic activity of azoxyglycosides. *Nature (Lond.)* **207**, 632 (1965).

Sakshaug, J., Sögnen, E., Hansen, M. A., and Koppang, N., Dimethylnitrosamine, its hepatotoxic effect in sheep and its occurrence in toxic batches of herring meal. *Nature (Lond.)* **206**, 1261—1262 (1965).

Schoental, R., Kwashiorkor-like syndrome and other pathological changes in rats as a result of feeding with senecio alkaloids (isatidine). *Voeding* **16**, 268—285 (1955).

— Liver lesions in young rats suckled by mothers treated with the pyrrolizidine (senecio) alkaloids, lasiocarpine and retrorsine. *J. Path. Bact.* **77**, 485—495 (1959).

— Liver disease and "natural" hepatotoxins. *Bull. Wld Hlth Org.* **29**, 823—833 (1963).

— Carcinogenesis by polycyclic aromatic hydrocarbons and by certain other carcinogens. In: E. Clar, *Polycyclic hydrocarbons,* vol. 1, p. 133—160. London: Academic Press 1964.

— Aflatoxins. *Ann. Rev. Pharmacol.* (in press) (1967).

Shrift, A., A selenium cycle in nature. *Nature (Lond.)* **201**, 1304—1305 (1964).

Skarzynski, B., An estrogenic substance from plant material *Nature (Lond.).* **131**, 766 (1933).

Staner, P., and Boutique, R., *Matériaux pour l'étude des Plantes Médicinales Indigènes du Congo Belge.* Bruxelles: Van Campenhout 1937.

Steyn, D. C., *The toxicology of plants in South Africa.* Johannesburg: Central News Agency 1934.

Trowell, H. C., Medical examination of 500 African railway workers. *Afr. med. J.* 311 bis 321 (1948).

WAGNER, J. C., SLEGGS, C. A., and MARCHAND, P., Diffuse pleural mesothelioma and asbestos exposure in the North Western Cape Province. *Brit. J. indust. Med.* **17**, 260—271 (1960).

WATT, J. M., and BREYER-BRANDWIJK, M. G., *The medicinal and poisonous plants of Southern and Eastern Africa.* Edinburgh: Livingstone 1962.

WEISS, U., Comments on chemistry of cycads. *Fed. Proc.* **23**, 1357—1360 (1964).

WESTON, HURST, E., and PAGET, G. E., Protoporphyrin, cirrhosis and hepatomata in the livers of mice given griseofulvin. *Brit. J. Derm.* **75**, 105—112 (1963).

WHITING, M. G., Toxicity of cycads. *Economic Bot.* **17**, 270—302 (1963).

— Food practices in ALS foci in Japan, the Marianas, and New Guinea. *Fed. Proc.* **23**, 1343—1345 (1964).

WOGAN, G. N., (edit.) *Mycotoxins in foodstuffs.* M.I.T. Press, Massachusetts Institute of Technology 1965.

WREN, R. C., *Potter's new cyclopaedia of botanical drugs and preparations* (re-edit. R. W. WREN). London: Potter & Clarke Ltd. 1956.

Discussion

Shabad: Experimental studies performed in our laboratory on the possible carcinogenic action of a new alkaloid, Sarrasin, with valuable antispasmodic activity, gave negative results. No tumours were seen in 89 rats or 122 mice after 2 years observation. Total dosage was 200 mg for rats and 100 mg for mice. The structure has no double bond, and Dr. SCHOENTAL, predicted from its chemical structure that it would not be carcinogenic. She was right.

Progesterone and Mammary Carcinogenesis

WILLIAM E. POEL

*Associate Professor, Director, Laboratory for Experimental Carcinogenesis,
Graduate School of Public Health, University of Pittsburgh,
Pittsburgh, Pa. U.S.A.*

Historical: The background for laboratory findings of a relationship between ovarian hormones and mammary cancer may be found in publications dating back to the turn of this century. The role of the functional corpus luteum in suppression of ovulation was suggested by BEARD, in 1898, and was demonstrated as a physiologic phenomenon by LOEB in 1911 [1, 2]. Later studies showed that the principal hormone of the corpus luteum is progesterone: in adequate amounts and in the presence of estrogen, it can prolong the luteal phase of the estrus cycle and suppress ovulation in the intact female. The physiologic effects of progesterone, synergized by estrogen in the intact animal, provide the basis for the current form of oral contraception, in which daily ingestion of a synthetic progestin plus a trace amount of estrogen is relied upon to suppress ovulation in the human.

There have been relatively few studies of humans or laboratory animals to show the long term biologic effects of the ingested synthetic progestins, or to clarify the long term effects of persistent disruption in the normal female cycle, induced by that practice. An impressive number of laboratory investigations do however, indicate direct relationships between excessive doses of ovarian hormones and mammary carcinogenesis.

On the one hand, LATHROP and LOEB, in 1916, observed that ovariectomy at an early age lowered the incidence, or completely prevented the appearance of mammary tumors in mice [3]. The work of these investigators provided a laboratory demonstration of BEATSON's observation in 1896 [4] that ovariectomy of premenopausal women with breast cancer induced regression of the malignancy in some patients. A more positive indication of the dependence of mammary tumors upon ovarian hormones was reported by LACASSAGNE in 1932, when he induced mammary tumors in male mice by means of estrogens [5], while CANTAROW and his associates in 1948 described the enhancement of mammary carcinogenesis by administering progesterone to rats fed the carcinogen precursor, 2-acetylaminofluorene [6]. More recent studies by HUGGINS have demonstrated the same phenomenon in rats fed the carcinogen 20-methylcholanthrene (MCA) [7]. The consensus, arising from laboratory investigations since earlier studies, is that ovarian hormones play a major role in the growth of mammary tumors, and are essential for the induction of mammary tumors with a polycyclic carcinogen [8, 9, 16].

Since the etiology of mammary cancer in the human is still unknown, even though man is affected by carcinogens in his every-day environment, there is a practical rationale for studying the joint effects of known carcinogens and progestins in experimental animals. The study now reported describes the effects of a prolonged progestational state, induced by repeated injections of progesterone, on the development of mammary cancers in sexually mature mice predisposed to those malignancies.

the virus alone, and to test the role of progesterone on their development, the experimental plan, shown on the next slide, was employed (Table I).

With reference to Table I, earlier studies had shown that methylcholanthrene, fed to this strain, enhanced mammary tumor development. Consequently, in the first group, mice received approximately 0.5 mg. of MCA in Tween-60 by

Table I. *Experimental plan to ascertain the effect of progesterone on mammary tumor induction in C_3H virgin ♀ mice*

Group		Treatment
I	a) Prog /P.O.	2.5 mg. progesterone in 0.05 ml. peanut oil, subcutaneously, $5\times$/week for 19 weeks
	b) MCA/Tw-60	0.5 mg. 20-methylcholanthrene in 0.1 ml. Tween-60, by gavage, $2\times$/wk, starting 2 weeks after "a"
II	a) (C) P.O.	0.05 ml. peanut oil, subcutaneously. $5\times$/wk for 19 weeks
	b) MCA/Tw-60	0.5 mg. MCA in 0.1 ml. Tween-60, by gavage, $2\times$/wk, starting 2 weeks after "a"
III	a) Prog/P.O.	2.5 mg. progesterone in 0.05 ml. peanut oil, subcutaneously, $5\times$/wk for 19 weeks
	b) (C) Tw-60	0.1 ml. Tween-60 by gavage, in lieu of "b"
IV	a) (C) P.O.	0.05 ml. peanut oil, subcutaneously. $5\times$/wk for 19 weeks
	b) (C) Tw-60	0.1 ml. Tween-60 by gavage, in lieu of "b"
V_1	a) (C) P.O.	0.05 ml. P.O., subcutaneously, as control treatment in lieu of "a"
V_2	b) (C) Tw-60	0.1 ml. Tween-60 by gavage, in lieu of "b"
V_3	0 (C)	Untreated

Materials and Methods: C_3H female mice, bought from the Jackson Laboratory, harbor a virus, the Mammary Tumor Agent (MTA) which may induce mammary adenocarcinomas in approximately 10% of virgin females by the time they are 39 weeks of age [10]. The histology of a typical mammary adenocarcinoma found in such animals is shown in the first slide. Here we see a characteristic tumor, with acinar, duct-like, and cystic structures. It may be hemorrhagic or necrotic in some areas. A portion of this tissue is shown on the next slide at higher magnification. To insure a greater incidence of mammary tumors than would be elicited by

stomach tube, twice a week, concurrent with a daily injection of Progesterone, to ascertain the effects of both agents. The second group was treated with MCA, but did not receive progesterone, while the third group received progesterone but no MCA. The fourth group was treated with the solvents, peanut oil and Tween-60; while the fifth group was treated to show the effects, if any, of each solvent individually, and to ascertain the characteristics of tumors in untreated females.

The results obtained are summarized in Table II. The most impressive observation here is the relatively rapid development of multiple mammary tumors in all effectively exposed mice of Group I (treated with MCA and progesterone). The acceleration of tumor genesis and growth in this group is striking, since all effectively exposed animals (23/23) had large, multiple tumors before the 25th week, when the first tumor was observed in the group treated with MCA only. By contrast, in Groups IV and V, we see that none of the control animals developed a palpable tumor during the same period of time. With reference to Group III, the earlier development of mammary tumors in two mice treated with progesterone, as compared with the controls, suggested the possibility that the persistent progestational state in those animals may have enhanced viral mammary carcinogenesis. Further observations in our laboratory to date have confirmed this possibility [15].

tumors in the animal treated solely with MCA, we see prominent masses in the one on the right. These tumors are seen better on the next slide, where it is apparent that mammary glands 1 through 5 are involved, on one or both sides of the body, in the progesterone — MCA treated mouse.

Histology: The histology of the induced tumors is interesting, insofar as the

Table II. *Effect of Progesterone on mammary carcinogenesis in C_3H/Jax V ♀ mice*

Treatment of C_3H ♀'s*	No. with MTs No. exposed > 13 wks.	% MTs by 27th week	Weeks preceding development of a tumor > 6 mm in diameter			
			No. of mice with tumors			
			17—19	20—22	23—25	26—27
I Prog'n MCA	23/23	(100)	6	15	2	0
II P.O. MCA	5/24	(21)			1	4
III Prog'n Tw-60	2/25	(8)			1	1
IV P.O. Tw-60	0/25	(0)				0
V P.O.	0/8					
Tw-60	0/7	(0)				0
None	0/10					

* Prog'n — 2.5 mg. progesterone in 0.05 ml. peanut oil, subcutaneously, 5×/week for 19 weeks.
   MCA— 0.5 mg. 20-methylcholanthrene in 0.1 ml. Tween-60, by gavage, 2×/wk, starting two weeks after"Prog'n", until a tumor developed.
P.O. — 0.05 ml. peanut oil, subcutaneously, 5×/week for 19 weeks.
Tw-60 — 0.1 ml. Tween-60, by gavage, 2×/week, until death.

The next slide shows a gross comparison of a mouse on the left, treated only with MCA, and one on the right that received Progesterone concurrently with MCA during the same period of time. By contrast with the absence of morphology suggests a relationship between the tumor and the primary viral or chemical carcinogen, rather that with the hormone. The next slide shows a section of adenocarcinoma in a mouse treated only with progesterone. The structure is uniformly acinar, and the basic tumor cells are cuboidal, arranged to form small duct-like cavities or cyst-like spaces. The supporting connective tissue in this instance is quite prominent, although not malignant. Secretory activity and cyst formation may be a striking characteristic, as seen in portions of this slide. The next slide is of a portion that was predominantly cystic; yet, there are papillary ingrowths into the cystic cavity. The tumor cells may also proliferate to form solid masses or bands of cells, with no glandular structure.

Let us now consider the capacity of these tumors to metastasize spontaneously as an index of their malignancy. The first shows the primary tumor of a progesterone treated mouse; its acinar structure is not as well organized as in the preceding example. The next slide shows metastasis to the lungs by way of the pulmonary arteries. The entire lumen is obliterated, while the vasculer wall shows a small portion infiltrated by malignant cells. A similar metastasis in an adjacent area, at higher magnification, shows a more solid growth of tumor cells in the blood vessel: as in the preceding example, a few areas suggest duct or cyst formation and secretory activity.

The way in which the tumor cells reach the lungs is suggested by the next two slides: the first shows a micronodule, or tumor clump within the right ventricle of the heart; a peripheral portion of the lung in the lower left field shows an established metastasis of the same acinar structure. The malignant embolus in the heart is seen at slightly higher magnification in the next slide. The lungs of the same animal are seen with pulmonary arteries obliterated by tumor growth. The metastasis, obviously, is a structural duplicate of the primary tumor.

To this point, we have seen examples of the tumors developed in Group III by mice that received repeated injections of progesterone only. The tumors were typical mammary adenocarcinomas; they are basically the same tumors as those developed by untreated animals of the same strain, but of an older age.

By contrast, we will now review tumors induced in mice treated with Progesterone and MCA.

The first slide of this group is of a primary malignancy — obviously a bizarre secretory mammary adenocarcinoma, seen surrounding a lymph node. The lymph node itself has been involved by direct extension of the neoplasm. A further indication of the malignant capacity of the tumors in this animal is seen in the metastatic mass in a pulmonary artery. The metastasis usually reflects the structure of the primary tumor: consequently, the primary source of this metastasis probably was not the same as the primary shown on the preceding slide, of the same animal. I make this point to emphasize that methylcholanthrene, fed to these mice may produce many structurally different mammary tumors in the same mouse, as compared with the more uniform pattern of adenocarcinoma induced in this strain by the MTA (virus) acting either alone, or in combination with progesterone. The variety of mammary tumors induced by the chemical carcinogen, MCA, are suggested by the following examples, (Table III) all taken from the same case. The first is of a papillary adenocarcinoma: the next, from the same animal, shows a nodule of a keratinizing epidermoid carcinoma. Between it and the overlying skin we see small patches of intraductal carcinoma. The next slide shows an adjacent area of a more typical mammary keratinizing epidermoid carcinoma. This obviously malignant carcinoma contains a core of connective tissue cells that are very suspicious looking. And the next slide shows that these are indeed malignant fibroblasts, in an area of collision between a carcinoma and a sarcoma. The next slide shows a higher power view of both malignancies: the sarcoma is apparently infiltrating and outgrowing the carcinoma.

Areas of collision between histogenetically different malignancies were quite common in these mice. From the same case, we see, on the next slide, a sarcoma in collision with, and infiltrating, an adenocarcinoma; on the next slide a carcinosarcoma infiltrating a keratinizing epidermoid carcinoma, and on the next slide, an epidermoid carcinoma infiltrating and destroying an adenocarcinoma.

In another case of this same group, treated with MCA and progesterone, we

the presence of a primary secretory intraductal carcinoma.

Obviously then, tumors in these animals may metastasize either by the intravascular, or lymphatic route; or they may infiltrate through the vascular wall and spread by both routes.

The role of progesterone in mammary carcinogenesis: Let us return now, to consider the tumors elicited in Group III,

Table III. *Mammary tumors induced in virgin female C₃H/Jax mice*

Tumor type	Carcinogenic agents	
	MTV*	MTV + MCA**
Adenocarcinoma (acinar, papillary, cystic, solid, misc.)	+	+
Epidermoid carcinoma (keratinizing and nonkeratinizing)	±	+
Adeno-acanthoma	—	+
Anaplastic carcinoma	—	+
Carcino-sarcoma	—	+
Fibro-sarcoma	—	+
Sarcoma, $\bar{c}$ or $\bar{s}$ giant cells	—	+

* Endogenous mammary tumor virus.
** MTV+20-Methylcholanthrene by gavage.

+ seen frequently; ± rarely seen; — not observed.

find an adenoacanthoma in the cervical region. The adenomatous and acanthomatous structures are seen in the next slide, at slightly higher magnification. In another area of the same animal is an anaplastic carcinoma, which, we see in this slide, has infiltrated the dermis, panniculus carnosis, and subcutaneous tissue. In a kidney of this animal a few suspicious microfoci were seen (Point out at least 3 areas). Higher magnification of two foci shows that these are indeed tumor cell emboli, from the same anaplastic primary carcinoma; each embolic clump is apparently in a perivascular lymphatic space.

By contrast, in a perivascular lymphatic space, in the lungs of this animal, we see a metastatic nidus, that suggests

in the animals treated with progesterone. All that developed in this group, before and after Table II was compiled, were typical mammary adenocarcinomas, of a basic acinar structure, with areas composed of fluid filled cysts, papillary invaginations, and glandular or solid cords, bands, and nests of cells. Adenocarcinomas of this type have been reported frequently in mice with the MTA [11]. By contrast, those elicited in Group I, in the animals treated with MCA and progesterone, comprised a wide spectrum of types and variants (Table III), identical in pattern and histogenesis to those of Group II, treated only with MCA. The obvious effects of progesteron were therefore associated with a profoundly more rapid development andae higher incidence of mammary tumors, but with no change in the histologic appearance of the tumors induced in its absence.

The question may be raised as to whether the effects of progesterone enhance the malignant capacity of the induced tumors. The capacity for metastasis of the induced adenocarcinomas was obvious and frequent, as shown in earlier slides, of Group III. Yet they were probably the least invasive of the tumors induced; for in the areas of collision with other tumors they were infiltrated and outgrown by epidermoid carcinomas, which, in turn were infiltrated and outgrown by the sarcomatous neoplasms. Whether progesterone played a role in enhancing the incidence, the variety, and the local or metastatic invasiveness of the tumors induced is yet to be ascertained. That possibility is not to be over looked, in view of a report in the literature that exogenous progesterone, administered daily, may enhance the metastasis of a transplantable pituitary tumor in mice [12].

The role of progesterone, or the anovulatory state induced by it may be considered in mammary carcinogenesis by reviewing the concept of a "cocarcinogen", as originated by SHEAR in 1938. The term was originally meant to designate a class of agents not carcinogenic per se, which enhanced the effect of a carcinogen, especially when the carcinogen was weak or administered under conditions otherwise inadequate for tumor development [13]. Later studies demonstrated that most if not all substances designated as "co-carcinogens" or "promoters" were either tumor-inducing agents that were tested under conditions which, at first, did not disclose their full carcinogenic potential, (i.e., croton oil, urethane), solvents that

increased the solubility and penetrability of residual carcinogens applied to the skin of mice (i.e., Tween-60), or crude solvents, totally inactive for tumor genesis, that were contaminated with trace amounts of laboratory or industrial carcinogens (i.e., phenol, or the basic oil fraction of high temperature coal tar or creosote oil [14]). An adequate definition for a hypothetical substance was thus created, which persisted in the literature. Since neither in this nor any study published to date is there conclusive evidence that progesterone per se is carcinogenic, progesterone, tentatively, might be considered a co-carcinogen for mammary carcinogenesis; possibly the first co-carcinogen to fit the definition proposed by SHEAR.

Whether the synthetic progestins currently available for human contraceptive purposes have co-carcinogenic effects similar to those of exogenous progesterone is yet to be established. The co-carcinogenicity of 2 oral contraceptives has since been reported. [POEL, W., Pituitary tumors in mice after prolonged feeding of synthetic progestins. Science 154, 402—403 (1966).] GRUENSTEIN and co-workers (1964) reported that the synthetic progestin, Norethynodrel, (in "Enovid") neither enhanced nor retarded mammary carcinogenesis evoked in rats by gastric intubations of MCA; they also found that progesterone did not increase the incidence of mammary tumors, although the mean tumor appearance time may have been shortened. Preliminary studies in our laboratory with the same, and another commercially available oral contraceptive showed each to be ineffective in altering the estrus cycle; they could not inhibit ovulation even when fed to mice at dose levels up to 25 times that effective in the human female: they were equally ineffective in altering mammary tumor induction in those animals. It may be that an adequate test of these synthetic progestins requires a test animal other than mouse or rat.

The divergence in reported findings may be more apparent than real, in view of differences in experimental test animals, agents, and test conditions. They do not necessarily represent conflicting observations: they do represent the need for further investigations to clarify our present limited understanding of hormone-carcinogenesis relationships. Laboratory results to resolve these and related questions with experimental animals should be available long before adequate epidemiologic studies give definitive answers pertinent to man. Although narrow limits must be imposed on the interpretation of laboratory data, and those should not be extrapolated directly to man, such data may suggest a parallel hazard for the human which may require decades to evolve. In that sense, the observations now reported for at least one experimental animal system suggest, in part, the need for greater caution than has been demonstrated to date in the indiscriminate human consumption of newer oral contraceptives and synthetic progestins, and the need for clinico-epidemiologic explorations for a possible human parallel to those seen experimentally.

Summary

A prolonged anovulatory state was induced in C_3H female mice by daily injections of progesterone. One group of animals so treated was also fed the polycyclic carcinogen 20-methylcholanthrene (MCA), by gavage. A striking acceleration in mammary tumor genesis and tumor growth was obtained in the animals treated with MCA and progesterone, as compared with those subjected solely to MCA feedings. An acceleration in mammary tumor growth was also indicated for those mice treated with progesterone, as compared with those that were acted upon solely by the mammary tumor virus endogenous in this strain. The histology of the induced tumors was associated with the primary chemical or viral carcinogen, rather than with the carcinogen-enhancing effects of progesterone. In light of the laboratory findings, the role of exogenous progesterone is described to be that of a potent co-carcinogen.

The absence of comparable epidemiologic data indicates the need for clinical and epidemiologic studies to ascertain the long term effects of a prolonged progestational state in the human, and suggests greater caution than has been demonstrated to date in the use of oral contraceptive agents for the induction of prolonged anovulatory periods.

References

[1] Beard, J., The rhythm of reproduction in mammalia. *Anat. Anz.* 14, 97—102 (1898).

[2] Loeb, L., Über die Bedeutung des Corpus luteum für die Periodizität des sexuellen Zyklus beim weiblichen Säugetierorganismus. *Dtsche. med. Wschr.* 37, 17—21 (1911).

[3] Lathrop, A., and Loeb, L., Further investigations on the origin of tumors in mice. III. On the part played by internal secretion in the spontaneous development of tumors. *J. Cancer Res.* 1, 1—19 (1916).

[4] Beatson, G. T., On the treatment of inoperable cases of carcinoma of the mamma. Suggestions for a new method of treatment, with illustrative cases. *Lancet* 1896 II, 104, 162.

[5] Lacassagne, A., Apparition de cancers de la mamelle chez la souris male, soumis a des injections de folliculine. *C.R. Acad. Sci.* (Paris) 195, 630—632 (1932).

[6] Cantarow, A., The influence of sex hormones on mammary tumors induced by 2-acetaminofluorene. *Cancer Res.* 8, 412—417 (1948).

[7] HUGGINS, C., BRIZIARELLI, M. D., and SUTTON, H., Rapid induction of mammary carcinoma in the rat and the influence of hormones on the tumors. *J. exp. Med.* **109**, 25—42 (1959).

[8] DAO, T., and SUNDERLAND, H., Mammary carcinogenesis by 3-methylcholanthrene. I. Hormonal aspects in tumor induction and growth. *J. nat. Cancer Inst.* **23**, 567—585 (1959).

[9] FURTH, J., Influences of host factors on the growth of neoplastic cells. *Cancer Res.* **23**, 21—34 (1963).

[10] MURRAY, W. S., Biological significance of factors influencing the incidence of mammary cancer in mice. *J. nat. Cancer Inst.* **34**, 21—41 (1965).

[11] DUNN, T., Morphology of mammary tumors in mice. *Physiopathology of Cancer*, 2nd ed. (F. Homberger, ed.), p. 38. 1959.

[12] POEL, W. E., Progesterone and tumour metastasis. *Lancet* **1963** II, 970—972.

[13] SHEAR, M. J., Studies in carcinogenesis V. Methyl derivatives of 1:2-benzanthracene. *Amer. J. Cancer* **33**, 499—537 (1938).

[14] POEL, W. E., Carcinogens and minimal carcinogenic doses. *Science* **123**, 588, 589 (1956).

[15] — The co-carcinogenic effect of exogenous progesterone in C₃H ♀ mice. *Proc. Amer. Ass. Cancer Res.* **1**, 56, 1966.

[16] KIRSCHBAUM, A., [*Ca. Res.* **17**, 432 (1957)] described estrogen to be a carcinogen comparable to methylcholanthrene for the development of mouse mammary cancer. As indicated by BERN [*Science* **131**, 10—39 (1960)], estrogen has been considered the prime hormonal inducer of mouse mammary cancer since the pioneering studies of LOEB [2].

Discussion

Della Porta: May I ask Dr. POEL why he used a strain of mice which carries the BITTNER virus and which develop mammary tumours in 100% of cases if the mice are kept long enough? It is known that hormonal manipulations, including oestrogen and progesterone administration, may influence the development of mammary tumours induced by viruses or chemical carcinogens, and therefore I think it would have been better to use an agent-free animal. I congratulate you on your beautiful histological demonstration, but I feel it is difficult to attach importance to different microscopic pictures in mammary tumours, particularly since you are comparing 28 methylcholanthrene-induced tumours with only 2 progesterone-induced tumours. Finally, in relation to the relevance of your experiment to oral contraception in humans, would you like to comment on the physiological differences in hormone-control in the two species and the likely effect of these differences on mammary tumour development.

Davey: The dose of progesterone used in your studies, namely 2.5 mg./mouse is so excessive that I doubt whether your results have any practical significance.

Poel: A much lower dose, say 0.5 mg./mouse, would probably have given the same result.

Kreyberg: May I call attention to two points. Firstly, it is well known that a single carcinogen may produce many types of tumours and that a single type of tumour may

be produced by many different carcinogens. In the present case the tumour type may not be primarily decided by the carcinogen but secondarily influenced by the hormonal factors. Secondly, I think it is permissible to use the term "carcino-sarcoma" as a pet name, provided that we have it in mind that we are most probably dealing with a purely epithelial tumour, an "epidermoide fuso-cellulare" as G. ROUSSY termed it in the early days of tar cancer. There are similar human tumours in the mouth, oesophagus, lung and other sites.

Doll: The present subject is one of the most important in this symposium — and one of the most complex. It is difficult enough to predict from animal experiments that a substance is likely to be a local carcinogen in man; but it is doubly difficult to predict the effect of a hormone. Thus it is doubtful whether Dr. POEL's experiments have relevance to predicting the effect of oral contraceptives in women. Some element in the menstrual cycle is probably responsible for the high rate of breast cancer in women, since the rate of increase of breast cancer incidence declines sharply after the menopause and the total incidence is reduced by the induction of an artificial menopause. Relevant animal tests of substances that disturb the menstrual cycle should, therefore, be made on mammals that have a corresponding cycle. Whether oral contraceptives can be regarded as having a primarily progesterone effect is also doubtful. The progestens used are not identical with progesterone; human progesterone secretion is diminished and the principal effect of the substances may be due to their oestrogen content. On theoretical grounds they are at least as likely to reduce breast cancer incidence as to increase it.

Chassagne: I should like to ask a practical question. What information is there on the effects of oral contraceptive preparations administered *orally* to experimental animals?

Poel: We saw no effects in mice fed oral contraceptive drugs. The mouse and the rat apparently metabolize oral contraceptives in a different way from man: oral administration of these agents did not alter the estrus cycle of the rodent.

Frazer: Oral contraceptives appear to be remarkably efficacious. They may, therefore, be the drug of choice in a patient to whom pregnancy is a serious risk. In such a patient, the cancer risk, if one exists at all, may be relatively unimportant. The use of oral contraceptives for family planning is another matter, especially if it involves relatively young people taking these drugs regularly over long periods. This problem is more akin to that associated with the use of food additives. An adequate evaluation of any possible cancer risk is essential. It is difficult, however, to plan suitable animal tests, since the biological effects in different species, especially in small laboratory animals, bear little or no resemblance to those produced in human subjects. The problem is a real and an urgent one, and calls for more research.

Shabad: I should like to draw attention to two points; firstly, the tumours produced are of a great histopathological variety, the range being similar to that seen in response to methylcholanthrene. What then is the role of progesterone in these experiments? Are you sure that it is a co-carcinogenic role, is it not possible that like croton oil and other so-called co-carcinogens it may be a weak carcinogen? Secondly, your report, though very interesting and stimulating, is really only the beginning of a research programme. It is necessary to conduct experiments in other species of animal at various dose levels and using various protocols. I see the need in experimentation to increase the exposure to a potential carcinogen to levels above normal human exposure, but in the present case it would be more realistic to test doses actually used in life.

Poel: In answer to Dr. DELLA PORTA, we used C_3H female mice because we wanted an experimental model, or a laboratory counterpart for the human female who is bound to develop mammary cancer It is a popular misconception that 100% of C_3H females with the Bittner mammary tumour virus develop mammary tumours. In our laboratory the incidence of tumours in control animals of the C_3H/Jax line varies from 8% to 25%. We wanted as high a tumour incidence as possible in order to determine the effect, if any, of progesterone treatment. Therefore we administered a chemical carcinogen that would insure mammary tumour development in all animals. Progesterone hastened the appearance of mammary tumours and increased their incidence: all progesterone-plus-carcinogen treated animals had mammary tumours by the time the first tumour developed in the group treated with carcinogen only. We now have studies under way in which mice, presumably free of the mammary tumour virus, are used.

I should like to emphasize that there is no evidence in this report nor in any report I could find in the literature that progesterone *per se* is a carcinogen. For this reason, I referred to the effect of progesterone as a *co-carcinogenic* effect.

With regard to the differences between the hormonal or physiological constitutions of rodents and humans, and to the influence of these differences on mammary tumour development, I should like to point out that although the differences are obvious, the similarities are unknown. We know that in mice mammary tumour development depends on at least three factors: (a) the biological or genetical background of the animal, (b) the hormonal status, and (c) the presence of carcinogenic agents which, in the C_3H mouse, include a late-acting virus and an exogenous chemical agent. We know also that radiation may induce mammary cancer experimentally. By contrast we are totally ignorant of the factors responsible for breast cancer in the human.

Ignorance of the factors responsible for mammary cancer development in the human is not a valid basis for saying that the causes of mammary cancer are not the same in mouse and man. It would be prudent however, to work from the known to the unknown; to use the information gained from the mouse as a basis for investigating whether a parallel situation exists for the human. It would also be prudent to avoid the error of saying mouse cancer is not like human cancer when we know so little about the determinants of human breast cancer, and to insist on greater caution than has been exercised in the past in the widespread use of potent progestational pills when so little is known of the long term effects of those pills in the human.

In response to Dr. DAVEY's comment that the dose of progesterone used in our study was grossly in excess of the physiological dose: it might be well to remember that the daily ingestion of a potent progestational agent for the purpose of inducing a persistent anovulatory state in the human also imposes a daily dose grossly in excess of the physiological one. As for why we used a 2.5 mg. dose per mouse: in a small pilot study we found that some mice became pregnant whilst receiving daily doses of 0.5 mg. or less of progesterone. There were no pregnancies in the group given daily doses of 2.5 mg. The optimally effective dose is somewhere between 0.5 and 2.5 mg. This study was a preliminary one, and does not answer all questions. Experiments to explore a dose-response relationship with progesterone or another progestational agent, either alone or in combination with exogenous oestrogen, are certainly indicated. I agree with Dr. SHABAD completely that these findings merely indicate a limited beginning.

Dr. SHABAD asked, "What is the role of progesterone in these experiments?" In essence, he has also asked, "What is the role of a co-carcinogen, in the process of carcinogenesis?" I do not know. These are excellent questions that can be answered by laboratory investigations, if further work should indeed support the present indications that progesterone is a co-carcinogen for mammary carcinogenesis.

In general I agree with Professor KREYBERG's first point. However from our experience in this and other experiments, and from the results of earlier investigators, whereas we expect methylcholanthrene, given by gavage to C_3H virgin females, to induce a wide variety of tumours, we can predict that the tumours that develop in C_3H mice not treated with an exogenous carcinogen will have a more limited histological pattern. Keratinizing carcinomas, sarcomas, etc. are relatively rare in such animals, and the administration of progesterone does little to increase the range of histological types of tumour which occur.

As to the use of the terms carcinosarcoma and sarcoma, I used these terms for their descriptive value. The term "spindlizing undifferentiated sarcomatoid carcinoma" may be more accurate but for the sake of brevity I prefer the term "sarcoma".

In reply to Dr. DOLL let me emphasize that I did not present the findings as a basis for predicting the effect of oral contraceptives in women. These are preliminary experimental findings which suggest that manipulation of the hormonal status of a mouse may have profound effects on the speed and incidence of development of tumours that would otherwise develop late in the life of the animal.

I agree with Professor FRAZER that the investigation of the physiological and physio-pathological effects of hormones, calls for far more research than is currently in progress, by experimental, clinical, and epidemiological investigators. Then, we may begin to understand whether or not, and how much, we can extrapolate from the laboratory animal to man. Meanwhile, we are in no position to ignore indications of potential carcinogenic hazard for man derived from animal experimentation.

On Blastomogenic Effect of Antithyroid Drugs

N. P. NAPALKOV

Chief, Laboratory of Experimental Tumours, The N. N. Petzov Research Institute of Oncology of the U.S.S.R. Ministry, of Public Health Leningrad, U.S.S.R.

The discovery of thyreostatic effect inherent to some naturally occurring substances and the subsequent development of numerous synthetic preparations with the same action gave an opportunity for systematic experimental investigation of thyroid tumours.

Besides the long-term administration of the so-called antithyroid (thyreostatic, goitrogenic) substances, thyroid tumours were induced when the gland was subjected to intensive external or internal irradiation with considerable damage of thyroid parenchyma, as well as when the animals had been kept for a long time on a low-iodine diet. In all above cases the experimental animals, mainly rats and mice, developed thyroid tumours of various morphological patterns and degree of malignancy. Detailed data on special features of experimental thyroid tumours are summarized in the relevant reviews (H. P. MORRIS, 1955; N. P. NAPALKOV, 1958).

As a result of the numerous investigations a sufficiently consistent conception of experimental thyroid tumour pathogenesis was formed, generally accepted and given a comprehensive description in the summarizing papers by F. BIELSCHOWSKY (1955) and J. FURTH (1959).

According to this concept, the origin and development of thyroid tumours are due to primary inhibition of hormonal production of the thyroid tissue (as a result of treatment with thyreostatic substances, radiation and iodine deficiency) and to the secondary stable intensification of synthesis and release of the pituitary thyreostimulating hormone (TSH). In this case the continuous intensive secretion and release of the pituitary TSH is assumed to be the basic pathogenic factor responsible for origination and development of the tumour growth.

Such factors of thyroid tumorigenesis as ionizing radiation and low iodine diet are not considered in this report and should be referred for special discussion. The effect of thyreostatic substances in the process of blastomogenesis is limited, according to the above mechanism, to inhibition of thyroid hormone production only and, thus, to the secondary stimulation of hormonal activity of the anterior pituitary.

However, some data have been obtained which do not fit into the said concept and call for careful consideration. It is quite probable that the effect of thyreostatic substances in the process of blastomogenesis is not limited to a shift in the hormonal balance only.

The problem of the rôle of antithyroid substances in carcinogenesis is not of solely theoretical importance.

A wide range of substances with thyreostatic action pertaining to various groups of chemical compounds were applied on a large scale in industry, agriculture, and, this being very important, in medicine within the last 20 years. Detailed information on this question indicating the specific groups of population which may be influenced by these compounds is contained in the comprehensive paper of W. C. HUEPER (1963). Suffice it to recall that thiourea, propylthiouracil, methylthiouracil, mercazolil, aminotriazole, potassium perchlorate and many other antithyroid drugs are (or were) used in clinical practice in treatment of hyperthyreoidism.

Hazards involved in use of antithyroid substances due to their ability of producing tumour growth in the thyroid were the object of numerous discussions in the literature in recent years, particularly, in connection with aminotriazole applications. Some additional experimental data have to be considered which could help to clarify the matter.

It is necessary to answer at least the following questions to be able to appraise the blastomogenic activity of thyreostatic substances.

1. Is it true that tumour development in the thyroid is caused by the continuous intensified TSH-secretion of the pituitary exclusively, when the antithyroid drugs are used?

2. Does tumour growth not occur in some organs and tissues other than thyroid and pituitary in cases of various routes of administration of thyreostatic compounds?

3. If tumours of other localizations arise is their appearance not associated with the developing hypofunction of the thyroid and intensified secretion of TSH as well?

What data are available to provide answers to these questions?

The investigations of B. V. ALESHIN and N. S. DEMIDENKO (1959) showed that following approximately 6-month continuous administration of 6-methylthiouracil (MTU) in doses sufficient for inducing tumours in rats the thyroid structure is morphologically restored back to normal. Basal metabolism intensity returned to usual values, colloid reappeared in the follicular lumina and the height of thyroid epithelial cells decreased. R. GRASSO (1946) recorded the same picture when thiourea was used. While studying the successive stages of thyroid blastomogenesis in rats treated with MTU, we also had the opportunity of observing the morphological evidences of change in the thyroid epithelium reaction and the development of refractory state to this thyreostatic substance (1959).

Following continuous MTU treatment the thyroid epithelium cells either underwent changes in some way and regained their ability for hormone production, despite the antithyroid agent administration, or the hormone synthesis was inhibited as before but the reaction to TSH changed.

In the first case one might have expected that the reappeared contents of the follicles possessed hormonal activity and TSH secretion decreased, whereas, in the second case, one might have expected the thyroid hormonal activity remained at the same low level, TSH secretion being intensive.

Our biological tests in tadpoles of blood, thyroid and putuitary tissue from rats which had been treated with MTU for long periods revealed that the thyroid tissue metamorphogenic activity reduced, while that of the anterior pituitary was increased at all stages of the experiment as compared with the samples of corresponding tissue taken from control animals and of similar weight.

As far as the pituitary gland is concerned, our findings are in full agreement with the observations of B. V.
Aleshin and N. S. Demidenko but somewhat differ from the results obtained by
Chen Hann-yuan (1963) who did not
observe substantial differences in TSH
contents in the pituitary of control rats
and of those treated with propylthiouracil.

But according to the data of even
this author, a considerably higher concentration of TSH in the pituitary of the
rats treated with thyreostatic substances
was observed in the sixth month of the
experiment, as compared with control
animals. The thyreostimulating activity of blood serum, however, was always more intense in rats treated with
the antithyroid drug.

Hence, it is possible to believe that
the partial morphologically detectable
normalization of the thyroid structure
brought about approximately six months
after the beginning of continuous administration of thyreostatic substances is
due to changes in the thyroid epithelial
cell reaction to TSH under the conditions of intensified production of this
hormone. Moreover, we have found
that it is in the period of changing of the
epithelium reaction to TSH that the first
focal proliferates appear which give rise
to the subsequent thyroid adenomas.

The experiments of Chen Hann-
yuan and N. S. Halmi and B. N. Spirtos (1954) permit to suggest that propylthiouracil either contributes to the
effect of TSH or suppresses some TSH
inhibitor in blood whose presence has
been discussed for many years.

Hence, when thyreostatic compounds
are administered for prolonged period of
time, the thyroid tissue is under such
conditions that its metabolic processes
are significantly disturbed by the above
substances while epithelial cells are stimulated intensively by the pituitary
TSH.

Due to simultaneous treatment of
rats with methylthiouracil and carbon
tetrachloride which is known to interfere with the liver enzymatic systems
responsible for inactivation of thyroid
hormones (G. Amelotti, 1954; A. Nakagawa, 1957) and, thus, to lower the
TSH secretion (K. Kowalewsky, G. E.
Edwards, 1957), we succeeded in inhibiting the diffuse hyperplasia of the
thyroid and pituitary to a considerable
degree. Thus, there was no typical reaction to the continuous intensified production of TSH. The incidence of thyroid tumour development, however,
was the same both when MTU had been
used only and when it had been combined with injections of carbon tetrachloride (1962).

Therefore, when MTU is administered, a continuous hypersecretion of TSH
proves not to be the obligatory prerequisite for tumour development even
in the thyroid.

Moreover, attempts of thyroid tumour induction due to the influence of
TSH increased secretion alone resulted
in appearance at later stages of the experiments of only benign hormone-de-
pendent tumours which could be transplanted successfully only in combination
with transplantation of the pituitary tumours which was the source of considerable amounts of TSH (N. Haran-
Ghera, P. Pullar and J. Furth, 1960).

In numerous experiments on intrasplenic autoimplantation of the thyroid
tissue in thyroidectomized animals it was
also possible to observe the irregular
hyperplasia only and a few benign nodular proliferates, though in this case the
implanted tissue had been subjected to
the continuous intensive stimulation
with the pituitary TSH (P. K. Bondy,
1951; D. Brachetto-Brian and R. Grin-

BERG, 1951; P. DESAIVE, 1959; M. GABE and L. ARVY, 1947; *et al.*).

In this connection we carried out an experiment involving the combination of the intrasplenic autoimplantation of the thyroid with MTU treatment. It was found that rats which had received MTU developed large tumours in intrasplenic implants, many of the tumours being characterized by the malignant growth pattern. The control animals developed only irregular hyperplasia in the intrasplenic implants within the same period of time. The mean weight of the hypophysis, TSH activity of pituitary tissue and blood serum in the animals of both groups were increased to a similar degre. It turned out that additional treatment with thyreostatic substance in conjunction with hormonal stimulation accelerated the tumour development in such experiments as well.

Summarizing the above observations it is possible to draw a conclusion that as far as a number of thyreostatic substances are concerned, their rôle in the process of blastomogenesis in the thyroid is not limited to secondary stimulation of TSH secretion by the pituitary only. The direct injury of the thyroid epithelial cells by these substances is, apparently, of significant importance.

Is the blastomogenic effect of antithyroid compounds limited to their ability of causing tumour growth in the thyroid only?

While studying the effect of 6-methylthiouracil in long-term experiments, we never failed to observe that, when sufficiently large doses of the substance (10—12 mg. per day) were administered, degeneration and cirrhotic changes developed in rat's liver. Similar changes were observed when other substances with the antithyroid effect—acetamide (F. I. DESSAU and B. JACKSON, 1955) and thioacetamide (J. R. RÜTTNER and R. RONDEZ, 1960)—were used. Therefore in our experiments an attention was attracted by the fact that sarcomas frequently arose near the wall of parasitic cysts in rats' liver affected with parasitic invasion (*Cysticercus fasciolaris*). When more than forty such observations were compared with the experimental conditions, it was revealed that sarcomas originated from the parasitic cyst wall developed only in the livers of rats which had been treated with MTU for long period of time and were not observed in nontreated or thyroidectomized animals. Hence, under conditions of reactive proliferation of the connective tissue cells near the cyst wall the additional effect of MTU stimulated the tumour growth.

Liver tumours in rats were induced as a result of feeding with thiourea and thioacetamide in the experiments of O.G. FITZHUGH and A. A. NELSON (1948). The same observations in experiments with thioacetamide were also described by D. N. GUPTA (1956) and H. C. GRANT and K. R. REES (1958).

J. SEIFTER *et al.* (1946—49) observed hepatoma development when rats were fed with bis-(4-acetaminophenyl)selenium dihydroxide for a long time.

It should be noted that all above mentioned antithyroid substances were rather highly toxic and, as a rule, were used in long-term experiments, in relatively small doses. Therefore, the results of our experiments aimed at investigation of the blastomogenic activity of the thyrostatic substance — 3-amino-1,2,4-triazole (AT) are of particular interest. The toxicity of AT is low and it was possible to keep rats on a diet containing up to 500 mg. of the substance per day for each animal during one year and longer.

Administration of small doses of AT in the experiments of T. H. JUKES and C. B. SHAFFER (1960) showed its ability of inducing thyroid adenomas in mice.

This brought about a lively discussion on possible hazardous effect of AT use as a herbicide.

In the first series of our experiments it was established that when 125 mg. of AT were injected subcutaneously twice a week or 25,250 and 500 mg. per rat were administered orally six days a week, nearly all the animals developed hepatomas or carcinomas of hepatocellular or hepatocholangiocellular origin one year since the beginning of the experiments. Almost in all animals were found thyroid tumours. Two rats developed polymorphocellular sarcomas originating from the subcutaneous connective tissue and in two other cases were observed mammary gland cancer (1962). The further investigation of AT confirmed its ability of inducing liver tumours not only in rats but in mice as well.

Thus, the marked blastomogenic activity of another thyrostatic substance was established.

Among neoplasms of other localizations, Zymbal gland (ear duct) carcinomas and tumours of the orbit and eyelids obtained due to treatment of rats with thiourea should be mentioned (A. Rosin and M. Rachmilewitz, 1954; A. Rosin and H. Ungar, 1957; H. Ungar and A. Rosin, 1960).

In 1962 R. N. Akimova discovered the ability of MTU to cause benign and malignant tumours in rat's kidneys.

All these data indicate that a number of substances producing the antithyroid effect can induce tumour growth not only in the pituitary and thyroid glands but in other organs and tissues as well. Development of tumours of other localizations is particularly distinct when large doses of antithyroid compounds are applied.

The extent to which the blastomogenic effect of thyreostatic substances depends on their inhibition of the thyroid functioning and intensification of the pituitary thyrostimulating activity should be considered separately.

As to the thyroid tumours it can be accepted that increased secretion of TSH is an important factor promoting the realization of the blastomogenic effect of thyreostatic substances. As far as tumour growth in organs other than thyroid is concerned, it should be taken into account that thyroidectomy and inhibition of the thyroid function retard the development of liver tumours induced, for instance, with N-2-fluorenylacetamide and its derivatives (S. R. Pai, R. S. Yamamoto and J. H. Weisburger, 1963—1964; J. H. Weisburger and E. K. Weisburger, 1963).

It is similar conditions that arise when thyreostatic substances are applied. It is possible to suppose that the ability of inhibiting the thyroid activity and intensifying the TSH output of the pituitary does not stimulate, but, on the contrary, reduces to a certain degree, carcinogenic effect of antithyroid substances on the liver.

In order to ascertain the rôle of hypofunction of the thyroid and intensified TSH output of the pituitary in development of tumours induced by aminotriazole the following experiments were carried out in our laboratory.

Rats of one group were treated for a long time with aminotriazole only, while in the other group administration of this compound was combined with daily injections of physiologic doses of thyroxine compensating for thyroid hormone deficiency. It has been found by now that normalization of the TSH secretion and compensation of thyroid deficiency do not prevent the development of liver tumours induced by aminotriazole.

The data presented above show that a number of substances possessing the antithyroid effect can induce tumour growth in various tissues and organs. The blastomogenic action of the said compounds cannot be explained by and limited to the secondary effect of hormonal imbalance caused by them alone. The direct injury of cells of various tissues and organs by these substances seems to be of considerable importance.

We are far from suggesting an unconditional prohibition of using all antithyroid substances in all cases on the basis of the above data and considerations. However, the discovery of blastomogenic activity of some antithyroid compounds calls for particular caution when prescribing their application.

It would be desirable to continue the search for antithyroid but non-carcinogenic agents, because there are no evidences to state that the ability of inhibiting the thyroid function always associates with the blastomogenic activity of the substance.

References

AKIMOVA, R. N., On development of renal tumours in rats. *Vrachebnoje Delo* **6**, 7 (1962).

ALESHIN, B. V., and DEMIDENKO, N. S., Reaction of the thyroid to 6-methylthiouracil as compared with that to thyreostimulating hormone. In: *Nervnaya regulatsia endokrinnikh funktsij*, p. 140. Kiev 1959.

AMELOTTI, G., Ricerche morfofunzionali su alcune glandole endocrine, nel corso dell' avvelenamento da tetracloruro carbonio (CCl_4). *Ormonologia* **14**, 6, 339 (1954).

BIELSCHOWSKY, F., Neoplasia and internal environment. *Brit. J. Cancer* **9**, 1, 80 (1955).

BONDY, P. K., Maintenance of normal thyroid activity after transplantation of thyroid gland into spleen or kidney. *Proc. Soc. exp. Biol. (N.Y.)* **77**, 4, 638 (1951).

BRACHETTO-BRIAN, D., y GRINBERG, R., Processo histologico de los autoinjertos intraesplenicos de tiroides en ratos tiroidectomizados. *Rev. Soc. argent. Biol.* **27**, 2, 199 (1951).

CHEN-HANN-YUAN, Studies on experimental rat thyroid tumour. *Acta Biol. exp. sin.* **6**, 1, 37 (1958).

— Rôle of thyreotropin inhibiting factor in Thyroid tumour induction. *Science (Chinese)* **3**, 59 (1963).

DESAIVE, P., Evalution des implants intraspléniques de thyroïde chez la lapine adulte. *Bull. Soc. int. Chir.* **18**, 4, 433 (1959).

DESSAU, F. I., and JACKSON, B., Acetamide-induced liver cell alternations in rats. *Lab. Invest.* **4**, 387 (1955).

FITZHUGH, O. G., and NELSON, A. A., Liver tumours in rats fed thiourea or thioacetamide. *Science* **108**, 626 (1948).

FURTH, J., A meeting of ways in cancer research: thoughts on the evolution and nature of neoplasms. *Cancer Res.* **19**, 241 (1959).

GABE, M., et ARVY, L., Les effects de l'autotransplantation preportale de la thyroide chez la rate. *Experientia (Basel)* **3**, 5, 193 (1947).

GRANT, H. C., and REES, K. R., The precancerous liver; correlations of histological and biochemical changes in rats during prolonged administration of thioacetamide and "butter yellow". *Proc. Roy. Soc. B.* **148**, 117 (1958).

GRASSO, R., The action of thiourea on the intracellular colloid of the thyroid gland. *Anat. Rec.* **95**, 365 (1946).

GUPTA, D. N., Nodular cirrhosis and metastasizing tumours produced in the liver of rats by prolonged feeding with thioacetamide. *J. Path. Bact.* **72**, 415 (1956).

HALMI, N. S., and SPIRTOS, B. N., Analysis of action of propylthiouracil on pituitary-thyroid axis of rats. *Endocrinology* **55**, 613 (1954).

HARAN-GHERA, N., PULLAR, P., and FURTH, J., Induction of thyrotropin-dependent thyroid tumors by thyrotropes. *Endocrinology* **66**, 694 (1960).

HUEPER, W. C., Environmental carcinogenesis in man and animals. *Ann. N.Y. Acad. Sci.* **108**, 3, 963 (1963).

JACKSON, B., and DESSAU, F. I., Liver tumours in rats fed acetamide. *Lab. Invest.* **10**, 909 (1961).

JUKES, T. H., and SHAFFER, C. B., Antithyroid effects of aminotriazole. *Science* **132**, 296 (1960).

KOWALEWSKY, K., and EDWARDS, G. E., Effect of thyrotropin (TSH) on the thyroid radio-iodine uptake in C_3H mice with experimental liver injury. *Acta endocr. (Kbh.)* **25**, 285 (1957).

MORRIS, H. P., Experimental development and metabolism of thyroid gland tumors. In: GREENSTEIN and HADDOW (Eds.), *Adv. Cancer Res.* **3**, 52 (1955).

Nakagawa, A., The experimental study of the metabolism of I$_{131}$ labelled diiodotyrosin. *Jap. J. med. Progr.* **44**, 5, 282 (1957).

Napalkov, N. P., Experimental tumours of thyroid gland. *Vop. Onkol.* **4**, 738 (1958).

— Morphological properties of experimental thyroid tumours induced in rats with 6-methylthiouracil. *Vop. Onkol.* **5**, 578 (1959).

— Blastomogenic effect of 3-amino-1,2,4-triazole. *Gig. Tr. prof. Zabol.* **6**, 48 (1962).

— Influence of carbon tetrachloride on appearance and development of changes in the thyroid of rats treated with methylthiouracil. *Vop. Onkol.* **8**, 10, 49 (1962).

Pai, S. R., Yamamoto, R. S., and Weisburger, J. H., Rapid liver tumour induction by concerted action of N-hydroxy-2-acetamidofluorene and hormonal stimulation. *Nature (Lond.)* **199**, 1299 (1963).

Rosin, A., and Rachmilewitz, M., The development of malignant tumours of the face in rats after prolonged treatment with thiourea. *Cancer Res.* **14**, 494 (1954).

—, and Ungar, H., Malignant tumors in the eyelids and auricular region of thiourea-treated rats. *Cancer Res.* **17**, 4, 302 (1957).

Rüttner, J. R., u. Rondez, R., Zur formalen Genese der Thioacetamid-Zirrhose der Ratte. *Path. et Microbiol. (Basel)* **23**, 113 (1960).

Seifter, J., Ehrich, W. E., and Hudyma, G. M., Effect of prolonged administration of antithyroid compounds on the thyroid and other endocrine organs of the rat. *Arch. Path.* **48**, 6, 536 (1949).

—, and Mueller, G., Thyroid adenomas in rats receiving selenium. *Science* **103**, 762 (1946).

Ungar, H., and Rosin, A., The histogenesis of the thiourea-induced carcinoma of the auditory duct sebaceous (Zymbal's) glands in rats. *Arch. Vecchi.* **31**, 419 (1960).

Weisburger, J. H., Pai, S. R., and Yamamoto, R. S., Pituitary hormones and liver carcinogenesis with n-hydroxy-n-2-fluorenylacetamide. *J. nat. Cancer Inst.* **32**, 881 (1964).

—, and Weisburger, E. K., Pharmacodynamics of carcinogenic azo dyers, aromatic amines and nitrosamines. *J. clin. Pharm. Ther.* **4**, 1, 110 (1963).

Discussion

Druckrey: Have you tested antithyroid compounds for carcinogenicity in young and pregnant animals as well as in adult rats and mice?

Napalkov: We have performed two types of experiments with methylthiouracil (MTU). First, we compared the results of treating young rats with those of treating adult animals. There was no difference either in tumour incidence or in the tumour induction time. Treatment of pregnant rats with MTU during pregnancy did not result in the development of thyroid tumours in the progeny. If animals were treated with MTU continuously for several successive generations (including periods of prenatal ontogenesis) an increased incidence of thyroid tumours was seen in some generations.

Schoental: Please could you give us more details of Dr. Akimova's experiments, on kidney tumour development in rats treated with MTU?

Napalkov: The method of treatment with MTU used by Dr. Akimova was practically the same as that used in our experiments. The fact that she saw a high incidence of renal tumours whereas we saw none is probably attributable to a difference in susceptibility in the two strains of rat used.

Boyland: Have you tested naturally occuring antithyroid substances, such as the ones which are present in Brassica seeds?

Napalkov: No.

Van Esch: We carried out experiments with aminotriazole (AT) at much lower dose levels, namely, 50 and 100 ppm, continuously throughout life. At the same time we fed rats with 200 ppm intermittently. The periods of intermittent feeding lasted for 7 days, 14 days or 20 days. At the end of the experiment the numbers of animals with thyroid tumours in the group fed 100 ppm AT continuously and in the three groups given intermittent treatment were not significantly different. Other experiments at present in progress suggest that AT may not act only via the pituitary gland.

In our experiments with doses of AT, lower than those used by Dr. Napalkov, no liver tumours were found.

Napalkov: I agree that your findings with AT suggest a mechanism of carcinogenesis which does not involve the pituitary.

Taylor: We can be grateful that experimental animals are different from human beings. Antithyroid drugs have been used clinically for 20 years. Has there been any increase in tumour incidence of the thyroid or other localizations? My impression is that there has been no increase which could be related to the use of antithyroid drugs. These drugs are usually used for 6 to 8 weeks before surgical treatment. Do you consider that the MTU doses were rather high in your long term experiments as compared to those given to humans? You administered 10—12 mg of MTU per day, while for humans one uses 300—400 mg.

Napalkov: There are so many other factors influencing the tumour development in patients treated with antithyroid drugs for thyroid lesions that it is impossible at present time to evaluate precisely the role of the above substances in carcinogenesis in human beings. The possibly long duration of the latent period of carcinogenesis in man has to be taken into consideration. It is difficult to make any definite statement on the carcinogenic risk in man from the use of goitrogens until sufficient statistical data are available. At the same time the possibility that goitrogens act in combination with other agents used in clinics has to be kept in mind. The main purpose of our communication is to attract attention of doctors to the fact that there are experimental data on the carcinogenic action of antithyroid drugs, that this effect is not necessarily related to their ability to increase TSH secretion, and that they can induce tu-

mours not only in thyroid but also in liver and other localizations. In passing it should be noted that some substances with antithyroid activity are used in industry and agriculture and thus may constitute a cancer hazard other than by use as drugs.

Schoental: Have you explored single dose treatment with antithyroid substances?

Napalkov: In experiments with a single dose treatment with antithyroid drugs we did not observe tumour development.

Napalkov: In reply to Dr. SHUBIK, animals of species other than mice and rats were not used in our experiments. Combined treatment with MTU and synestrol [4,4'-(1,2-diethyl-ethylene) diphenyl; hexestrol] did not influence liver tumour development but decreased the incidence of thyroid tumours. Simultaneous treatment with AT and l-thyroxine showed that normalization of TSH secretion did not inhibit liver tumour production in rats. More experiments are needed to clarify the role of the pituitary in liver tumorigenesis.

On Potential Carcinogenicity of Some Hydrazine Derivatives Used as Drugs

J. Juhász

*I. Department of Pathological Anatomy and Experimental Cancer Research,
Medical University, Budapest, Hungary*

The research of the carcinogenic risk of the more and more widespread chemical environment is one of the important aims of the investigations of carcinogenesis, also from a practical point of view. The large number of compounds makes it almost impossible to have an exact knowledge of the eventual carcinogenic effect of all new compounds. This refers also to those used in the therapy. The list about drugs with a potential carcinogenic effect, made known by Truhaut [43] in the Conference held at Lausanne (1964), clearly shows how large the number of compounds among drugs is which endanger the organism. We think that as a result of the experimental research this list will still be complemented. Experts in experimental carcinogenesis have a clear understanding of the importance of this question. Clinicians, unfortunately, pay only little attention to findings relating to the cancerogenic effect of drugs. Even in great, detailed special works dealing with the side effects of drugs we may hardly find even sporadic hints in this respect.

To make our choice for the examination it is very important to lay stress, before all, upon the examination of drugs which get into the organism during a long period and in large doses.

That is why our attention was directed to isonicotinic acid hydrazide which as an efficacious antituberculous drug will be administered to hundreds of thousand patients. Shortly after the introduction of isoniazid into the therapy Hein and Stefani [20] have observed that in lungs of individuals treated with INH, adenoma-like areas of hyperplasia developed in an uncommon large number. The epithelial hyperplasia first showed itself in the wall of the bronchioli or in the alveolar epithelium. Already they presumed that such epithelial proliferations may develop tumours after a longer period. Berencsy et al. [7] observed the uncommonly rapid progression of one patient's lung cancer following INH-therapy. According to Tiboldi et al. [42] the Brown-Pearce carcinoma produced more and larger metastases than usual in animals treated with INH.

These few data are giving a hint to the necessity of studying the carcinogenic effect of INH. The present work aims at giving a short summary of the experimental investigations regarding the carcinogenic effect of INH and is endeavouring to report of the present situation of this problem.

Though it is also an important question wether INH is able to promote the growth of tumours, in our experiments we wished to determine if INH by itself has a tumourigenic effect. In our first experiment we examined a substance produced in Hungary. In course of the preliminary toxicological tests we found that, when white mice were given a daily dose of 0.2 ml intraperitoneally from a 1 per cent solution

and that in 1 case Kupffer-cell sarcoma of the liver developed.

As controls, 50 white mice of both sexes and the same breeding were used and there occurred not a single spontaneous tumour during the above period. The aforesaid experiments published in 1957 presented the first evidence of the cancerogenic effect of INH [21].

Table I. *Tumours induced by INH-administration*

Tumours	Period of survival days	Total amount of INH mg
1. Lung adenoma (multiple)	61	46
2. Lung adenoma (solitary)	187	82
3. Lung adenoma (multiple)	225	82
4. Lung adenoma (solitary)	225	82
5. Lung adenoma (solitary)	225	82
6. Lung adenoma (multiple)	225	82
7. Lung adenoma (solitary)	225	82
8. Lymphatic leukemia	91	79
9. Lymphatic leukemia and mediastinal tumour	75	55
10. Lymphatic leukemia and mediastinal tumour	102	82
11. Myeloid leukemia	187	82
12. Histiocytic leukemia	71	46
13. Histiocytic leukemia	175	82
14. Reticulum cell sarcoma of the liver	203	82

of the in water easily soluble compound, the animals were able to tolerate it without any side-effects for a long time. So we administered this dose to 50 white mice of both sexes having an average weight of 20 g every other day. After 8 injections the daily dose has been raised to 0.3 ml. The previous dose corresponded to 2 mg, the latter to 3 mg INH. Intraperitoneal injections have been given on 30 occasions in all so that the treated animals got 82 mg INH altogether. After an observation period of $7^1/_2$ months we noticed in 14 of the treated animals the growth of a tumour. It appears from Table I that in 7 cases lung adenomas and in 6 leukemias

Two years later MORI and YASUNO [28] in Japan made known that INH proved to be carcinogenic in strain dd mice even when orally administered. From INH added to the food 1.5—3 mg got daily into the organism of the animals. In 134—210 days a lot of lung adenomas developed as well as such hyperplastic foci which corresponded to the early stage of tumourous growth. When the amount of INH, added to the food, was elevated, lung tumours were much earlier engendered. They were able to demonstrate an actual relationship between the amount of INH and the frequency of tumours too. The cancerogenic effect of INH was manifest not only in case of oral administration but also when subcutaneously given.

After our own investigations and those of Mori et al. [29], mentioned above, Wolfart [48] has critically analysed, from a clinical point of view, the results of these investigations. In view of the importance of the question

method affords the most accurate dosing. Inbred white mice of both sexes, weighing on an average 20 g were given every other day 2 mg, later 1 mg INH in a 1 per cent physiological saline solution. In this experiment 55 mg of INH were given in all. The period of observation lasted 400 days. Whereas in the control group of 50 non-treated and for the

Table II. *Tumours induced by INH-administration (2nd experiment)*

Tumours	Period of survival days	Total amount of INH mg
1. Lung adenoma (multiple)	187	55
2. Mediastinal lymphosarcoma	145	40
3. Mediastinal lymphosarcoma	169	49
4. Mediastinal lymphosarcoma	171	50
5. Mediastinal lymphosarcoma	173	51
6. Mediastinal lymphosarcoma	188	55
7. Mediastinal lymphosarcoma	400	55
8. Mediastinal reticulum cell sarcoma	201	55
9. Reticulum cell sarcoma of the mesenterium	223	55
10. Reticulum cell sarcoma of the mesenterium	400	55
11. Myeloid leukemia	95	40
12. Myeloid leukemia	157	44
13. Myeloid leukemia	157	44
14. Myeloid leukemia	258	55
15. Myeloid leukemia	291	55

he emphasized that there are a lot of tuberculous patients living who have been given much more INH in course of an antituberculous therapy as the quantity (body weight/kg) used in the experiments.

The question has been raised too that perhaps some contamination arose in the drug during the production of INH and that it might be responsible for the carcinogenic effect. Therefore, we studied in our next experiment a preparation placed at our disposal by Prof. G. Domagk. Tests were carried out under the same circumstances as previously i.e. we applied intraperitoneal injections for we had found that this

same period observed animals there were no tumours, the treated 50 animals showed tumours and leukemias in 15 cases. So we were able to prove the results of our former investigations through this proceeding too. The tumours and leukemias produced during the experiment are summarized in Table II.

Further evidence has been furnished by Schwan [36, 37] in Poland, who in two series of experiments observed the appearance of lung adenomas and leukemias in strain R_3 mice after they had been intraperitoneally treated with INH. Weinstein and Kinosita [47] equally verified the experimental cancerogenic effect of INH in strain A and C57bl female mice. It is worth mentioning that ARFFMANN [3] compared the INH-effect with the known cancerogenic hydrocarbons using the newt skin test applied by NEUKOMM [30] and has ascertained that isonicotinic acid hydrazide brought forth epidermic hyperplasia and epithelial infiltration on the newt skin of equal intensity as caused by chrysen. Out of all experiments published in the literature only in those of VIALLIER and CASANOVA [44] didn't

that isonicotinic acid alone doesn't produce tumours whereas hydrazine sulphate has an equally intense cancerogenic effect as isonicotinic acid hydrazide. They mean this would be developed by the hydrazine group. Examining the metabolism of INH, KRÜGER-THIEMER [24] has ascertained that this drug will be split in the organism in isonicotinic acid and hydrazine. In the opinion of MORI et al. [29] the carbamyl-group is responsible for the carcinogenic effect.

Table III. *Experiments proving the carcinogenic effect of INH in different inbred mice strains*

JUHÁSZ, BALÓ and KENDREY (1957)	albino mice from own breeding, males and females
MORI and YASUNO (1959)	dd strain, males and females
MORI and co-workers (1960)	dd strain, males and females
SCHWAN (1961)	R_3 strain, males and females
SCHWAN (1962)	R_3 strain, males and females
BIANCIFIORI and RIBACCHI (1962)	BALB/C, females
JUHÁSZ, BALÓ and SZENDE (1963)	albino mice from own breeding, males and females
RIBACCHI and co-workers (1963)	BALB/c, males
BIANCIFIORI and co-workers (1963)	CBA strain, males and females
WEINSTEIN and KINOSITA (1963)	A strain, females
WEINSTEIN and KINOSITA (1963)	C 57 bl strain, females
ARFFMANN (1964)	NEUKOMM's newt skin test

appear any carcinogenic effect; they have used Swiss strain mice.

Table III. shows the summary of the experiments proving the carcinogenic effect of INH in mice coming from different inbred mice strain.

A research group in Italy headed by BIANCIFIORI [9, 10, 11, 17, 27, 34] is dealing with the problem. In several of their experiments INH proved to be cancerogenic in strain BALB/c mice. It is worth mentioning that besides lung adenomas malignant and metastazing lung tumours and leukemias were observed as well. Upon the effect of INH hepatomas were observed in strain CBA mice with males at 62 per cent and with females at 71 per cent which brought forth lung metastases too. BIANCIFIORI and RIBACCHI [11] also ascertained

In our own last experiment we studied the potential carcinogenic effect of the pure hydrazine (NH_2—NH_2). It is present in the watery solution in the form of mono- or dihydrate. We intraperitoneally administered to 30 male and 30 female white mice 0.5 mg hydrazine in a 0.5 ml physiological saline solution every other day, later every third day. Sixteen intraperitoneal injections were given in all which correspond to 400 mg/body weight kg hydrazine. In the first period of the experiment focal liver necroses were engendered in one part of the animals. The hepatotoxical effect of hydrazine has been several times observed in course of experiments (BROIHAN [16]; GARDNER [18]; WEATHERBY and YARD [46]) but also in men liver damages were found after the administration of drugs containing hydrazine (ALEXANDER [2]; BEER and SCHAFFNER [6]; SHAY and SUN [38]). Tumours and leukemias were produced in 13 cases out of the 34 surviving mice in 100 to 313 days from the beginning of the experiment. The tumours developed in

hydrazine sulphate in the experiments of BIANCIFIORI and RIBACCHI [11]. Hydrazine is perhaps the substance of the simplest chemical structure which is able to produce tumours in animals. The study of carcinogenic agents having such a simple structure may be of im

Table IV. *Tumours induced by hydrazine treatment*

Tumours	Period of survival days	Total amount of hydrazine mg/kg
1. Myeloid leukemia	108	400
2. Myeloid leukemia	110	400
3. Myeloid leukemia	111	400
4. Myeloid leukemia	171	400
5. Myeloid leukemia	183	400
6. Reticulum cell sarcoma of the mediastinum	183	400
7. Reticulum cell sarcoma of the mediastinum	190	400
8. Reticulum cell sarcoma of the mediastinum	211	400
9. Myeloid leukemia	215	400
10. Reticulum cell sarcoma of the mediastinum	216	400
11. Myeloid leukemia	238	400
12. Myeloid leukemia	287	400
13. Myeloid leukemia	302	400

the mediastinum showed a local invasiveness and proved to be reticulum cell sarcomas evidencing a metastatic spread in the lungs, pleura and liver. In cases of myeloid leukemias hepatosplenomegaly and an enlargement of all lymph nodes were occurred; histologically in immature myeloid cell infiltration could be observed in the aforesaid organs and bone marrow. There was only 1 case of spontaneous thymic lymphoma in 60 control mice. We displayed the tumours produced by hydrazine in Table IV.

On the basis of the hydrazine experiments we are of the opinion that the hydrazine group plays an important role in the tumour-producing effect of INH. The same has been proved with

portance theoretically too. Studies of such a tendency are but at their first stage.

It is well known that tumour-inhibiting agents may produce tumours in experimental animals; on the other hand, by tumour-inducing compounds it is possible to influence the progression of tumours. In connection with the hydrazine experiments it is worth mentioning that BOLLAG and co-workers [12, 13, 14, 35] in 1963 discerned a new class of cytotoxic agents. The new tumour inhibiting compounds are methylhydrazine derivatives which in animal and cytological experiments gave evidence of a very significant antiblastic effect. On the human tumours in cases of malignant lymphomas there has been experienced a favorable effect (D'ALESSANDRI *et al.* [*1*]). On the other hand, KELLY and co-workers [*23*] engendered through oral and intraperitoneal administration of the same methylhydrazine derivative in strain CD_2F_1 as well as in noninbred albino mice multiple lung tumours and leukemias. Such a paradoxical effect in connection with INH has been observed in experiments by several investigators, in whose opinion INH is able to inhibit the growth of transplantable animal tumours and the development of metastases (SIEGEL [*39*]; SIEGEL and IWAINSKY [*40*]; SIMON [*41*]; GROSS [*19*]; WAGNER and MORITZ [*45*]; BRAMBILLA and BALDINI [*15*]). MATSUMOTO and co-workers [*26*] succeeded in significantly inhibiting the hepatocarcinogenic effect of p-dimethylaminoazobenzene by simultaneously administering INH. We think the aforesaid examinations also support the importance of the searching activity connected with the hydrazine compounds.

In INH-experiments the drug affected normal tissues. In clinical practice this drug will be applied at high daily doses and for a long time, even for years. It has been proved many a times that tuberculosis by itself may provide favourable conditions for the development of tumours in tissues not only in those of the lung but of other organs too (BALÓ [*4*]). The spontaneous or by drugs promoted healing up of a tuberculous process happens through the fibrous transformation of the tissues. The scar tissue of non-specific origin may also further the development of

epithelial proliferations and tumours (BALÓ, JUHÁSZ and TEMES [*5*]). During the INH-therapy the mentioned alterations of the tissue may promote the engendering of tumours also in humans. Though the very few clinical data (POMPE [*32*]; RANDAZZO [*33*]) didn't provide sufficient proof for the cancerogenic effect of this drugs in humans, nevertheless, the hitherto gathered experimental findings point to the possibility of a severe danger. Further investigations may be indicated by the fact that isonicotinic acid hydrazide isn't the only drug which may liberate hydrazine during the metabolic processes. Among the anti-hypertonic drugs as well as the antidepressant ones, which will be widely applied in the neuro-psychopharmacology in the last years, there are also many hydrazine derivatives to be found. The antidepressant drugs containing hydrazine group are the inhibitors of monoaminooxidase and these compounds are able to develop severe pathological alterations in the nervous system of dogs (PALMER and NOEL [*31*]). Their eventual carcinogenic effect has not been examined yet. The anti-hypertensive and anti-depressant drugs are also compounds which will be applied in humans for a long time and there may also be potential carcinogenic compounds among them. The hitherto performed investigations seem to justify our endeavours to go on thoroughly studying the potential carcinogenic action of drugs containing hydrazine group.

References

[*1*] D'ALESSANDRI, A., KEEL, H. J., BOLLAG, W., u. MARTZ, G., Erste klinische Erfahrungen mit einem neuen Cytostaticum. *Schweiz. med. Wschr.* **93**, 1018 (1963).

[*2*] ALEXANDER, H. L., *Reactions with drug therapy.* Philadelphia and London: W. B. Saunders Co. 1955.

[*3*] ARFFMANN, E., Studies on the newt test for carcinogenicity. 4. Supplementary experiments on specificity. *Acta path. microbiol. scand.* **60**, 13 (1964).

[*4*] BALÓ, J., Lungenkarzinom und Lungenadenom. Budapest: *Verlag der Ungarischen Akademie der Wissenschaften*, 1959.

[5] Baló, J., Juhász, J., and Temes, J., Pulmonary infarcts and pulmonary carcinoma. *Cancer* (Philad.) **9**, 918 (1956).

[6] Beer, D. T., and Schaffner, F., Fatal jaundice after administration of beta-phenyl-isopropyl-hydrazine. Report of a case. *J. Amer. med. Ass.* **171**, 887 (1959).

[7] Berencsy, Gy., Entz, A., and Vajkóczy, A., Isonikotinsavhydrazid (INH)-kezelés és tüdörák. *Tuberk. Kérd.* **8**, 84 (1955).

[8] Berneis, K., Kofler, M., Bollag, W., Kaiser, A., and Langemann, A., The degradation of deoxyribonucleic acid by new tumour inhibiting compounds: the intermediate formation of hydrogen peroxide. *Experientia* (Basel) **19**, 132 (1963).

[9] Biancifiori, C., Bucciarelli, E., Clayson, D. B., and Santilli, F. E., Induction of hepatomas in CBA/Cb/Se mice by hydrazine sulphate and the lack of effect of croton oil on tumour induction in BALB/c/Cb/Se mice. *Brit. J. Cancer* **18**, 543 (1964).

[10] — — Santilli, F. E., e Ribacchi, R., Cancerogenesi polmonare da idrazide dell'acido isonicotinico (INI) e suoi metaboliti in topi CBA/Cb/Se substrain. *Lav. Anat. Pat. Perugia* **23**, 209 (1963).

[11] —, and Ribacchi, R., Pulmonary tumours in mice induced by oral isoniazid and its metabolites. *Nature (Lond.)* **194**, 488 (1962).

[12] Bollag, W., The tumor-inhibitory effects of the methylhydrazine derivative RO 4-6467/1. (NSC-77213). *Cancer Chemother. Rep.* **33**, 1 (1963).

[13] — Suppression of the immunological reaction by methyl-hydrazines, a new class of antitumour agents. *Experientia (Basel)* **19**, 304 (1963).

[14] —, and Grunberg, E., Tumour inhibitory effects of a new class of cytotoxic agents: methylhydrazine derivatives. *Experientia (Basel)* **19**, 130 (1963).

[15] Brambilla, G., et Baldini, L., Azione inibitrice dell'acido isonicotinico sullo sviluppo del sarcoma Galliera del ratto. *Boll. Soc. ital. Biol. sper.* **35**, 1169 (1959).

[16] Broihan, F., Über die Giftwirkung des Hydrazins. *Zbl. Arbeitsmed.* **7**, 62 (1957).

[17] Di Leo, F. P., e Milia, U., Problemi biochimici nella tumorigenesi polmonare sperimentale da isoniazide e idrazina. *Lav. Anat. Pat. Perugia* **23**, 129 (1963).

[18] Gardner, D. L., The response of the dog to oral l-hydrazino-phthalazine (hydralazine). *Brit. J. exp. Path.* **38**, 227 (1957).

[19] Gross, W., Ein Beitrag zur cytostatischen Wirkung des Isonicotinsäurehydrazids (INH). *Klin. Wschr.* **34**, 495 (1956).

[20] Hein, J., u. Stefani, H., Die gewebliche Reaktion der Lungentuberkulose bei Isonicotinsäurehydrazid-Behandlung. *Z. Tuberk.* **101**, 180 (1952).

[21] Juhász, J., Baló, J., u. Kendrey, G., Über die geschwulsterzeugende Wirkung des Isonikotinsäurehydrazid (INH). *Z. Krebsforsch.* **62**, 188 (1957).

[22] — — u. Szende, B., Neue experimentelle Angaben zur geschwulsterzeugenden Wirkung des Isonikotinsäurehydrazid (INH). *Z. Krebsforsch.* **65**, 434 (1963).

[23] Kelly, M. G., O'Gara, R. W., Gadekar, K., Yancey, S. T., and Oliverio, V. T., Carcinogenic activity of a new antitumor agent, N-isopropyl-α-/2-methyl-hydrazino/-p-toluamide, hydrochloride (NSC-77213). *Cancer Chemother. Rep.* **39**, 77 (1964).

[24] Krüger-Thiemer, E., Isonicotinic acid hypothesis of the antituberculous action of isoniazid. *Amer. Rev. Tuberc.* **77**, 364 (1958).

[25] Martz, G., D'Alessandri, A., Keel, H. J., and Bollag, W., Preliminary clinical results with a new antitumor agent RO 4-6467 (NSC-77213). *Cancer Chemother. Rep.* **33**, 5 (1963).

[26] Matsumoto, K., Mori, K., and Yasuno, A., Effect of isonicotinic acid hydrazid on hepatocarcinogenesis. *Gann* **51**, 91 (1960).

[27] Milia, U., Gaetani, M., e Biancifiori, C., Azione carcinogenetica dell'acido 4-/isonicotinil-idrazone (pimelico/4-INIP) in topi BALB/c/b/Se subtrain. *Lav. Anat. Pat. Perugia* **24**, 39 (1964).

[28] Mori, K., and Yasuno, A., Preliminary note on the induction of pulmonary tumors in mice by isonicotinic acid hydrazide feeding. *Gann* **50**, 107 (1959).

[29] — —, and Matsumoto, K., Induction of pulmonary tumors in mice with isonicotinic acid hydrazid. *Gann* **51**, 83 (1960).

[30] Neukomm, S., Un test sensible et ultra rapide du pouvoir cancerigène de certaines substances chimiques. *Oncologia (Basel)* **10**, 107 (1957).

[31] PALMER, A. C., and NOEL, P. R., Neuropathological effects of prolonged administration of some hydrazine monoamine oxidase inhibitors in dogs. J. Path. Bact. 86, 463 (1963).

[32] POMPE, K., Einfluß von Isonicotinhydrazid auf die Lupuskarzinomentstehung. Derm. Wschr. 133, 105 (1956).

[33] RANDAZZO, S. D., Eventuale influenza dell'idrazide dell'acido isonicotinico sull'insorgenza di neoplasie in processi tubercolari cronici. G. Med. Tisiol. 8, 667 (1959).

[34] RIBACCHI, R., BIANCIFIORI, C., MILIA, U., DI LEO, F. P., e BUCCIARELLI, E., Cancerogenesi polmonare da idrazide dell'acido isonicotinico in topi maschi BALB/c, con e senza MTV. Lav. Anat. Pat. Perugia 23, 103 (1963).

[35] RUTISHAUSER, A., and BOLLAG, W., Cytological investigations with a new class of cytotoxic agents: methylhydrazine derivatives. Experientia (Basel) 19, 131 (1963).

[36] SCHWAN, S., Hydrazid kwasu izonikotynowego (H.K.I.N.) jake czynnik „rakotwórczy" u myszy. Pat. pol. 12, 53 (1961).

[37] — Hydrazid kwasu izonikotynówego (INH) jako czynnik „rakotworczy" u myszy. Donieienie II. Pat. pol. 13, 185 (1962).

[38] SHAY, H., and SUN, D. C. H., Massive necrosis of the liver following iproniazid. Ann. intern. Med. 49, 1246 (1958).

[39] SIEGEL, D., Kernmorphologische Veränderungen an Ehrlich-Ascites-Tumorzellen durch Iso-Nicotinsäure-Hydrazid (INH). Arch. Geschwulstforsch. 18, 295 (1962).

[40] SIEGEL, D., u. IWAINSKY, H., Über den Einfluß von Iso-Nicotinsäure-Hydrazid (INH) auf die Metastasierungsquote des Ehrlichschen Ascitescarcinom der Maus. Klin. Wschr. 38, 769 (1960).

[41] SIMON, K., Untersuchung von Derivaten des Hydrazins auf ihre cytostatische Wirkung am Ascitestumor der Maus. Z. Naturforsch 7b, 531 (1952).

[42] TIBOLDI, T., DÁVID, M., KOVÁCS, K., u. MOLNÁR, P., Die Wirkung des Isonikotinsäurehydrazid auf das Brown-Pearce-Karzinom des Kaninchens. Z. Tuberk. 106, 257 (1955).

[43] TRUHAUT, R., The risk of cancerisation arising from the therapeutic use of certain chemical agents. Excerpta med. (Amst.), Int. Congr. Ser. 75, 107 (1964).

[44] VIALLIER, J., et CASANOVA, F., L'isoniazide a-t-il des propriétés cancerigènes? Essai sur l'animal. C.R. Soc. Biol. (Paris) 154, 985 (1960).

[45] WAGNER, H., u. MORITZ, R., Beeinflussung des Tumorwachstums durch INH in Tierversuch und Gewebekultur. Arch. Geschwulstforsch. 19, 123 (1962).

[46] WEATHERBY, J. H., and YARD, A. S., Observations on the subacute toxicity of hydrazine. Arch. industr. Hlth 11, 413 (1955).

[47] WEINSTEIN, H. J., and KINOSITA, R., Isoniazid and pulmonary tumors in mice. Amer. Rev. resp. Dis. 88, 124 (1963).

[48] WOLFART, W., Ruft Isonikotinsäurehydrazid Tumoren hervor? Dtsch. med. Wschr. 85, 1655 (1960).

Plastics Carcinogenesis, Some Experimental Data and Its Possible Importance for Clinic and Prophylaxis of Cancer

L. M. SHABAD

Institute of Experimental and Clinical Oneology of the Academy of Medical Sciences of the USSR, Moscow, Kashirskoye Shosse, 6, USSR

Investigations of possible carcinogenic effect of introduction of various polymers into the organism are of great practical importance because polymers are being widely used in bone and maxillofacial surgery, in operations on large vessels, etc.

FIRST, TURNER (1936, 1938) occasionally discovered fibrosarcoma formation in rats at sites where bakelite plates had been introduced, subcutaneously. Then OPPENHEIMER et al. (1948) observed sarcomas also in rats after a cellophane capsule had been applied to the kidney (with a view to obtain experimental hypertension) as well as in cases when cellophane had been implanted subcutaneously. A considerable amount of experimental investigations followed these casual observations and they confirmed and substantially contributed to basic factual material. OPPENHEIMER and his co-workers in the U.S.A. (1953—1964), DRUCKREY (1952) and NOTHDURFT (1955, 1959) in FRG, ALEXANDER and HORNING (1959) in England, A. H. KOGAN (1954—1964) and L. V. OLSHEVSKAYA (1961, 1962) in the USSR and many other authors furnished the findings of numerous experiments which confirmed that introduction of plates of various materials subcutaneously or into pararenal tissue of rats resulted in a certain

percentage of sarcoma formation. We are not going to dwell upon all published papers but we shall underline the main well established facts and consider certain data of the experiments of A. H. KOGAN (approx. on 1,500 rats) and L. V. OLSHEVSKAYA (on 600 rats) which were carried under our consultation.

The first of the well established results is the fact that introduction of various polymers such as, for instance, cellophane, polyethylene, polyvinyl chloride, tephlon, nylon, dacron, polymethylmetacrylat, etc., as well as foils of different metals, such as tantalum, silver, gold, platinum and even ivory under the skin leads to sarcoma formation.

Thus, it has led to the conclusion that the chemical composition of the substance introduced has nothing to do with tumour formation in this case.

Another basic fact is that blastomogenesis in this case is determined by the physical shape of the implanted material. Sarcomas occur approximately in 30—40% of rats bearing subcutaneously the whole plates and only approximately in 10% cases when plates were perforated. When capron fibres (my previous experiments in 1940—1941) or dacron and nylon fibres were introduced under the skin, the tumours did not occur at all. Tumours were not induced when powders or finely-ground cellophane and other polymers were introduced, whereas the same materials induced tumours when they were implanted as plates. In other words, pulverization of the plate removes its carcinogenic properties.

The size of the implanted plate is of much importance — the bigger the plate, the more tumours and faster the rate of their development. For instance, when cellophane plates measuring 1×3 cm. were introduced under the skin, sarcomas occurred in 33.3% of rats which survived over 9 months since the beginning of the experiment, while with plates measuring 2×3 cm. tumours occurred in 51.1% (experiments of L. V. OLSHEVSKAYA). With larger plates the average latent period dropped from 15 to 12 months. Introduction of pulverized cellophane did not cause tumours in a single animal (140 rats which survived over 9 months since the beginning of the experiment; they were under control for two and a half years, experiments of L. V. OLSHEVSKAYA).

The rates of tumour formation when whole plates are implanted under the skin or into pararenal tissue are approximately the same and average about 35% according to A. H. KOGAN and OPPENHEIMER.

Tumours are less frequent when polyethylene discs are implanted into abdominal cavity. For instance, according to DRUCKREY they occur in one rat out of 28. DRUCKREY explains this by shifting of the discs due to the peristaltic movement of the intestine. An extremely long (especially as compared with carcinogenic hydrocarbons) latent period of not less than 10 months (according to OPPENHEIMER) or 12 months (according to L. V. OLSHEVSKAYA) is the general and important feature of polymer blastomogenesis.

Rats seem to be the most suitable animals for experimental study of blastomogenesis caused by polymers. Therefore, the majority of the experiments have been conducted on them. Mice, as it was shown by TOMATIS (1963) and hamsters (BERING and HANDLER, 1957) may be also used for this purpose though tumours arise in fewer cases.

The above basic features of blastomogenesis caused by polymers call for a particularly careful study of tumour formation mechanism in this case. The apparent dependence of blastomogenesis on the shape of implanted material and the seeming independence on its chemical composition contradict, on the face of it, many testimonies of correlation between blastomogenic activity and chemical structure of cancer inducing substances.

It was not without reason that the well known biochemist O. WARBURG who presided over one of the meetings of the International Symposium on Carcinogenesis (Berlin, 1959) referred to plastics carcinogenesis as one of the most puzzling problems of contemporary experimental oncology.

Is it possible to consider formation of tumours in sites where polymer plates were introduced as a result of mere nonspecific chronic "irritation" caused by a foreign body? Or, is it some certain mechanism of carcinogenesis familiar to us according to other experimental oncologic models? Is it not a case of relatively specific chemical carcinogenic influence? Such are the questions which have naturally arisen before us and we shall try to throw at least some light on them drawing upon the data obtained in our experiments.

We shall begin with the results of systematic morphologic and histo-chemical study of reactions of connective tissue around the implanted plate. It is known that such plate is always encapsulated but our knowledge of the capsule structure has been insufficient. Therefore, many authors as well as OPPENHEIMER believed that the capsule around the polymer plate is "quiet" during the latent period, that all active processes cease in it and that "suddenly", many months later, a tumour begins to grow in it. Investigations of L. V. OLSHEVSKAYA and later L. V. OLSHEVSKAYA and N. T. RAIKHLIN have shown that it is absolutely not true.

As quickly as 1 month since the beginning of the experiment, the structure of the connective tissue capsule embedding the whole cellophane plate is characterized by massiveness, thickness and heterogenicity. The three following layers can be traced in it:

1. internal layer consisting of young fibroblasts;

2. intermediate layer consisting of dense collagenous bundles and a great number of mature fibroblasts, and

3. external layer consisting of loosely arranged elements of connective tissue and a large quantity of blood vessels. Within the first 6—7 months of its life the connective tissue capsule is constantly in active condition. It takes the form of constant proliferation of young fibroblasts in the internal layer, increased thickness of the intermediate collagenous layer, and the most important of it, the persistant presence of metachromatic mucopolysaccharides indicating a long-term continuous process of noncompleting collagen formation. Constant hyperaemia of capsule external layer vessels is apparent. Later, beginning from the 7th or 8th month particularly significant morphologic and histochemical changes are observed in the capsule. First of all, the following considerable changes occur in the intermediate layer: collagenous fibres take irregular staining, form separate swellings and look like a homogeneous mass which does not produce typical histochemical reactions characteristic of normal collagen. In other words, the process of collagen formation is upset which is accompanied by disorganization of collagen; collagen is converted to an atypical protein mass. On the other hand, the internal layer displays a still more distinct proliferation of cells which spreads diffusely at first but then becomes non-uniform. This results in irregular hyperplasia of fibroblasts in the internal layer which serves as the background for subsequent development of focal proliferates. The cells of these proliferates become less differentiated and atypical eventually. At later stages focal proliferates look like isolated formation and their own stroma consisting of argyrophilic fibres can be traced in them. Cells of such proliferates tend to grow infiltratively into the surrounding parts of the capsule. The morphological pattern of such focal proliferates largely coincides with that of the so-called "presarcoma" foci (according to L. M. SHABAD) observed when carcinogenic hydrocarbons are introduced (Y. M. VASILJEV, 1955, 1961). It is true that morphological and histochemical changes in connective tissue capsule around a whole polymer plate (cellophane) are similar in many respects to those occurring around paraffin pellets which contain carcinogenic hydrocarbons — in both cases one can observe an accumulation of many fibroblasts which get less and less differentiated gradually. Nodular proliferates appear on the diffuse hyperplasia background. Subsequently these proliferates become isolated and form foci of "presarcoma". Finally, in both cases one observes profound disturbance of collagen formation, its disorganization and accumulation of atypical intermediate substance. This substance contains separate fibroblasts or their clusters which conse-

quently find themselves under conditions significantly differing from normal ones.

Slower development of the entire process and a kind of delayed changing of its stages when polymer plates are introduced constitute a substantial distinctive feature, as compared with carcinogenic hydrocarbone effect.

When minced polymer is introduced, the process is quite different. Reactive inflammation observed in this case at early stages takes acute and, as a rule, more rapid form, than in the case of the whole plate. Separate particles of the polymer are encapsulated rather quickly and then the process of proliferation of connective tissue cell is completed. The capsule embedding separate polymer particles remains thin during the whole term of observation, i.e. during the whole life of the animal; collagen retains the normal fibrous structure and conventional staining properties. Proliferation of fibroblasts in such capsule does not differ from usually observed one in normal connective tissue; atypical cells and formation of focal cellular proliferates are not observed. At much later stages a great number of cells-phagocytes were observed around the pulverized polymer in the capsule; they must have been involved in resorption of newly-formed collagen. It is worth mentioning that such phagocytes are not observed, as a rule, in the capsule around the whole polymer plate. A comparative study of the reaction of connective tissue to the whole polymer plate (in our case-cellophane) and to particles obtained by pulverization of the same has revealed very substantial distinctions. Introduction of fine particles causes a distinct inflammation and results in encapsulation without further pathological consequences, whereas introduction of a whole plate results in atypical tissue growth and after a number of successive stages

(which are well known with carcinogenic hydrocarbon effect, by the way) in a sarcoma. The above data provides a vivid illustration of possible mechanisms of blastomogenesis in this case. One can suppose that disorganization of intermediate substance, atypization of collagen interspersed with dividing and dedifferentiating fibroblasts play the most important part in tumorigenesis. The long-term fibroblastic proliferation takes place undoubtedly under conditions of considerable disturbance of oxidative and other types of metabolism. It is possible that it is these conditions that contribute to selection of those fibroblasts which will give rise to clones of tumour cells.

How are these conditions brought about? Undoubtedly, they are connected with the shape and size of introduced material.

The results of research done by To-MATIS are an eye-opener in this respect. In 1963 the author reported that, unlike other investigators, he succeded in inducing sarcomas in mice by subcutaneous introduction of minute fragments of teflone. Thanks to his courtesy I could get first-hand knowledge of his microscopic slides, while I visited the Shubik Laboratory in Chicago, 1964. The changes were discovered which were identical with those observed in the slides of L. V. OLSHEVSKAYA in her experimental series on implantation of whole plates in rats, the changes being fully described above. In this case as well the process started with disorganization of collagen formation and with irregular fibroblastic hyperplasia. Rather large (0.5—1 square mm) cut pieces of minced polymer in TOMATIS experiments were the same factor in case of the mice organism as whole plates — in the case of rats. Therefore, the concept of the size of introduced plate needs to be limited to an extent depending on the size of experimental animal. Hence, it refers us back to what we believe is the most important factor of blastomogenesis of this type — to the role of organism and its metabolism. It is natural that the similarity of the so-called polymer blastomogenesis to sarcoma induction with carcinogenic hydrocarbons demonstrated by us should suggest an idea that in this case some chemical carcinogenic influences take place too. As they are not apparently connected with the introduced material, the idea of their possible origin in the experimental animal organism itself and mere accumulation on the implanted plate seems natural. One can imagine that some metabolites capable of acting as endogenous carcinogenic substances concentrate on its surface. Such metabolites may be steroids and some derivatives of tryptophane (Boyland et al.). It should be reminded that similar phenomena of peculiar adsorption and deposition of the endogenous agent occur in the genesis of cysticercous sarcomata of liver in rats, i.e. in those animals which were used in the overwhelming majority of polymer experiments.

Certain findings of the experiments of A. H. Kogan fit the framework of the above hypothesis very well. Let us consider them.

A. H. Kogan was the first to show that application of a polymer capsule to the kidney may induce in rats not only a sarcoma but a carcinoma as well. We mean papillary carcinomas originating from pelvic epithelium which were observed 4 times in experiments with capron, cellophane, polyvinyl chloride and tephlon. But it is of particular interest that advanced hyperplasia and marked papillomatosis of pelvic epithelium, obvious precancerous changes, were found in 20 other rats (experiments with polyethylene, lavsan, tephlon, polystyrene, capron and cellophane). It should be noted that pelvic epithelium was not

in direct contact with the polymer capsule applied to the kidney. In such case one cannot but think about the carcinogenic effect of some endogenous metabolites (possibly, derivatives of tryptophane) which could be retained and accumulated in the pelvis because the kidney was squeezed by the polymer capsule. In special check experiments (capsule was not applied to the kidney) when the ureter was tied up and urinary metabolites were kept in the pelvis for a long time, no cancer was induced, but hyperplasia of pelvic epithelium was observed in some animals.

A. H. Kogan's experiments on minced cellophane and urinary metabolites are especially interesting. Initially, these experiments confirmed again the well-established fact-subcutaneous introduction of minced cellophane does not cause tumours in rats. Then, in a special series of experiments minced cellophane was incubated in vitro with urine of normal intact rats under sterile conditions for 30 months, i.e. during a term equal to the longest life expectancy of the rat and exceeding by far the latent period of plastics blastomogenesis. Introduction of minced cellophane which had been incubated with the urine resulted in sarcomata in 10 out of 31 rats during terms ranging from 11.5 to 21.5 months, i.e. as far as blastomogenic activity is concerned it had the same effect as introduction of cellophane whole plates. As check measures, both rat's pure urine and rat's urine in which cellophane had been steeped were introduced into rats subcutaneously during 5 months, but no tumours were obtained.

In another series of experiments minced cellophane was introduced into a kidney with the ureter tied up. As a result pelvic carcinomas were obtained in 5 out of 39 rats which survived from 7.5 to 18.5 months. Besides, papillomatosis of the pelvis was observed in another 6 rats. In check experiments when minced cellophane was introduced into the kidney but the ureter was not tied up or when the ureter was tied up but cellophane was not introduced, no tumours were induced.

Thus, it is possible to prove under certain experimental conditions that a polymer can adsorb blastomogenic urinary metabolites, i.e. endogenous carcinogenic substances. This makes the explanation of plastics blastomogenesis given by us above probable, but, of course, it does not exhaust the problem.

But, whatever is our idea of the causes and mechanisms of tumour origin following introduction of various polymer materials into organism, no matter how difficult it may be to give a comprehensive explanation of mechanism of sarcoma formation at sites of implantation of different plates, the experimental data available may and must be taken into consideration for practice.

On the basis of numerous experimental data we can propose a number of concrete suggestions concerning uses of polymer materials in surgery, orthopedics, in reparative and plastic operations.

Introduction of whole plates into organism for long periods (for years) should be avoided. It is preferred to introduce perforated plates; shapes like sieves, interlaced threads and "matting" would be still better.

The shape of the prosthesis may be an important factor the more streamlike it will be, the better. The prosthesis and any foreign body introduced into the organism should be as small as possible.

When materials are selected for introduction into organism, natural and, if possible, easy-resolvable materials should be preferred. No tumours were induced in the experiments of A. H. KOGAN, when such natural polymers as rubber, procollagen (from rat's skin) and fibrin (from dog's plasma) were applied on the rat's kidney as a capsule.

When polymers are introduced into organism, any combination with chemical carcinogenic substances, endogenous ones included, should be avoided. In this connection, special care should be taken when polymers are applied in surgery of urinary and probably, biliary ducts.

Similarly, a combination of polymers which can induce a focus of chronic inflammation with irradiation should be avoided.

It was long ago that LACASSAGNE showed that irradiation of an inflamed tissue may result in sarcoma formation, and A. H. KOGAN reported 2 cases of leucosis in rats which had had cellophane capsules around the kidneys and had been exposed to the total X-ray dose of 350 r; no leucosis was obtained in control experimental series.

Finally, we should point out the harmless effect of introduction of pulverized substances and threads. The latter is of special importance for medical practice.

Thus, we come to the conclusion that in this particular field of blastomogenesis, like in many others, results of experimental research work may be used not only for the study of etiology and pathogenesis of tumours but for their prophylaxis as well.

References

ALEXANDER, P., and HORNING, E., *The Oppenheimer method of inducing tumours by subcutaneous implantation of plastic films*. In: Ciba Fundation Symposium on carcinogenes mechanisms of action. London 1958, 12—22 (1959).

BERING, B. A., and HANDLER, A. H., The production of tumors in hamsters by implantation of polyethylene films. *Cancer (Philad.)* **10**, 414 (1957).

Boyland, E., *Aromatische Amine als endogene Carcinogene.* Berl. Symposium über Fragen der Carcinogenese. Dezember, 1959, Berlin, 165—166 (1960).

Druckrey, H., Hamperl, H., u. Schmähl, D., Cancerogene Wirkung von metallischem Quecksilber nach intraperitonealer Gabe bei Ratten. *Z. f. Krebsforsch.* **61**, 511—519 (1957).

—, u. Schmähl, D., Cancerogene Wirkung von Kunststoff-Folien. *Z. Naturforsch.* **7**, 353—356 (1952).

— — Cancerogene Wirkung von Quarz bei Implantation an Ratten. *Naturwissenschaften* **41**, 534 (1954).

— u. Mecke, R., Cancerogene Wirkung von Gummi nach Implantation an Ratten. *Z. f. Krebsforsch.* **61**, 55—64 (1956).

Golbert, Z. V., and Shabad, L. M., *Presarcoma* [in Russian]. In: Zlokachestvennyye opukholi, p. 23—27. Moscow 1948.

Kogan, A. H., Über die blastomogene Wirkung makromolekularer Verbindungen [in Russian]. *Pat. Fiziol. éksp. Ter.* **3**, 74—80 (1959).

— *Die blastomogene Wirkung einer Kunststoffe im Experiment.* Berl. Symposium über Fragen der Carcinogenese. Dezember 1959, Berlin, 90—97 (1960).

— *Experimental carcinogenesis induced by synthetic polymers* [in Russian]. In: Carcinogenesis; mechanisms of action, p. 215—236. Moscow 1965.

—, and Beryozov, T. T., *Dynamics of transaminases activity of conjunctive tissue capsules, developing around film implants, in the process of malignization.* In: 8. Internat. cancer congr. 1962 Abstracts of papers, p. 465.

— Chechulin, A. S., u. Aliev, M. A., Über die blastomogene Wirkung von Cellophan bei experimenteller Nierenhypertonie bei Ratten [in Russian]. *Arkh. Pat.* **17**, 65—66 (1955).

— — Vedrova, N. N., and Filimonova, M. V., Analysis of significance of the mechanical factor in the blastomogenic effect of compressive cellophane capsules placed on the kidneys [in Russian]. *Arkh. Pat.* **20**, 44—49 (1958).

—, and Tugarinova, V. N., On the blastomogenic action of polyvinylchloride [in Russian]. *Vop. Onkol.* **5**, 540—545 (1959).

Nothdurft, H., Experimentelle Sarcome durch reizlos einheilende Fremdkörper. *Strahlentherapie* **100**, 192—210 (1956).

Nothdurft, H., *Tumorerzeugung durch Fremdkörperimplantation.* Berl. Symposium über Fragen der Carcinogenese. Dezember 1959, 80—89. Berlin 1960.

Olshevskaya, L. V., Early morphological changes in rat connective tissue around implanted cellophane films [in Russian]. *Bull. exp. Biol. Med.* **51**, 116—120 (1961).

— Changes in the connective tissue of rats during the process of tumour development caused by the implantation of cellophane film [in Russian]. *Bull. exp. Biol. Med.* **52**, 79—84 (1961).

— Comparative study of the changes in the connective tissue of rats developing around cellophane imbedded subcutaneously. *Acta Un. int. Cancr.* **19**, 612—614 (1963).

Oppenheimer, B. S., Oppenheimer, E. T., Danishefsky, I., and Stout, A. P., Carcinogenic effects of metals in rodents. *Cancer Res.* **16**, 439—441 (1956).

— — — —, and Eirich, F. R., Further studies of polymers as carcinogenic agents in animals. *Cancer Res.* **15**, 333—340 (1955).

— —, and Stout, A. P., Sarcomas induced in rodents by imbedding various plastic films. *Proc. Soc. exp. Biol. (N.Y.)* **17**, 366—369 (1952).

— — — Carcinogenic effect of imbedding various plastic films in rats and mice. *Surg. Forum* **4**, 672—676 (1953).

— — — Danishevsky, T., and Eirich, F. R., Malignant tumors and high polymers. *Science* **118**, 783 (1953).

— Stout, A. D., Oppenheimer, E. T., and Willhite, M., Study of the precancerous stage of fibrosarcomas induced by plastic films. *Cancer Res.* **2**, 237 (1957).

Oppenheimer, E. T., Willhite, M., Danishefsky, T., and Stout, A. P., Observations on the effects of powder polymers in the carcinogenic process. *Cancer Res.* **21**, 132—138 (1961).

Shabad, L. M., Olshevskaya, L. V., and Vasiliev, Yu. M., On the tumor development in rats following polymer films insertion (Bulgary). *Khirurgiya (Sofiya)* **15**, 325—333 (1962).

Tomatis, L., Studies in subcutaneous carcinogenesis with implants of glass and teflon in mice. *Acta Un. int. Cancr.* **19**, 607—611 (1963).

Turner, F. C., Sarcomas at sites of subcutaneous implanted Bakelite disk in rats. *J. nat. Cancer Inst.* **2**, 81—83 (1941).

VASILIEV, YU. M., Experimental histological study of neoplastic processes in connective tissue [in Russian]. *Vop. Onkol.* **1**, 5—16 (1955).
— Early changes in the subcutaneous connective tissue of rats after implantation of pellets containing carcinogenic polycyclic hydrocarbons. *J. nat. Cancer Inst.* **23**, 441—486 (1959).

VASILIEV, YU. M., *Connective tissue and neoplastic growth in experiment* [in Russian]. Moscow 1961.
— OLSHEVSKAYA, L. V., RAIKHLIN, N. T., and IVANOVA, O. YU., Comparative study of alterations induced by 7,12-Dymethylbenz (a)anthracene and polymer films in the subcutaneous connective tissue of rats. *J. nat. Cancer Inst.* **28**, 515—559 (1962).

Plastic Carcinogenesis; Suggestions for the Use of Plastics in Surgery, Orthopedics, etc...

G. J. VAN ESCH

Head, Laboratory of Toxicology, Rijks Instituut voor de Volksgezondheid, Utrecht, The Netherlands

Plastics are macromolecules with long chains and molecular weights ranging from 10^4 up to 10^6. These polymers are formed by the chemical addition or condensation of a great number of units: the monomers. The chemical process of polymerization is highly dependable upon factors as temperature, pressure, solvents, catalysts, inhibitors and other factors.

The following type of polymers are produced: straight single polymers, polymers with side chains and polymers with a three dimensional structure. Furthermore the following types of polymerization may be distinguished: homopolymerization (one kind of monomer), copolymerization (different types of monomers) and heteropolymerization (one of the monomers is not capable of polymerization, but becomes activated by another monomer).

The chemical composition of the polymers is of primary importance and the molecular units estimate the physical properties of the polymers. The chemical properties are determined by the functional groups at the end of the chains and side-chains and also by the low molecular compounds which have been added. It must be mentioned that in industrial practice however, the polymerization end-products hardly contain any active functional group.

The various plastics have complete different properties, and they can be divided in 3 main groups:

1. Thermohardening polymers: during heating chemical reaction takes place and a threedimensional structure is formed. These polymers can not longer be remodelled.

2. Thermoplastic polymers. Plastics which are softened by heat and hardened on cooling. These polymers of linear arrangement are important *for the use in surgery*.

3. Rubbers, characterized by elasticity.

There is a great variety of plastics which differ widely in chemical composition.

In processing or adapting the end-products to fullfill the special requirements of the plastics as flexibility, toughness, rigidity and temperature stability, a great number of additives is used. These additives modify the physical and chemical properties of the plastics. Polymers are often sold under trade-names. In general only the basic manufacturer knows precise details of the used additives because these data are kept secret. The intermediate manufacturer who supplies the surgeon and other users with their appliances, will have only a general idea of the nature of the material in question. The users often does not have the knowledge to choose and handle the appropriate plastic.

The number of additives which are available to the producer is enormous and the main groups of additives are:

catalysts, inhibitors, curing agents, accelerators, stabilizers, antioxidants, plasticizers, fillers, brighteners, antistatics, emulsifiers, foaming agents, lubricants, solvents, colorants and fungicides.

In general the total quantity of these additives and monomers which did not react does not exceed 4%, exclusive fillers and plasticizers which can range up to 50%. All these low-molecular substances can migrate out of the polymer into the surrounding tissue after implantation.

The chemical composition of the polymer can be changed for instance by gammaradiation. Links, as $-\overset{|}{\underset{|}{C}}-Cl$ and $-\overset{|}{\underset{|}{C}}-O-\overset{|}{\underset{|}{C}}-$ are broken permanently, while other links are only broken temporary and sometimes reform. This can be very important if, for instance, gammaradiation is used as means of sterilization or when implanted material is irradiated in situ.

Other influences which can change the chemical structure of polymers are for instance temperature, chemical treatment and stretching. In all cases the results will be permanent or temporary changes in the properties of the polymers.

TURNER (1941) was the first author, who described the induction of fibrosarcoma in rats after subcutaneous implantation of bakelite. After this finding, other authors published results with polymers and other substances which confirmed the results of TURNER. In experiments with rats, rabbits, hamsters and other species, which were carried out

during the last 20 years, the following type of polymers are tested:

cellophane (a polysaccharide), dacron (a linear polyester), polyethylene, polyvinylchloride, silastic (dimethylpolysiloxane), pliofilm (a caoutchouc), nylon (a polyamide), perspex (polymethylmethacrylate), polystyrene, saran (mixpolymer of polyvinylidene chloride and polyvinylchlorid), ivalon (polyvinylalcohol), Kel-F (polytrifluorochloroethylene, teflon (polytetrafluoroethylene) and others (table I).

From these experiments it is clear that the shape of the implant is of great importance: films, squares or discs induce a higher percentage of subcutaneous tumours than sticks, textile (fibers woven into textile), small pieces, grain or powder. The induction of tumours decreases in the mentioned order. Imperforated films induce more tumours than perforated ones and also the size of the pores is important, the smaller the diameter of the pore, the more tumours are induced. The same was found for the pores of sponges. Also the size of the implant is of importance. A number of authors established correlation between the size of the implant and the number of induced tumours; the bigger the size, the more tumours and as you know the shorter the latency-period.

STINSON (1960) showed in experiments with perspex discs of different diameter implanted intramuscularly, that there seems to be a minimal size, a sort of threshold value, which is necessary to induce tumours. This can perhaps be explained by the fact that, in this case, the latency-period is longer as the lifetime of the animal.

Also the thickness of the implant is important, the thicker the implant the more tumours are induced. On the contrary, the roughness of the surface of the implant seems to have no influence on

Table I. Units of a number of homopolymers, copolymers and heteropolymers

$$\left[\begin{array}{c} \text{OH} \quad \text{OH} \\ | \quad | \\ \text{CH—CH} \\ \text{—HC} \diagdown \quad \diagup \text{CH—O—} \\ \text{CH—O} \\ | \\ \text{CH}_2\text{OH} \end{array}\right]_n \quad \text{(Cellophane)}$$

$$[\text{—CH}_2\text{—CH—}]n \quad \text{(Polystyrene)}$$
(with phenyl group)

$$\left[\text{—CH}_2\text{—}\underset{\text{COOCH}_3}{\overset{\text{CH}_3}{\underset{|}{\overset{|}{\text{C}}}}}\text{—}\right]_n \quad \text{(Perspex)}$$

Polymers

$$[\text{—CH}_2\text{—CH}_2\text{—}]\,n \quad \text{(Polyethylene)}$$

$$\left[\underset{\text{COOCH}_3}{\overset{}{\text{—CH—CH}_2\text{—}}}\underset{\text{CN}}{\overset{}{\text{CH—CH}_2\text{—}}}\right]_n \quad \text{(Vinyon N)}$$

$$[\text{—CH}_2\text{—CHOH—}]\,n \quad \text{(Ivalon)}$$

Polycondensates

$$[\text{—CHCl—CH}_2\text{—}]\,n \quad \text{(PVC)} \qquad \text{—HN(CH}_2)_6\text{—NH—CO—(CH}_2)_4\text{—CO—} \quad \text{(Nylon-66)}$$

$$\left[\text{—CH}_2\text{—}\underset{}{\overset{\text{CH}_3}{\underset{|}{\overset{|}{\text{CCl}}}}}\text{—CH}_2\text{—CH}_2\text{—}\right]\,n \quad \text{(Pliofilm)}$$

Polyesters

$$[\text{—CF}_2\text{—CFCl—}]\,n \quad \text{(Kel-F.)} \qquad \left[\text{—O—}\underset{\text{O}}{\overset{}{\text{C}}}\text{—C}_6\text{H}_4\text{—}\underset{\text{O}}{\overset{}{\text{C}}}\text{—OCH}_2\text{—CH}_2\text{—}\right]n \quad \text{(Dacron)}$$

$$[\text{—CF}_2\text{—CF}_2\text{—}]\,n \quad \text{(Teflon)}$$

Silicone

$$[\text{—CCl}_2\text{—CH}_2\text{—CHCl—CH}_2\text{—}]\,n \quad \text{(Saran)} \qquad \left[\text{—}\underset{\text{CH}_3}{\overset{\text{CH}_3}{\underset{|}{\overset{|}{\text{SI}}}}}\text{—O—}\right]_n \quad \text{(Silastic)}$$

tumour induction, since Brunner (1959) did not find differences between pieces of perspex with 50% of fibrin, which give a very rough polymer.

Oppenheimer, Oppenheimer, Stout, Willhite and Danishefsky (1958) studied the necessity of the presence of the implant for the induction of tumours by experiments in which the implant or the implant and pocket were removed at different times. It appears necessary that the implants are left in the pocket for a minimal period. After this critical period its removal does not affect the production of tumours. If the implant is removed earlier no tumours are induced. When the pocket also is removed, no tumours are induced, regardless of the times of removal. From other experiments it

seems that the critical period during which the implant must be present is different depending on the type of material implanted in the rat.

From experiments in which implantation of polymers or other substances was combined with treatment by X-rays or carcinogenic substances, an increase of tumour production was found (Vollmar and Ott, 1961; Tomatis and Shubik, 1963).

Grindlay and Waugh (1955) were struck by the apparent "inertness" of polyvinylalcohol sponge because tissue adopts and uses it as a framework for the ingrowth of fibrous tissue. For this reason these sponges have often been used by plastic surgeons, especially during the past ten years. The question is studied by a number of authors (BERING, McLAURIN, LLOYD and INGRAHAM, 1955; ARONS, SABESIN, SMITH, 1961; DUKES, and MITCHLEY, 1962; and ARONS, 1963) as to whether these implanted sponges influences the formation and spread of metastasis. The results of the experiments are till now not decisive, and further studies are necessary.

From the results of all these experiments, which were carried out in the past 25 years, the necessity emerges to draw up requirements for polymers which may be used safely in plastic surgery.

SCALES published in 1953 already the following requirements for an "ideal" polymer:

1. It must be possible to fabricate the polymer in the desired form and the end-product of the polymerization process must be resistent to mechanical strains.

2. It must be possible to sterilize the polymers, without inducing chemical changes.

3. The polymer must be chemically inert.

4. The polymer may not be modified physically by tissue-fluids.

5. The polymer may not excite an inflammatory of foreign-body reaction or give hypersensitivity.

6. The polymer may not be carcinogenic.

To which extend it is possible to meet at the moment these "ideal" requirements or what can be done to meet them.

Ad 1. This is a pure technical problem and can be left to the producer. It is however necessary that the producer discusses the requirements with the user before fabricating the polymer, so that the most suitable polymer is produced for a certain application.

Ad 2. From the introduction it is clear that sterilization by heat or irradiation can introduces important chemical changes in the polymer and consequently changes the properties of the polymer. Also in this case the producer must give directions for the sterilization of the different types of polymers.

Ad 3. The polymer must be inert means that when the polymer is implanted it may not change. In practice it will be difficult to prove that a polymer is inert. In any way it will be necessary to lay down requirements for the purity of the polymer and the migration of additives and other low molecular compounds. This can be done in the same way as for packaging materials, for which legal regulations are drafted at the moment in the Netherlands and some other countries.

Ad 4. About this point little is known, but there is some evidence that tissue-fluids attact or change a number of polymers. Clearly more research is desired.

Ad 5. All polymers which seem to be chemically and physically suitable for implantation should be studied biologically to show which of them give no or only a slight tissue reaction so that the best type of polymer can be chosen for clinical use. For this purpose different types of biological test methods are developed:

a short-term test with rabbits, in which the tissue-reaction is studied after subcutaneous implantation of the polymers; influence of the polymer on embryo or other tissue cultures; a test to study the influence of the polymer on the respiration of skin coupes of guinea-pigs; experiments with bacteria.

The results of these tests are till now very difficult to understand and more research is necessary, so that the meaning of these tests becomes better defined.

Ad 6. This question, as it is put by SCALES, is very diffcult to answer at the moment, because the mechanism of the subcutaneous carcinogenesis is still not understood. For this reasons, at the moment, it is necessary to met as good as possible the requirements of the "ideal" one, it still will be necessary to handle the polymers in practice with special precautions. A number of these precautions are already mentioned in 1961, by VOLLMAR and OTT. They are summarized below and some other suggestions are added.

1. In each case the indication to implantation must be discussed critically, especially for children. When it concerns people of the age of 50 years and older a number of objections can be neglected (except when future experiments would show that implants (sponges) promote metastasizing).

2. When polymers are implanted, then as possible, not in massive form, but with pores or perforations. It is necessary to choose pores or perforations of optimal size.

3. The implant must be as small as possible.

4. When the implant is not longer necessary, it must, if possible, be taken out, including the pocket which is formed around the implant.

5. When polymers are implanted, the person should not be exposed to syn-carcinogenic noxes, for instance carcinogenic substances and X-rays.

6. When implants are removed, they must be studied histologically to get informed about the tissue reactions in man, so that these can be compared with the reactions found in the animal experiments.

7. It is necessary to registrate details of material which is used in practice, such as: type of material, size, shape, weight, perforation, pore size, etc. There must be a carefull registration of the incidence of tumours in man so that possibly more can be learned about the risks of the use of polymers in surgery, orthopedics etc. in future.

References

ARONS, M. S., SABESIN, S. M., and SMITH, R. R., Experimental studies with etheron sponge. Effect of implantation in tumor-bearing animals. *Plast. reconstr. Surg.* **28**, 72 (1961).

— Plastic in plastic surgery; a review of the cancerogenic problem. *Tex. Rep. Biol. Med.* **21**, 163 (1963).

BERING, E. A., McLAURIN, R. L., LLOYD, J. B., and INGRAHAM, F. D., The production of tumors in rats by the implantation of pure polyethylene. *Cancer Res.* **15**, 300 (1955).

BRUNNER, H., Experimentelle Auslösung von Tumoren durch Implantation von Polymethylmethacrylat bei Ratten. *Arzneimittel-Forsch.* **9**, 396 (1959).

DUKES, C. E., and MITCHLEY, B. C. V., Polyvinyl sponge implants: experimental and clinical observations. *Brit. J. plast. Surg.* **15**, 225 (1962).

GRINDLAY, J. H., and WAUGH, J. M., Plastic sponge which acts as a framework for living tissue (experimental studies and preliminary report of use to reinforce abdomal aneurysms). *Arch. Surg.* **63**, 288 (1951).

OPPENHEIMER, B. S., OPPENHEIMER, E. T., STOUT, A. P., WILLHITE, M., and DANISHEFSKY, I., The latent period in carcinogenesis by plastics in rats and its relation to the presarcomatous stage. *Cancer (Philad.)* **11**, 204 (1958).

SCALES, J. T., Tissue reactions to synthetic materials. *Proc. roy. Soc. Med.* **46**, 647 (1953).

STINSON, N. E., Tissue reaction to polymethylmethacrylate in rats and guinea-pigs. *Nature (Lond.)* **188**, 678 (1960).

TOMATIS, L., and SHUBIK, P., Influence of urethane on subcutaneous carcinogenesis by teflon implants. *Nature (Lond.)* **198**, 600 (1963).

TURNER, F. C., Sarcomas at sites of subcutaneously implanted bakelite disks in rats. *J. nat. Cancer. Inst.* **2**, 81 (1941).

VOLLMAR, J., and OTT, G., Experimentelle Geschwulstauslösung durch Kunststoffe aus chirurgischer Sicht. *Langenbecks Arch. klin. Chir.* **298**, 729 (1961).

Discussion of Papers by Professor Shabad and Dr. van Esch

Boyland: We have heard two interesting papers on the so-called Oppenheimer effect. Incubation of the plastic in urine for 30 months might allow formation of fungal or bacterial metabolites. If the effect depends upon absorption of materials from urine, then 1 hr. should be sufficient. It would be interesting to determine how long exposure to urine is necessary for the minced plastic to become carcinogenic. Plastics could be treated with urine and also with those tryptophan metabolites which are known to be carcinogenic. Although the carcinogenicity of plastics is considered to be physical, there may be chemical mechanisms involved in the carcinogenic process.

Shabad: Whilst I cannot exclude the possibility that mould or bacterial products played a part in the induction of tumours, I think it unlikely because of the uniformity of the results. I cannot say how long the period of incubation needs to be. Our first problem was to induce cancer. Having done this we can begin to study the mechanism.

Roe: There can be no doubt that the long list of chemicals which may be present in plastic materials is disturbing. This point has been made most convincingly by Dr. van Esch. However, the fact that a wide variety of chemical agents, including reactive substances, may be present in these materials is not of itself sufficient evidence for preferring a chemical to a physical explanation of the tumour induction which follows their implantation. Where tumours result from the implantation of large pieces of a plastic material, but not from the same amount of material after it has been broken up into small pieces, it is difficult to believe that a physical mechanism is not more likely than a chemical one.

With reference to the general review of the subject so admirably presented by Professor Shabad, I should like to report an experiment from our laboratories. Solid glass beads, either with smooth surfaces or with roughened surfaces, were implanted into the lumen of the bladder of mice and left there for 40 weeks. The rough beads accumulated more calcarious material around them than the smooth ones. One benign, one malignant and one probably malignant bladder tumour were seen in 67 mice bearing rough glass beads, but no tumours were seen in those bearing smooth beads. The oral administration of urethane markedly increased the incidence of bladder tumours in response to the implantation of rough glass beads (see Ball et al., 1964).

Finally, I should like to ask a general question. If these chemically inert materials induce cancer as a result of their physical presence at a site for a prolonged period, should we not encourage plastic surgeons to use, for implantation, materials which can be, at least slowly, absorbed?

Reference

Ball, J. K., Field, W. E. H., Roe, F. J. C., and Walters, M., The carcinogenic and co-carcinogenic effects of paraffin wax pellets and glass beads in the mouse bladder. *Brit. J. Urol.* 36, 225 (1964).

Schoental: The fact that, regardless of chemical composition, certain materials such as plastics, glass or metals induce fewer tumours when introduced as finely powdered solids than when implanted as large pieces, suggests that their carcinogenic action is more likely to be related to their physical presence than to their chemical constituents. By the use of newly developed electron spin resonance methods, it would be instructive to compare the signals due to free radicals in tissues adjacent to solid and powdered plastics implanted subcutaneously.

Hueper: Dr. van Esch suggested that manufacturers of plastics might be persuaded to produce special plastics for implantation. They are not interested in such small business. They would prefer to see the use of plastics in surgery discontinued rather than make the effort to develop suitable materials.

In California there are thousands of women with plastic implants in both breasts. I suggested that this kind of medicine was bad, but was told that the psychic trauma due to flat chestedness was worse than the cancer risk.

Van Esch: I am more optimistic than Dr. Hueper with regard to the co-operation of industry in producing safe plastics for surgery, because I believe that in the near future the requirements for polymers, for instance, in the field of packaging materials will be also much more strict, this means that a more careful choice of additives must be made before the polymer is fabricated. When the requirements are more stringent the manufacturer will become interested in manufacturing special polymers for surgery and orthopaedics, because the purity of the polymers for the different purposes will not differ very much.

Druckrey: There is no doubt that sarcomas which develop at the site of subcutaneous implantation are mainly due to physical effects, however it would be dangerous to generalise. After the intraperitoneal implantation of plastics, rubber or metallic mercury we observed multiple sarcomas, although there was no formation of a fibrous capsule.

Studying the patent literature, we found a number of patents for the use of substances to initiate, accelerate, or stop polymerization processes, or as stabilizers. Some of these are suspected or known to be carcinogenic, e.g. certain N-nitroso-compounds and aromatic amines. It is necessary therefore to consider not only the main compounds but also substances added during the production of the finished article or material. In this respect we should warn against the use of dangerous additives, especially for materials to be used in surgery.

Finally it may be relevant to refer to the induction of sarcomas by the implantation of asbestos, for in this case there is ample evidence that asbestos is carcinogenic for sites remote from the implantation site; also it is known to produce cancer in man.

Higginson: There appears to be a discrepancy between the ease with which the Oppenheimer effect can be demonstrated in animals and the rarity of sarcoma development at the site of implanted plastics in man. Sarcomas form only a small group of all human tumours and it should be relatively easy to form a sarcoma register in order to determine whether an aetiological relationship to any stimulus can be demonstrated. In a review of our material at the University of Kansas, covering over 16.000 tumours at all sites, I was unable to show that the distribution of sarcomas was more related to the usual sites of injection than would be anticipated on the basis of chance.

It should never be forgotten that where plastics are implanted in man, in the majority of cases their use is essential to maintain life.

Shabad: I think your suggestion with regard to a sarcoma register should be followed.

Saffiotti: I was very interested to hear Professor SHABAD's interpretation of the pathogenesis of the subcutaneous sarcomas around implants as due to a selection mechanism, because I had come to the idea of selection as a possible causative mechanism by looking at the problem from a different angle and starting from considerations derived from tissue culture work. Dr. L. HAYFLICK of the Wistar Institute recently presented his studies on the *in vitro* transformation of certain cell strains into cell lines with neoplastic characteristics: the environmental conditions and many aspects of the morphology

of these flattened out cell layers, growing *in vitro* on a smooth surface in which foci of transformed cells suddenly appear and grow, struck me as being somewhat similar to the conditions of the cells forming the "pocket" around subcutaneous implants of smooth films. If one assumes that the aetiology of transformation may be a spontaneous mutation or even an induced change (e.g. by a latent virus or by a minimal "contamination" with a carcinogen), then the hypothesis can be suggested that the special cellular environment represented by a layer of cells flattened out over an impermeable membrane is selectively favourable to the growth of these transformed cells, which develop into a tumour, while in normal tissues this transformation does not represent a competitive advantage and is not followed by growth of the transformed cell line. Following a stimulating discussion with Drs. HAYFLICK and H. M. TEMIN of the McArdle Memorial Laboratory, it was felt that experimental studies could be made to test this hypothesis. I find it at present the most satisfying theoretical explanation available for the phenomenon of sarcoma induction by implants. I think that the selected character (e.g. an enzymatic requirement) which gives the transformed cells a competitive advantage in the special conditions of growth, might well be retained in the whole tumour and be detectable in it by biochemical methods.

Truhaut: I should like to mention a particularly serious type of toxic effect in the production of which both physical and chemical factors are implicated. I refer to the effect produced by silica and certain silicates in the lungs. The physical form is important since only crystalline particles are active. On the other hand the chemical structure is also important since silicotic lesions are only produced by particles which consist chemically of silica or silicates.

Boyland: If the suggestion of Dr. SHABAD that plastics which are absorbed are not carcinogenic is correct, then attempts should be made to develop plastics which are absorbed for surgical use.

Van Esch: This may introduce further difficulties in that one will have to consider the toxicity of polymer breakdown products and a great number of low molecular weight compounds which become free.

Druckrey: We should distinguish between the scientific and the practical aspects. When the implantation of plastic materials produces tumours in 30—35% of rats after 1 to 2 years, this is only a weak effect. One to two years in rats would correspond to 30—60 years in humans. There is no objection to the implantation of plastics in adults whose life expectation is short, however with young people it is different.

At present we cannot argue that man is not susceptible to the induction of sarcoma by the implantation of plastics on the grounds that no cases have been described. It may well take 30 to 60 years to induce such cancers in man and this time has not elapsed since the use of many of these materials was introduced.

Roe: We had the opportunity of studying a large polyvinyl (Ivalon) sponge implant removed from the breast of a 22 year old woman. The sponge had been implanted between the mammary gland and pectoral muscles for cosmetic reasons. Within 10 months of the operation the region of the implant became hard, heavy and uncomfortable so that the sponge had to be removed. Histological examination showed that the interstices of the sponge had filled with collagen-producing fibrocytes, phagocytes and multinucleate giant cells. This is precisely the picture which precedes sarcoma formation in laboratory animals following implantation of the same material. Another point of interest is that separate particles of sponge were found lying in a portion of mammary gland overlying the implant, indicating that there is a possibility of adverse effects at sites at a distance from the implantation site.

Biochemical Aspects of Carcinogenesis with Special Reference to Alkylating Agents and Some Antibiotics

E. BOYLAND

Chester Beatty Research Institute, London, Great Britain

That many of the methods used in the control of cancer can themselves induce cancer, may appear as a paradox. An early example of an agent producing the two effects is radiation. Soon after their discovery, X-rays were used to treat cancer and within a decade of the discovery it was recognised that X-rays caused cancer in men exposed to the radiation. Other forms of radiation used in the control of cancer and leukaemia have been found to cause cancer. In some cases the biochemical processes involved in carcinogenesis and inhibition of growth are probably similar.

Thirty years ago HADDOW (1935) found that many cancer-producing compounds, particularly the polycyclic hydrocarbons such as benzopyrene and 1,2,5,6-dibenzanthracene inhibited the growth of animal tumours. The carcinogenic polycyclic hydrocarbons have been used occasionally for the control of cancer and leukaemia in patients. These hydrocarbons probably act by forming complexes with cellular nucleic acids (BOYLAND and GREEN, 1962).

The parallelism between growth inhibition and carcinogenic activity has important consequences in research. Biological tests for growth inhibition can be carried out much more rapidly than tests for carcinogenicity and some-

times give indications of cancer-producing activity. The discovery of the carcinogenic aminostilbene derivatives depended in part on the use of tests for growth inhibition.

Growth inhibition and carcinogenic activity of chemical compounds are two examples of biological actions which are also produced by radiation. There are many other radiomimetic effects caused by chemical substances, but in some cases the biological actions of the chemicals are more specific than those of radiation. Because of the close association between carcinogenesis and therapy of cancer, fundamental research on the two problems is closely associated. It is probable that the biochemical lesions caused by nitrogen mustard and other alkylating agents used either in controlling malignant disease or inducing cancer are similar. Recent work has shown that the essential reaction of alkylating agents is the introduction of alkyl groups into the guanine residues of deoxyribonucleic acid within the cells (BROOKES and LAWLEY, 1964). Many of the active compounds are bifunctional and act as crosslinking agents. The ethylenimine compounds such as TEM (SHIMKIN, 1954) are also carcinogenic to mice. TEM was used as a crosslinking agent in the textile industry and later in the treatment of HODGKIN's disease.

The original nitrogen mustards, HN2 or mustine and HN3, were found effective in the treatment of Hodgkin's disease and of lymphatic leukaemia when given by intravenous injection. Both these compounds have produced tumours on injection into animals (Boyland and Horning, 1949), and it would be surprising if they did not do so in human beings, given sufficient time. Following the wartime discovery of the chemotherapeutic effects of these simple nitrogen mustards, extensive research has revealed a number of derivatives which have some clinical advantages over the original compounds. Some four thousand chemical compounds, which can be considered as derivatives of nitrogen mustard, have been synthesised and tested against tumours in animals. Some of these are aromatic compounds and Haddow (1953) has shown that a number of these are carcinogenic on injection into rats. Two aromatic nitrogen mustards which are widely used today are Chlorambucil or Leukeran (4-bis(2-chloroethyl)-aminophenylbutyric acid) and melphalan or sarcolysin (4-bis-(2-chloroethyl)-aminophenylalanine). Leukeran acts as an initiator for skin tumours in mice (Salaman and Roe, 1956). Sarcolysin has induced mammary lymphadenomas in virgin rats (Presnov and Jushkov, 1964).

Some cancer chemotherapeutic agents are active only after metabolism. The Japanese nitrogen mustard N oxide Nitromin, the American triethylene thiophosphoramide, Thiotepa and the German Cyclophosphamide or Endoxan are compounds of this kind. Cyclophosphamide has induced embryonic abnormalities (Greenberg and Tanaku, 1964) leukaemia in mice (Vesela, 1962) and damage to the mucosa of the bladder in rats and dogs (Philips, Sternberg, Cronin and Vidal, 1961).

Myeleran, Busulfan or 1;4-dimesylbutane glycol is remarkably effective in the control of chronic myelocytic leukaemia. It has minor side effects causing depression of ovarian function and some skin pigmentation. Upton, Wolff and Sniffen (1961) found that although it decreased the incidence of myeloid leukaemia in mice it increased the incidence of thymic lymphomas.

Chloronaphazine, Erysan or CB1048 which is 2-bis(2-chloroethyl)aminonaphthalene, is a derivative of 2-naphthylamine, which is known to cause cancer of the bladder in men and in dogs. Danish workers (Thiede, Chievitz and Christensen, 1965; Viedebaek, 1964) have reported cases of bladder cancer occurring in patients between five and ten years after having been treated with CB1048. Manson (personal communication) has shown in the laboratory that CB1048 is converted to derivatives of 2-naphthylamine in rats. The bladder tumours produced in these patients were probably caused by 2-naphthylamine formed by metabolic dealkylation rather than by the original drug. Drugs of this type should not be used if the patients are likely to live for more than two or three years. In this case the chemotherapeutic action is probably due to the alkylating action of the drug itself and the carcinogenic effect to some metabolite excreted in urine.

CB 1151 (2-bis(2-chloropropyl)aminonaphthalene), also used clinically, is an alkylating agent and a derivative of 2-naphthylamine. This compound is given with urethane for the treatment of multiple myeloma, and as it can be metabolised to 2-naphthylamine it could induce bladder cancer in patients. Because of the risk of bladder cancer the urine of patients who have received either CB1048 or CB1151 should be examined for cancer cells by the

Papanicolaou technique, to facilitate early diagnosis of the disease.

Urethane, which as previously mentioned is used in the treatment of multiple myeloma, was shown to induce lung adenomata in mice by Nettleship and Henshaw in 1943, and as a result of quite independent researches, clinical trials with urethane in the treatment of cancer began about the same time. These led to the treatment of leukaemia with urethane by Paterson, Ap Thomas, Haddow and Watkinson, 1946). Since then it has been used less in leukaemia but has been used widely in multiple myeloma. Urethane is a multipotential carcinogen: it induces lymphomata in mice and rats and carcinomata of the forestomach in hamsters.

Urethane is metabolised by mammals to N-hydroxyurethane (Boyland and Nery, 1965) and the carcinogenic and antileukaemic effects are probably caused by this metabolite which reacts with the cytosine residues of RNA.

One of the most effective forms of chemotherapy of cancer is the treatment of cancer of the prostate with stilboestrol or other oestrogens. Oestrogens are also effective in some cases of breast cancer in women. Stilboestrol is carcinogenic, inducing kidney tumours in hamsters, mammary tumours in rats and mice, and pituitary tumours in rats. The carcinogenic hazard to man from the use of oestrogens in the treatment of prostatic or mammary cancer must be small, because most of the patients are old at the time when treatment is instituted, and although this form of therapy has been used for over twenty years there has been no convincing evidence that the treatment has caused cancer in human beings. The biochemistry of the mode of action of oestrogen is not known.

In addition to alkylating agents and hormones, antimetabolites and anti-

biotics are used in therapy. Mitomycin C is an antibiotic discovered in Japan (Hata, Sano, Sugawora, Matsumae, Kanamori, Shima and Hoshi, 1956). It can be considered as a derivative of ethyl carbamate or urethane and of ethylenimine. After metabolic activation mytomycin C crosslinks DNA through molecules of cytosine and guanine (Iyer and Szybalski, 1964). The ethylenimine group would be expected to react with the N7 atom of guanine, the ethyl carbamate group to condense with cytosine after metabolic oxidation to an N-hydroxycarbamate, as has been shown to occur with urethane. Actinomycin D is remarkable in its specific effect on Wilms' tumour of the kidney. Although Actinomycin D has not been tested for carcinogenic activity, other actinomycins have been shown to be carcinogenic (Kawamata, Nakabayashi, Kawai and Ushida, 1958). Actinomycin D in low concentrations inhibits synthesis of ribonucleic acid (RNA) controlled by DNA. This effect is probably due to the formation of complexes between DNA and Actinomycin D. These complexes may be similar to those formed with polycyclic hydrocarbons and DNA.

Griseovulvin is an antibiotic which is effective in systemic treatment of many skin infections. Oral administration of griseovulvin to mice has induced porphyria and hepatomas (Hurst and Paget, 1963). In view of this finding griseovulvin should be used only for treatment of conditions which will not respond to other treatment.

It must be accepted that it is justifiable to treat cancer with drugs which may themselves induce cancer. In many cases the patients are unlikely to survive long enough for the carcinogenic effect of the drugs to appear. These drugs should, however, not be used in other conditions unless they seem to offer great advantages.

Knowledge and understanding of the mechanism of action of the carcinogenic agents should help towards the solution of the cancer problem by eventually decreasing the human exposure to carcinogenic stimuli and in the discovery of improved methods of treating the disease.

References

BERENBLUM, I., BEN-ISHAI, D., HARAN-GHERA, N., LAPIDOT, A., SIMON, E., and TRAININ, N., Skin initiating action and lung carcinogenesis by derivatives of urethane (ethyl carbamate) and related compounds. *Biochem. Pharmacol.* **2**, 168—176 (1959).

BOYLAND, E., and GREEN, B., The interaction of polycyclic hydrocarbons and nucleic acids. *Brit. J. Cancer* **16**, 507—517 (1962).

—, and HORNING, E. S., The induction of tumours with nitrogen mustard. *Brit. J. Cancer* **3**, 118—123 (1949).

—, and NERY, R., The metabolism of urethane and related compounds. *Biochem. J.* **94**, 198—208 (1965).

BROOKES, P., and LAWLEY, P. D., Alkylating agents. *Brit. med. Bull.* **20**, 91—95 (1964).

GREENBERG, C. H., and TANAKU, K. R., Congenital anomalies probably induced by cyclophosphamide. *J. Amer. med. Ass.* **188**, 423—426 (1964).

HADDOW, A., Influence of certain polycyclic hydrocarbons on the growth of the Jensen rat sarcoma. *Nature (Lond.)* **136**, 868—869 (1935).

— In: Physiopathology of cancer, The chemical and genetic mechanisms of carcinogenesis. II. Biologic alkylating agents, 2nd ed. (ed. F. HOMBURGER), p. 602—685. London: Cassell 1953.

HATA, T., SANO, Y., SUGAWARA, R., MATSUMAE, A., KANAMORI, K., SHIMA, T., and HOSHI, T., Mitomycin, a new antibiotic from streptomyces. *J. Antibiot.* (Tokyo), Ser. A **9**, 141—146 (1956).

HURST, F. W., and PAGET, G. E., Protoporphyrin, cirrhosis and hepatomata in the livers of mice given griseofulvin. *Brit. J. Derm.* **75**, 105—112 (1963).

IYER, V. N., and SZYBALSKI, U., Mitomycins and porfiromycin: chemical mechanism of activation and cross-linking of DNA. *Science* **145**, 55—58 (1964).

KAWAMATA, J., NAKABAYASHI, N., KAWAI, A., and USHIDA, T., Experimental production of sarcoma in mice with actinomycin. *Med. J. Osaka* **8**, 753—762 Univ. (1958).

NETTLESHIP, A., and HENSHAW, P. S., Induction of pulmonary tumors in mice with ethyl carbamate (urethane). *J. nat. Cancer Inst.* **4**, 309—319 (1943).

PATERSON, E., AP THOMAS, I., HADDOW, A., and WILKINSON, J. M., Leukaemia treated with urethane compared with deep X-ray therapy. *Lancet* **1946** I, 677—683.

PHILIPS, F. S., STERNBERG, S. S., CRONIN, A. P., and VIDAL, P. M., Cyclophosphamide and urinary bladder toxicity. *Cancer Res.* **21**, 1577—1589 (1961).

PRESNOV, M. A., and JUSHKOV, S. F., The development of mastopathy and fibroadenoma in the rat mammary gland after intraabdominal sarcolysin injections. *Vop. Onkol.* **10** (5), 66—72 (1964).

SALAMAN, M. H., and ROE, F. J. C., Further tests for tumour-initiating activity: N,N-DI-(2-chloroethyl)-P-aminophenylbutyric acid (CB 1348) as an initiator of skin tumour formation in the mouse. *Brit. J. Cancer* **10**, 363—378 (1956).

SHIMKIN, M., Pulmonary-tumor induction in mice with chemical agents used in the clinical management of lymphomas. *Cancer (Philad.)* **7**, 410—413 (1954).

THIEDE, T., CHIEVITZ, E., and CHRISTENSEN, B. C., Chlornaphazine as a bladder carcinogen. *Acta med. scand.* **175**, 721—725 (1964).

UPTON, A. C., WOLFF, F. F., and SNIFFEN, E. P., Leukemogenic effect of myleran on the mouse thymus. *Proc. Soc. exp. Biol. (N.Y.)* **108**, 464—467 (1961).

VESELÁ, H., Induktion von Leukämie mit Phosphoramid bei Mäusen des C 57 B 1-Stammes. *Neoplasma (Bratisl.)* **9**, 75—80 (1962).

VIDEBAEK, A., Chlornaphazin (Erysan) may induce cancer of the urinary bladder. *Acta med. scand.* **176**, 45—50 (1964).

Discussion

Druckrey: We tested nitrogen mustard-N-oxide in rats. Even when high doses were administered continuously only weak carcinogenicity was observed. The parent nitrogen mustard, on the other hand, is a potent carcinogen. It follows that chemotherapeutic and carcinogenic activity do not necessarily go hand in hand.

Davey: I do not think that griseofulvin is carcinogenic in any specific way or that carcinogenesis is a hazard which will be encountered in the use of the drug. If relatively enormous doses are given to mice (more than 1% in the diet) porphyrin metabolism is excessively disturbed, deposits of protoporphyrin are laid down in the liver, liver damage and work hypertrophy ensue, and finally hepatomas are formed. I think the hepatomas are consequent on the excessive liver damage and that without it no tumours would appear.

Metabolism of Drugs in Relation to Carcinogenicity*

James A. Miller and Elizabeth C. Miller

McArdle Memorial Laboratory for Cancer Research, Medical School, University of Wisconsin, Madison, Wis. U.S.A.

The experimental production of cancer by chemicals was first accomplished with coal tar in Japan some five decades activities of these compounds are available [1—3]. An excellent treatise on chemical carcinogenesis has been published

3,4-Benzpyrene

2-Acetylaminofluorene

4-Dimethylaminoazobenzene

Dimethylnitrosamine

Ethionine

4-Nitroquinoline N-Oxide

Carbon Tetrachloride

Ethyl Carbamate

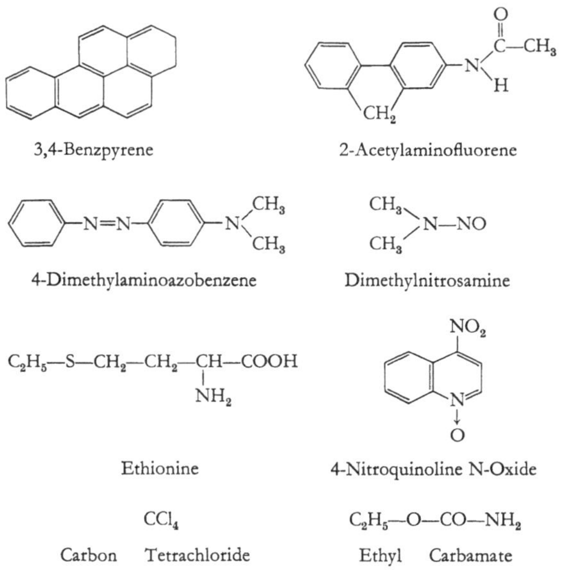

Fig. 1. Structural variety of synthetic chemical carcinogens [3]

ago. These observations provided the basis for the discovery of the first pure chemical carcinogens, the polycyclic aromatic hydrocarbons, in the early 1930's. Since that time numerous substances with diverse structures have been found to induce tumors in a variety of species and tissues. The majority of these substances are man-made or synthetic, and compilations of data on the carcinogenic recently by Clayson [3]. Some idea of the variety of structure that exists among the synthetic chemical carcinogens is

* Our work in this field is supported by Grant C 355 of the National Cancer Institute, U. S. Public Health Service; by a grant from the Jane Coffin Childs Memorial Fund for Medical Research; and by a grant from the Alexander and Margaret Stewart Trust Fund. This paper was published previously in the *Ann. N.Y. Acad. Sci.* **123**, 125—140 (1965).

apparent from Fig. 1. Some of these compounds (dimethylnitrosamine, ethionine, ethyl carbamate, 4-nitroquinoline N-oxide) appear to give rise to alkylating or arylating agents *in vivo;* Fig. 2 displays some of the variety in structure to be found among the known carcinogenic synthetic alkylating agents. Most of these compounds have proved to be less potent than the compounds depicted in Fig. 1. Furthermore, in recent years a number of natural products have been

be related to the diverse functional groups present in the nucleic acids and proteins of cells and thus to the variety of reactions possible between these macromolecules and the chemical carcinogens or their metabolites. In this way structurally diverse chemical carcinogens might react in different ways with these determinants of cell heredity and metabolism to bring about the same or similar irreversible changes responsible for the conversion of normal to malig-

CH_3—$N(CH_2CH_2Cl)_2$

Methyl
bis-(2-chloroethyl)amine

1-Ethylenoxy-
3,4-epoxycyclohexane

CH_3CO—$N\begin{smallmatrix}CH_2\\|\\CH_2\end{smallmatrix}$

N-acetyl ethylene imine

$CH_3SO_2O(CH_2)_4OSO_2CH_3$

1,4-Dimethanesulfonyl-oxybutane

β-Propiolactone

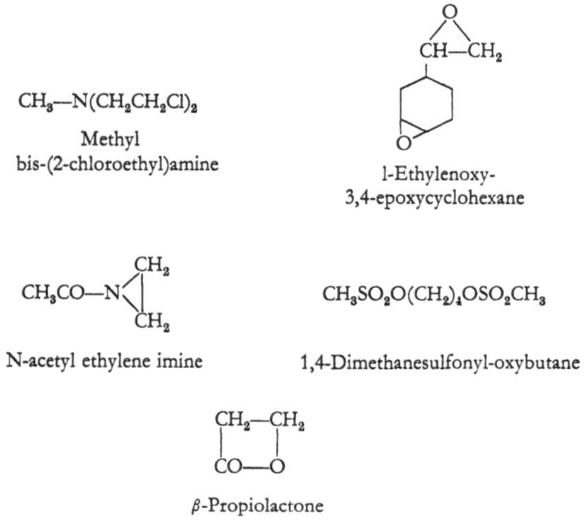

Fig. 2. Some carcinogenic alkylating agents [3]

found to be carcinogenic. The structures of several known and presumptive naturally occurring dietary carcinogens [4—8] are shown in Fig. 3. The compounds shown here or the crude natural source in which they occur all produce liver cancer when fed to the rat. The hepatocarcinogen ethionine, originally discovered as a synthetic chemical carcinogen, has recently been found as a metabolite of several bacteria [9].

No common structure is evident among the chemical carcinogens, nor is there any common metabolic pattern or metabolic derivative known for these agents. Our view is that this variety of structures for chemical carcinogens may

nant cells; in essence this conversion is characterized by a loss of or decrease in the control of the growth of these altered cells.

Man is susceptible to the carcinogenic action of certain chemicals, and indeed man was the species in which chemical carcinogenesis was first demonstrated. This finding came from numerous well-authenticated cases of cancer peculiar to small occupational groups [10—13] which were exposed to gross amounts of crude hydrocarbon mixtures such as tars and oils or to certain aromatic amines for long times. A variety of other chemicals are considered to pose carcinogenic hazards for humans [3]. Synthetic chemicals are widely and increasingly employed in the modern world, and this fact coupled with knowledge of chemical carcinogenesis has given rise to concern and to legislation on the carcinogenic hazards to man of the chemicals in our environment. As our knowledge of carcinogenic natural products increases, concern is also being expressed over this aspect of our environment. Hence, more attention is being paid to the induction of cancer as an important aspect of chronic toxicity tests [14—16]. Chemical carcinogens differ greatly in their potencies and toxicities, and no rapid test not

pounds to rats and mice at dosages up to maximally tolerated levels; large numbers of animals must be maintained throughout in reasonably good health.

Our present knowledge of the metabolism of chemical carcinogens, like that of their structures, is of no great predictive value in evaluating the possible carcinogenic hazards of a new chemical structure. However, information is available on some of the reactions which appear to be involved in either the activation or deactivation of carcinogens, and it may be hoped that with time these and other data can be helpful in

Pyrrolizidine alkaloids
(senecio and crotolaria genera)

Aflatoxin B
(aspergillus flavus strain)

β-Glucosyl-O—CH$_2$—N=N—CH$_3$

Cycasin (cycad nuts)

Safrole (oil of sassafras)

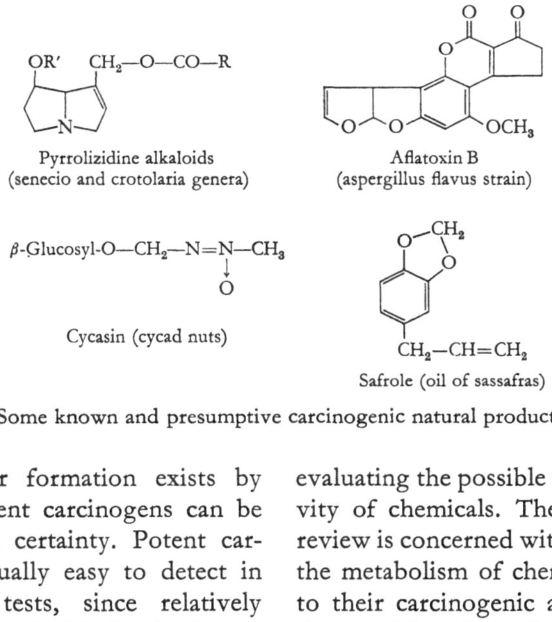

Fig. 3. Some known and presumptive carcinogenic natural products [4—8]

involving tumor formation exists by which even potent carcinogens can be recognized with certainty. Potent carcinogens are usually easy to detect in carcinogenicity tests, since relatively short times are required before high incidences of tumors are obtained; however, some compounds which are very active under one set of conditions may show little activity with another mode of administration or in another species. Detection of weak carcinogenic activity and, especially, the provision of reasonable evidence of noncarcinogenicity of chemicals are much more difficult to achieve. Such tests are generally considered to require lifetime administration of com-

evaluating the possible carcinogenic activity of chemicals. The following brief review is concerned with some aspects of the metabolism of chemicals in relation to their carcinogenic activity. Some of these problems have also been considered in a recent review by the WEISBURGERS [17].

Activation of Carcinogens In Vivo

A question commonly asked about drugs and their mechanisms of action applies to the chemical carcinogens as well, i.e. is a particular carcinogen active *in vivo* as such or must it be converted by one or more reactions into active or proximate carcinogens? A proximate carcinogen is here considered to be one which is identical with the final active carcinogen or is closer to it than the compound administered. Examples of both types appear to exist among the carcinogens. The carcinogenic alkylating agents [3] are often considered to be active per se and the reactivity of these agents with cellular constituents *in vitro* and *in vivo* [18—21] appears to support this view. The recent work, especially that of LAWLEY and BROOKES [21], on the ability of these agents to alkylate the ring nitrogen atoms in the constituent bases of the nucleic acids *in vitro* and *in vivo*, demonstrates the great progress being

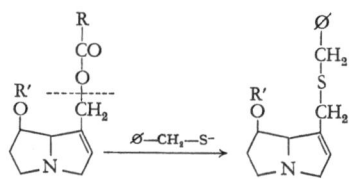

Fig. 4. Alkylating action of pyrrolizidine alkaloids [22]

made in this field. Similarly, the potent naturally occurring hepatocarcinogenic pyrrolizidine alkaloids [4] are probably alkylating agents per se *in vivo*, for CULVENOR et al. [22] have found these compounds to possess alkylating activity *in vitro* against nucleophilic reagents such as benzyl mercaptan (Fig. 4). Only the pyrrolizidine alkaloids with a sterically hindered allylic ester grouping have alkylating activity and hepatotoxic properties. It seems highly probable that the carcinogenic activity of these alkaloids in the liver of the rat also depends on this structural requirement.

The carcinogenic polycyclic aromatic hydrocarbons are also often considered to be carcinogenic as such and not to require activation *in vivo* [23—25]. This view is supported by the ability of microgram quantities of these carcinogens to produce tumors at sites of application

and by the inactivity of their known metabolites. Among the properties of these carcinogens that have been considered to be related to their carcinogenic activity per se are their abilities to act as electron donors and acceptors in charge-transfer reactions [26—27] and their structural resemblance to estrogens and to the guanine-cytosine base pair [28]. The PULLMANS [29], however, feel that no correlations exist between the carcinogenic activities of the hydrocarbons and other organic carcinogens and their electron-donor or electron-acceptor properties. Alternatively, as expressed by BOYLAND [30] some years ago, these hydrocarbons may be oxidized *in vivo* to reactive epoxides, particularly at the phenanthrene-like double bond or "K" region [31]. The syntheses of the proposed epoxy metabolites for direct tests in animals have not been achieved, but BOYLAND and SIMS have provided indirect evidence for epoxide formation in the metabolism of the noncarcinogen phenanthrene [32]. The alicyclic insecticides heptachlor [33] and aldrin [34] are similarly metabolized *in vivo* to epoxides; these epoxy metabolites were the first examples of their kind. A variety of synthetic carcinogenic epoxides are known [35—36], and these compounds are also alkylating agents [18, 35]. KOTIN and FALK [37] considered that the carcinogenic air pollutants they studied were free of aromatic hydrocarbons and that epoxides and peroxy compounds derived from olefins were probably responsible for the activity.

The carcinogenic aromatic amines, in contrast to the aromatic hydrocarbons, have long been considered to require activation *in vivo* since they produce tumors distant from sites of administration and since relatively large amounts of compound are required for tumor production. The *o*-hydroxy derivatives of the

carcinogenic amines were the first metabolites to be considered as proximate
carcinogenic metabolites. Some evidence
in favor of this hypothesis was obtained
from the carcinogenicity of several *o*-
hydroxy amines when implanted into the
lumen of the mouse bladder and from the
lack of activity of the parent amines in
this test [3]. However, the failure of a
number of *o*-hydroxy derivatives of other
carcinogenic amines to induce tumors in
this test system [38—40] and by other
methods of administration (discussed
in [41]) indicate that the *o*-hydroxy amine
hypothesis for the carcinogenicity of aromatic amines is not generally applicable.

Evidence has been obtained recently
to implicate the *N*-hydroxy metabolites
of certain carcinogenic aromatic amines
and amides as proximate carcinogenic
agents. The *N*-hydroxy derivatives are
carcinogenic at a number of sites and in a
number of species, and their activities are
usually considerably greater than those
of the parent carcinogens. The first data
on the formation and carcinogenicity of
a *N*-hydroxy metabolite were obtained
with the potent carcinogen 2-acetyl-
aminofluorene, which is active in a variety of species and tissues [42]. Following administration of this amide its *N*-
hydroxy derivative is excreted (in conju-
gation with glucuronic acid) in the urine
of several species (Fig. 5) [43—48], including all those known to be susceptible to
its carcinogenic action as well by man
and the rhesus monkey, whose susceptibility to the carcinogen is not known.
The guinea pig fails to excrete detectable
amounts of the *N*-hydroxy metabolite [44], and this species is very resistant
to the carcinogenic action of AAF [42].
N-Hydroxy-2-acetyl-aminofluorene is a
very potent carcinogen, which is not
only more active than the parent amide
at the usual sites of tumor formation in
the rat, but is active locally at three sites

where AAF is inactive (Fig. 5) [50—51].
The high activity of *N*-hydroxy-2-
acetylaminofluorene is in marked contrast to the lack of carcinogenic activity
of the phenolic metabolites of 2-acetyl-
aminofluorene which have been tested
[49—50]. Findings similar to those with
2-acetylaminofluorene have been made
for a variety of other carcinogenic amides

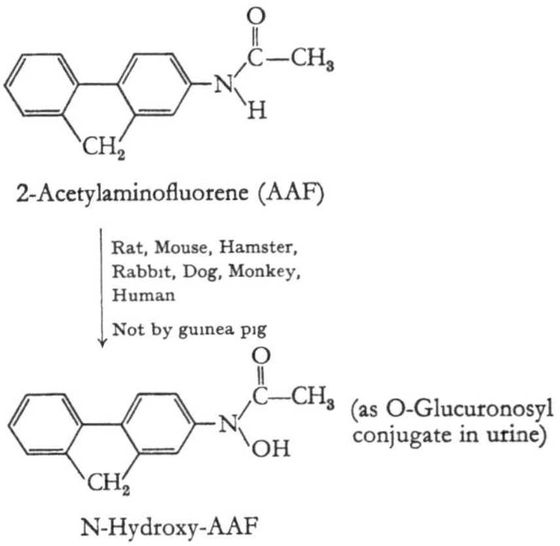

2-Acetylaminofluorene (AAF)

Rat, Mouse, Hamster,
Rabbit, Dog, Monkey,
Human

Not by guinea pig

N-Hydroxy-AAF

Fig. 5. The conversion of 2-acetylaminofluorene
to a proximate carcinogen [43—48, 50, 51]

and amines (Fig. 6). Each of these carcinogens is metabolized to *N*-hydroxy
derivatives which are more carcinogenic
than the parent compounds [38, 39, 41,
52—55]. The *N*-hydroxylation of these
carcinogens requires a reduced triphos-
phopyridine nucleotide (TPNH)-depend-
ent oxidase system which, in the rat,
occurs principally in the microsome fraction of the liver [56, 57]. The *N*-hydro-
xylation of aniline also occurs in this
site [58].

In this connection it is of interest that
BOYLAND et al. [59] recently detected the
N-hydroxylation *in vivo* of the carcinogenic aliphatic amide ethyl carbamate or
urethan. *N*-Hydroxy urethan and its *N*-
acetyl derivative were found in the urines
of rats, rabbits, and man after the administration of urethan. Ethyl mercapturic
acid was also detected in these urines,

and BOYLAND *et al.* suggested that the *N*-hydroxy metabolite may be acting as an alkylating agent *in vivo*. While these workers quoted BERENBLUM *et al.* [60] that *N*-hydroxy urethan has the same carcinogenic activity as urethan, the data published by BERENBLUM *et al.* and from this laboratory [44] showed that *N*-hydroxy urethan was clearly less active han urethan in mice for the induction of ung tumors and as an initiator of skin

xic and hepatocarcinogenic properties of dimethylnitrosamine by MAGEE and BARNES [61], a variety of analogous compounds were found to be carcinogenic in many tissues and in several species including the guinea pig [62—77]. For carcinogenic activity these compounds appear to require alkyl groups which contain hydrogen on the α-carbon atoms. *In vivo* or *in vitro* these dialkylnitrosamines undergo an oxidative dealkylation to

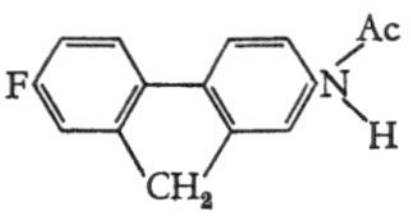

7-Fluoro-AAF

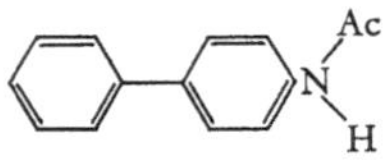

4-Acetylaminobiphenyl

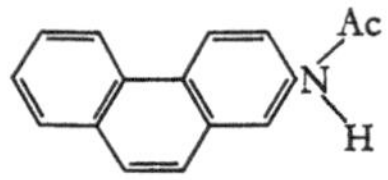

2-Acetylaminophenanthrene

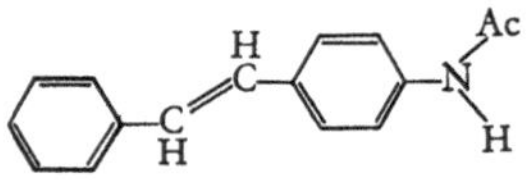

4-Acetylaminostilbene

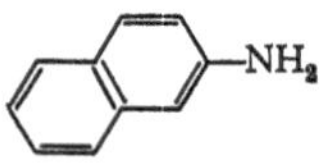

2-Naphthylamine

Fig. 6. Carcinogenic aromatic amides and amines which form *N*-hydroxy metabolites with increased carcinogenicity [38, 39, 41, 52—55]

papillomata. However, this does not exclude the strong likelihood that *N*-hydroxy urethan may be a proximate carcinogenic metabolite of urethan. *N*-Hydroxy urethan is considerably more carcinogenic than the many other possible metabolites of urethan that have been tested [60], and it may be too labile under the conditions used for accurate comparisons of its carcinogenicity with that of urethan.

The carcinogenic dialkylnitrosamines also appear to require activation *in vivo* before they can act carcinogenically. Following the discovery of the hepatoto-

monoalkylnitrosamines; this reaction requires TPNH and oxygen and occurs mainly in the liver microsomes [78,79]. Presumably the monoalkylnitrosamines then spontaneously lose water and nitrogen to yield reactive alkylating groups. Diazoalkanes may be intermediates in this process [67], and the probable sequence of reactions for dimethylnitrosamine is shown in Fig. 7. Direct evidence that dimethylnitrosamine acts as an alkylating agent has been obtained through the methylation of rat liver slice proteins *in vitro* [80] and of ribonucleic acid (RNA) and deoxyribonucleic acid

(DNA) in the livers of rats *in vivo* [*81*]. 7-Methylguanine was demonstrated in the hydrolysates of rat liver RNA. These observations on the methylation of RNA have recently been extended to a number of other rat tissues [*82*]. These alkylation reactions may have a mutagenic effect and thus play a major role in carcinogenesis by these compounds. Similarly, nitrous acid, which may also be a metabolic product of the nitrosamines, could play a mutagenic role [*83*]. The metabolism and carcinogenicity of the dialkylnitrosamines have recently been critically reviewed by MAGEE [*84*].

The toxic and carcinogenic properties of cycad nuts [*7*] are very similar to these properties of dimethylnitrosamine, and it is highly probable that the hepatotoxic aliphatic azoxy glycoside cycasin (Fig. 3) is the major active constituent in these nuts. The hepatotoxic aglycone, methylazoxymethanol, which can be derived from cycasin [*85*] is very unstable and decomposes to methanol, formaldehyde, and nitrogen. It seems likely that diazomethane or a reactive CH_2 group is an intermediate in this process and accounts for the hepatotoxicity of cycasin and the carcinogenicity of cycad nuts.

N-nitroso methylaniline has been found by DRUCKREY *et al.* [*86*] to produce tumors of the esophagus following prolonged feeding to rats. It is difficult to envision the formation of a diazoalkane or CH_2 group from this compound, and DRUCKREY *et al.* have proposed that the compound is oxidatively demethylated with the subsequent formation of a carcinogenic diazonium ion. Studies on the metabolism of *N*-nitroso methylaniline labeled with isotope in the methyl group or in the benzene ring and carcinogenicity tests on related diazonium compounds should clarify this problem.

The hepatocarcinogen ethionine appears to be incorporated as such into the proteins of several tissues of the rat *in vivo*, while its ethyl group is incorporated into the RNA and DNA of the liver [*87, 88*]. The incorporation of this foreign amino acid into protein probably requires carboxyl activation with adenosine triphosphate (ATP) according to the now familiar scheme for protein synthesis from amino acids. The incorporation of the ethyl

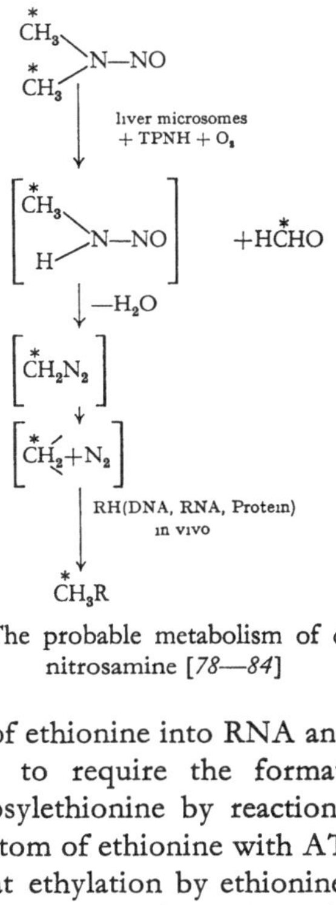

Fig. 7. The probable metabolism of dimethylnitrosamine [*78—84*]

group of ethionine into RNA and DNA appears to require the formation of *S*-adenosylethionine by reaction of the sulfur atom of ethionine with ATP. The fact that ethylation by ethionine *in vivo* occurs only in the liver, the only organ in the rat in which it induces tumors, leads to the attractive idea that the induction of hepatic cancer by ethionine is related to the formation of abnormal RNA and/or DNA molecules via the foreign alkylating agent *S*-adenosylethionine. This and other possibilities are discussed in the informative reviews by FARBER [*87*] and STEKOL [*88*].

Deactivation of Carcinogens In Vivo

The reactions which lead to the destruction of a carcinogen are possibly of less intrinsic interest than reactions which produce carcinogenic derivatives. However, processes which deactivate carcinogens *in vivo* are important in that they reduce the potential dose of the active agent with a resultant reduction in tumor incidence and an increased latent period. A number of metabolic reactions are known by which carcinogenic agents are converted to inactive derivatives, and these reactions are generally similar to those known for many other drugs [89]. Reference has already been made to

sible for the reduction of the azo linkage contains riboflavin-adenine dinucleotide as a cofactor, and the maintenance of the reductase activity by high levels of dietary riboflavin appears to explain at least a major part of the ability of this vitamin to delay the production of tumors by 4-dimethylaminoazobenzene [91]. The known metabolites of the carcinogenic polycyclic aromatic hydrocarbons, of which 1,2,5,6-dibenzanthracene and 3,4-benzpyrene have received the most attention, are formed through processes

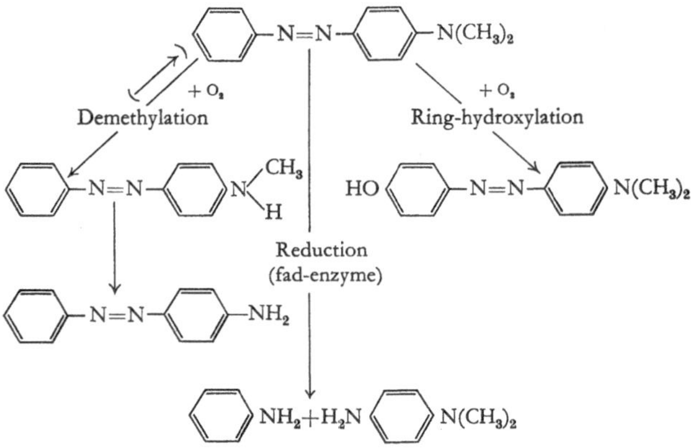

Fig. 8. Hepatic microsomal TPNH-dependent metabolism of
4-dimethylaminoazobenzene [91, 93]

the noncarcinogenic phenolic metabolites of 2-acetylaminofluorene which are formed by a TPNH-dependent microsomal system found principally in the liver [90]. Several similar systems are involved in the destruction of the carcinogenic properties of 4-dimethylaminoazobenzene (Fig. 8) and related dyes for the liver of the rat. Oxidative removal of both N-methyl groups, reduction of the azo linkage, or ring-hydroxylation of these hepatocarcinogens leads to noncarcinogenic metabolites [91, 92]. Each of these reactions is catalyzed by enzyme systems in the microsomal fraction of rat liver which require TPNH for activity; the two oxidative systems also require molecular oxygen [91, 93]. The system respon-

which are primarily oxidative in nature and result in deactivation or detoxification of the carcinogens (reviewed in [3]) [23—25, 94].

3-Methylcholanthrene and some related hydrocarbons are powerful inhibitors of the carcinogenic action of the aminoazo dyes and of 2-acetylaminofluorene when they are fed at a low level (0.003 per cent) in the diet with the amine carcinogens [95, 96]. Studies with the aminoazo dyes showed that administration of the hydrocarbons permits the maintenance of the normal levels of the microsomal deactivation enzymes in the rat liver in spite of the feeding of the dyes. When the dyes were fed without the hydrocarbons, the concentrations of these enzymes declined significantly over a period of weeks. Furthermore, the protective effect of 3-methylcholanthrene could be overcome by feeding a high level of the carcinogenic dye, which was lethal within a few weeks when it was fed without hydrocarbon.

This somewhat paradoxical inhibition of the carcinogenic activities of the amine carcinogens by carcinogenic hydrocarbons led to the discovery of the inducible nature of several of these hepatic microsomal enzyme systems in the rat [90, 94, 97]. Large increases in the concentrations of these enzymes in the livers of weanling rats occurred within hours after the intraperitoneal injection of 1 mg. or less of certain of these hydrocarbons (Fig. 9). These hydrocarbons had no effect *in vitro* on the enzyme systems and the *in vivo* enhancement was prevented by the administration of ethionine; the latter inhibition was removed by the injection of methionine. The induction of benzpyrene hydroxylase and of aminoazo dye *N*-demethylase in several extrahepatic tissues in the rat by benzpyrene or methylcholanthrene has also been observed [98—100]. A number of noncarcinogenic drugs such as phenobarbital [101, 102] also produce increases in the amounts of many TPNH-dependent enzymes in liver microsomes after administration *in vivo*. 3-Methylcholanthrene appears to be more selective than phenobarbital in the induction of synthesis of these microsomal enzymes. The inhibition by puromycin and actinomycin D [100, 102] of the induction of these enzymes by phenobarbital and 3-methylcholanthrene suggest that these inducers accelerate the DNA-directed synthesis of RNA molecules which then serve as templates for the synthesis of these enzymes on the ribosomes. These and other aspects of the induction of enzyme synthesis by these compounds are well re-

viewed in the recent papers by CONNEY and GILMAN [102] and by GELBOIN and BLACKBURN [100]. Recent electron microscopic and metabolic studies [103] have shown that phenobarbital stimulates the formation of the smooth membrane of the hepatic endoplasmic reticulum which contains these TPNH-dependent oxidative enzymes.

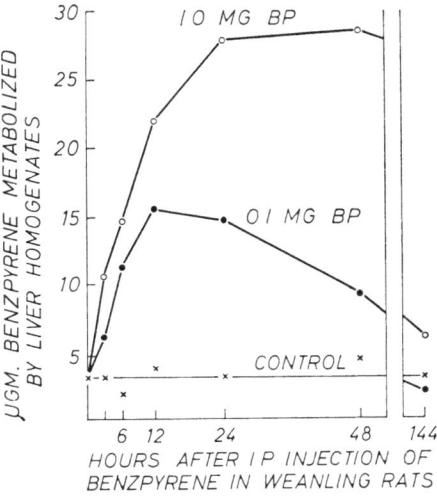

Fig. 9. The induction of benzpyrene hydroxylase synthesis by benzpyrene *in vivo* [94]

The enzyme-inducing properties of a series of polycyclic aromatic hydrocarbons were not correlated with the activities of these compounds as carcinogens [94, 97]. However, this property may represent a type of response to the carcinogenic hydrocarbons which is related to the carcinogenic processes induced by them in various tissues other than the liver.

Mechanisms of Action of Chemical Carcinogens

The cellular and molecular mechanisms of action are not known for any carcinogenic agent. Progress in this area depends in part on a sound knowledge of the histogenesis of cancer. This point has been reemphasized recently by FARBER

[87] who outlined the need for suitable *in vivo* and *in vitro* models for delineation of the sequence of morphological and metabolic alterations at the cellular and subcellular levels which are responsible for the conversion of normal cells to neoplastic cells. The heritable and apparently irreversible nature of this conversion is generally thought to involve changes in the hereditary apparatus of normal cells; through their phenotypic expressions these changes then account for the loss of control over their growth which would otherwise be exercised by the host. In the normal host controls and would eventually give rise to gross cancers. Indeed, it does not seem too early to suggest that all low molecular weight organic chemical carcinogens may initiate the neoplastic change through alkylating or arylating reactions. Furthermore, the possibility has long existed that viruses and latent viruses are involved in the chemical induction of some cancers; much further work on this aspect of chemical carcinogenesis is needed.

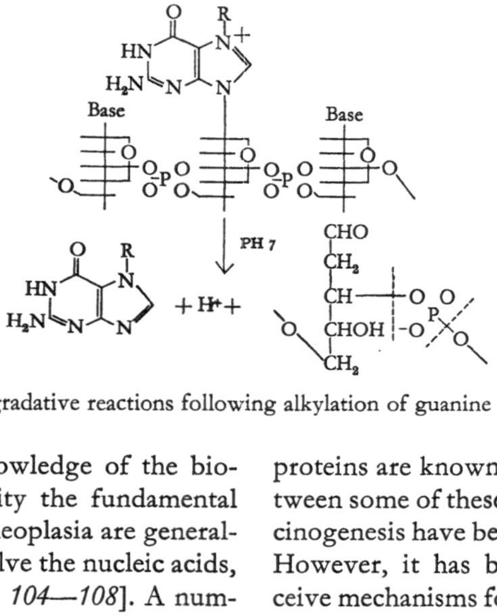

A number of interactions *in vivo* of carcinogens or their metabolites with

Fig. 10. Degradative reactions following alkylation of guanine in DNA [21]

light of present knowledge of the biochemistry of heredity the fundamental changes leading to neoplasia are generally conceived to involve the nucleic acids, especially DNA [87, 104—108]. A number of interactions of carcinogens and their metabolites with DNA and RNA are known, but few correlations of these interactions with carcinogenesis have been reported [87]. At the molecular level the reactions of carcinogenic alkylating agents with RNA and DNA *in vivo* seem to have the most direct implications (Fig. 10) for the nature of the carcinogenic process induced by these agents. In these instances it is not difficult to conceive how subtle mutations could be induced in somatic cells which would permit them some freedom from proteins are known, and correlations between some of these interactions and carcinogenesis have been obtained [91, 109]. However, it has been difficult to conceive mechanisms for the perpetuation of these changes in subsequent cell generations [87, 105]. Recently Pitot and Heidelberger [110] have utilized recent concepts of the control of enzyme synthesis to develop a speculative model of carcinogenesis in which the earliest steps involve protein-carcinogen interactions.

It is interesting to consider the concept that, given enough time, loss of growth control with the formation of cancer is inevitable in a few cells of every tissue. This biologically inevitable process of carcinogenesis could depend on either or both of an inherent instability of the cell genome and the presence of endogenous or exogenous carcinogens. If the points of genetic instability and the sites of action of carcinogens can be identified and studied, it may be possible to delay the process of carcinogenesis and, hopefully, to prevent cancer formation in some tissues within a normal life span.

References

[1] HARTWELL, J. L., *Survey of compounds which have been tested for carcinogenic activity*, 2nd ed. Washington, D. C.: U. S. Public Health Service 1951.

[2] SHUBIK, P., and HARTWELL, J. L., *Survey of compounds which have been tested for carcinogenic activity*, Suppl I. Washington, D. C.: 1957. U. S. Department of Health, Education, and Welfare.

[3] CLAYSON, D. B., *Chemical carcinogenesis*. Boston, Mass.: Little, Brown & Co. 1962.

[4] SCHOENTAL, R., HEAD, M. A., and PEACOCK, P. R., Senecio alkaloids: primary tumors in rats as a result of treatment with (1) a mixture of alkaloids from *S. jacobae* a Lin.; (2) retrorsine; (3) isatidine. *Brit. J. Cancer* 8, 458—465 (1954).

[5] ASAO, T., BÜCHI, G., ABDEL-KADER, M. M., CHANG, S. B., WICK, E. L., and WOGAN, G. N., Aflatoxins B and G. *J. Amer. chem. Soc.* 85, 1706 (1963).

[6] LANCASTER, M. C., JENKINS, F. P., and PHILP, J. McL., Toxity associated with certain samples of groundnuts. *Nature (Lond.)* 192, 1095—1096 (1961).

[7] LAQUEUR, G. L., MICKELSON, O., WHITING, M. G., and KURLAND, L. T., Carcinogenic properties of nuts from *Cycas circinalis* L. indigenous to Guam. *J. nat. Cancer Inst.* 31, 919—952 (1963).

[8] LONG, E. L., NELSON, A. A., FITZHUGH, O. G., and HANSEN, W. H., Liver tumors produced in rats by feeding safrole. *Arch. Path.* 75, 595—604 (1963).

[9] FISHER, J. F., and MALLETTE, M. F., The natural occurrence of ethionine in bacteria. *J. gen. Physiol.* 45, 1—13 (1961).

[10] HENRY, S. A., Occupational cutaneous cancer attributable to certain chemicals in industry. *Brit. med. Bull.* 4, 389—401 (1947).

[11] GOLDBLATT, M. W., Occupational carcinogenesis. *Brit. med. Bull.* 14, 136—140 (1958).

[12] — Occupational cancer of the bladder. *Brit. med. Bull.* 4, 405—417 (1947).

[13] WALPOLE, A. L., and WILLIAMS, M. H. C., Aromatic amines as carcinogens in industry. *Brit. Med. Bull.* 14, 141—145 (1958).

[14] SHUBIK, P., and SICÉ, J., Chemical carcinogenesis as a chronic toxicity test. *Cancer Res.* 16, 728—742 (1956).

[15] CARTER, H. E., CANNON, P. R., KENSLER, C. J., LEVIN, M. L., MILLER, J. A., NELSON, A. A., and SHUBIK, P., Problems in the evaluation of carcinogenic hazard from use of food additives. *Cancer Res.* 21, 429—456 (1961).

[16] JOINT FAO/WHO expert committee on food additives, fifth report. Evaluation of the carcinogenic hazards of food additives, 33 p. *Wld. Hlth. Org. Rep. Ser.* No 220 (1961).

[17] WEISBURGER, J. H., and WEISBURGER, E. K., Pharmacodynamics of carcinogenic azo dyes, aromatic amines, and nitrosamines. *Clin. Pharmacol. Ther.* 4, 110—129 (1963).

[18] HADDOW, A., The chemical and genetic mechanisms of carcinogenesis. II. Biologic alkylating agents. In: *The physiopathology of cancer*, 2nd ed. (F. Homburger, ed.), p. 602—685. New York, N. Y.: P. B. Hoeber, Inc. 1959.

[19] ROSS, W. C. J., *In vitro* reactions of biological alkylating agents. *Ann. N. Y. Acad. Sci.* 68, 669—681 (1958).

[20] WHEELER, G. P., Studies related to the mechanisms of action of cytotoxic alkylating agents: a review. *Cancer Res.* 22, 651—688 (1962).

[21] LAWLEY, P. D., and BROOKES, P., The action of alkylating agents on deoxyribonucleic acid in relation to biological effects of the alkylating agents. *Exp. Cell Res.* 9, 512—520 (1963).

[22] CULVENOR, C. C. J., DANN, A. T., and DICK, A. T., Alkylation as the mechanism by which the hepatotoxic pyrrolizidine alkaloids act on cell nuclei. *Nature (Lond.)* 195, 570—573 (1962).

[23] FALK, H. L., and KOTIN, P., Chemistry, host entry, and metabolic fate of carcinogens. *Clin. Pharmacol. Ther.* 4, 83—103 (1963).

[24] — —, LEE, S. S., and NATHAN, A., Intermediary metabolism of benzo(*a*)pyrene

in the rat. *J. Nat. Cancer Inst.* **28**, 699—724 (1962).

[25] KOTIN, P., FALK, H. L., and MILLER, A., Effect of carbon tetrachloride intoxication on the metabolism of benzo(a)pyrene in rats and mice. *J. nat. Cancer Inst.* **28**, 725—745 (1962).

[26] SZENT-GYÖRGYI, A., ISENBERG, I., and BAIRD jr., S. L., On the electron donating properties of carcinogens. *Proc. nat. Acad. Sci. (Wash.)* **46**, 1444—1449 (1960).

[27] ALLISON, A. C., and NASH, T., Electron donation and acceptance by carcinogenic compounds. *Nature (Lond.)* **197**, 758—765 (1963).

[28] HUGGINS, C., and YANG, N. C., Induction and extinction of mammary cancer. *Science* **137**, 257—262 (1962).

[29] PULLMAN, B., and PULLMAN, A., Electron-donor or electron-acceptor properties and carcinogenic activity of organic molecules. *Nature (Lond.)* **199**, 467—469 (1963).

[30] BOYLAND, E., The biological significance of the metabolism of polycyclic compounds. In: *Biological oxidation of aromatic rings* (R. T. Williams, ed.) (Biochem. Soc. Symp. No 5), p. 40—54. New York, N. Y.: Cambridge University Press 1950.

[31] PULLMAN, A., and PULLMAN, B., Electronic structure and carcinogenic activity of aromatic molecules. *Advanc. Cancer Res.* **3**, 117—169 (1955).

[32] BOYLAND, E., and SIMS, P., Metabolism of polycyclic compounds. 21. The metabolism of phenanthrene in rabbits and rats: dihydrodihydroxy compounds and related glucosiduronic acids. *Biochem. J.* **84**, 571—582 (1962).

[33] DAVIDOW, B., and RADOMSKI, J. L., Isolation of an epoxide metabolite from fat tissues of dogs fed heptachlor. *J. Pharmacol. exp. Ther.* **107**, 259—265 (1953).

[34] BANN, J. M., DECINO, T. J., EARLE, N. W., and SUN, Y, The fate of aldrin and dieldrin in the animal body. *J. Agr. Food Chem.* **4**, 937—941 (1956).

[35] WALPOLE, A. L., Carcinogenic action of alkylating agents. *Ann. N.Y. Acad. Sci.* **68**, 750—761 (1958).

[36] DURREN, B. L. VAN, NELSON, N., ORRIS, L., PALMES, E. D., and SCHMITT, F. L., Carcinogenicity of epoxides, lactones, and peroxy compounds. *J. nat. Cancer Inst.* **31**, 41—55 (1963).

[37] KOTIN, P., and FALK, H. L., The production of tumors in C57BL mice with atmosphere-extracted aliphatic hydrocarbons. *Proc. Amer. Ass. Cancer Res.* **2**, 30 (1955).

[38] BONSER, G. M., BOYLAND, E., BUSBY, E. R., CLAYSON, D. B., GROVER, P. L., and JULL, J. W., A further study of bladder implantation in the mouse as a means of detecting carcinogenic activity; use of crushed paraffin wax or stearic acid as the vehicle. *Brit. J. Cancer* **17**, 127—136 (1963).

[39] BRYAN, G. T., BROWN, R. R., and PRICE, J. M., Studies on the etiology of bovine bladder cancer. *Ann. N.Y. Acad. Sci.* **108**, 924—937 (1963).

[40] IRVING, C. C., GUTMANN, H. R., and LARSON, D. M., Evaluation of the carcinogenicity of aminofluorenols by implantation into the bladder of the mouse. *Cancer Res.* **23**, 1782—1791 (1963).

[41] ANDERSEN, R. A., ENOMOTO, M., MILLER, E. C., and MILLER, J. A., Carcinogenesis and inhibition of the Walker 256 tumor in the rat by *trans*-4-acetylaminostilbene, its *N*-hydroxy metabolite, and related compounds. *Cancer Res.* **24**, 128—143 (1964).

[42] WEISBURGER, E. K., and WEISBURGER, J. H., Chemistry, carcinogenicity, and metabolism of *N*-2-fluorenamine and related compounds. *Advanc. Cancer Res.* **5**, 331—431 (1958).

[43] CRAMER, J. W., MILLER, J. A., and MILLER, E. C., *N*-Hydroxylation: a new metabolic reaction observed in the rat with the carcinogen 2-acetylaminofluorene. *J. biol. Chem.* **235**, 885—888 (1960).

[44] MILLER, J. A., CRAMER, J. W., and MILLER, E. C., The *N*- and ring-hydroxylation of 2-acetylaminofluorene during carcinogenesis in the rat. *Cancer Res.* **20**, 950—962 (1960).

[45] ENOMOTO, M., LOTLIKAR, P., MILLER, J. A., and MILLER, E. C., Urinary metabolites of 2-acetylaminofluorene and related compounds in the rhesus monkey. *Cancer Res.* **22**, 1336—1342 (1962).

[46] POIRIER, L. A., MILLER, J. A., and MILLER, E. C., The *N*- and ring-hydroxylation of 2-acetylaminofluorene and the failure to detect N-acetylation of 2-aminofluorene in the dog. *Cancer Res.* **23**, 790—800 (1963).

[47] IRVING, C. C., N-hydroxylation of 2-acetylaminofluorene in rabbits. Cancer Res. 22, 867—873 (1962).

[48] WEISBURGER, J. H., GRANTHAM, P. H., VANHORN, E., STEIGBIGEL, N. H., RALL, D. P., and WEISBURGER, E. K., Activation and detoxification of N-2-fluorenylacetamide in man. Cancer Res. 24, 475—479 (1964).

[49] MORRIS, H. P., VELAT, C. A., WAGNER, B. P., DAHLGARD, M., and RAY, F. E., Studies of carcinogenicity in the rat of derivatives of aromatic amines related to N-2-fluorenyl-acetamide. J. nat. Cancer Inst. 24, 149—180 (1960).

[50] MILLER, E. C., MILLER, J. A., and HART-MANN, H. A., N-hydroxy-2-acetylaminofluorene: a metabolite of 2-acetylaminofluorene with increased carcinogenic activity in the rat. Cancer Res. 21, 815—824 (1961).

[51] MILLER, J. A., ENOMOTO, M., and MILLER, E. C., The carcinogenicity of small amounts of N-hydroxy-2-acetylaminofluorene and its cupric chelate in the rat. Cancer Res. 22, 1381—1388 (1962).

[52] — WYATT, C. S., MILLER, E. C., and HARTMANN, H. A., The N-hydroxylation of 4-acetylaminobiphenyl by the rat and dog and the strong carcinogenicity of N-hydroxy-4-acetylaminobiphenyl in the rat. Cancer Res. 21, 1465—1473 (1961).

[53] BOYLAND, E., DUKES, C. E., and GROVER, P. L., Carcinogenicity of 2-naphthylhydroxylamine and 2-naphthylamine. Brit. J. Cancer 17, 79—84 (1963).

[54] TROLL, W., and NELSON, N., N-hydroxy-2-naphthylamine, a urinary metabolite of 2-naphthylamine in man and dog. Fed. Proc. 20, 41 (1961).

[55] MILLER, J. A., and MILLER, E. C., Unpublished observations on 7-fluoro-2-acetyl-aminofluorene and 2-acetylaminophenanthrene and their N-hydroxy metabolites in the rat. 1963.

[56] IRVING, C. C., N-hydroxylation of the carcinogen 2-acetylaminofluorene by rabbit-liver microsomes. Biochem. biophys. Acta (Amst.) 65, 564—566 (1962).

[57] UEHLEKE, H., N-hydroxylation of carcinogenic amines in vivo and in vitro with liver microsomes. Biochem. Pharmacol. 12, 219—221 (1963).

[58] KIESE, M., u. UEHLEKE, H., Der Ort der N-Oxydation des Anilins im höheren Tier. Naunyn-Schmiedebergs Arch. exp. Path. Pharmak. 242, 117—129 (1961).

[59] BOYLAND, E., NERY, R., PEGGIE, K. S., and WILLIAMS, K., The metabolism and possible mode of action of urethane. Biochem. J. 89, 113 P—114 P (1963).

[60] BERENBLUM, I., BEN-ISHAI, D., HARAN-GHERA, N., LAPIDOT, A., SIMON, E., and TRAININ, N., Skin initiating action and lung carcinogenesis by derivatives of urethane (ethyl carbamate) and related compounds. Biochem. Pharmacol. 2, 168—176 (1959).

[61] MAGEE, P. N., and BARNES, J. M., The production of malignant primary liver tumours in the rat by feeding dimethylnitrosamine. Brit. J. Cancer 10, 114—122 (1956).

[62] ZAK, F. G., HOLZNER, J. H., SINGER, E. J. and POPPER, H., Renal and pulmonary tumors in rats fed dimethylnitrosamine. Cancer Res. 20, 96—99 (1960).

[63] DRUCKREY, H., PREUSSMANN, R., SCHMÄHL D., u. MÜLLER, M., Chemische Konstitution und carcinogene Wirkung bei Nitrosaminen. Naturwissenschaften 48, 134—135 (1961).

[64] — — — Erzeugung von Magenkrebs durch Nitrosamide an Ratten. Naturwissenschaften 48, 165 (1961).

[65] ARGUS, M. F., and HOCH-LIGETI, C., Comparative study of the carcinogenic activity of nitrosamines. J. nat. Cancer Inst. 27, 695—709 (1961).

[66] MAGEE, P. N., and BARNES, J. M., Induction of kidney tumours in the rat with dimethylnitrosamine (N-nitrosodimethylamine). J. Path. Bact. 84, 19—31 (1962).

[67] SCHOENTAL, R., and MAGEE, P. N., Induction of squamous carcinoma of the lung and of the stomach and esophagus by diazomethane and N-methyl-N-nitroso-urethane, respectively. Brit. J. Cancer 16, 92—100 (1962).

[68] DRUCKREY, H., u. PREUSSMANN, R., Erzeugung von Lungenkrebs durch subcutane Injektion von N,N-Diamylnitrosamin an Ratten. Naturwissenschaften 49, 111—112 (1962).

[69] DONTENWILL, W., u. MOHR, U., Carcinome des Respirationstractus nach Behandlung von Goldhamstern mit Diäthylnitrosamin. Z. Krebsforsch. 64, 305—312 (1961).

[70] — — u. ZAGEL, M., Über die unterschiedliche Lungencarcinogene Wirkung des

Diäthylnitrosamin bei Hamster und Ratte. *Z. Krebsforsch.* **64**, 499—502 (1962).

[71] DRUCKREY, H., PREUSSMANN, R., SCHMÄHL D., u. MÜLLER, M., Erzeugung von Blasenkrebs an Ratten mit *N,N*-Dibutylnitrosamin. *Naturwissenschaften* **49**, 19 (1962).

[72] — — AFKHAM, J., u. BLUM, G., Erzeugung von Lungenkrebs durch Methylnitrosourethan bei intravenöser Gabe an Ratten. *Naturwissenschaften* **49**, 451—452 (1962).

[73] — u. STEINHOFF, D., Erzeugung von Leberkrebs an Meerschweinchen. *Naturwissenschaften* **49**, 497—498 (1962).

[74] ARGUS, M. F., and HOCH-LIGETI, C., Induction of malignant tumors in the guinea pig by oral administration of diethylnitrosamine. *J. nat. Cancer Inst.* **30**, 533—551 (1963).

[75] DRUCKREY, H., PREUSSMANN, R., BLUM, G., and IVANKOVIC, S., Carcinogene Wirkung von Diazoessigester und von *N*-Nitroso-Sarkosinester als Beispiel für das Prinzip: Transport- und Wirk-Form. *Naturwissenschaften* **50**, 99—100 (1963).

[76] — — — u. AFKHAM, J., Erzeugung von Karzinomen der Speiseröhre durch unsymmetrische Nitrosamine. *Naturwissenschaften* **50**, 100—101 (1963).

[77] — — and SCHMÄHL, D., Carcinogenicity and chemical structure of nitrosamines. *Acta Un. int. Cancr.* **19**, 510—512 (1963).

[78] MAGEE, P. N., and VANDEKAR, M., Toxic liver injury. The metabolism of dimethyl-nitrosamine *in vitro. Biochem. J.* **70**, 600—605 (1958).

[79] BROUWERS, J. A., and EMMELOT, P., Microsomal *N*-demethylation and the effect of the hepatic carcinogen dimethylnitrosamine on amino acid incorporation into the proteins of rat livers and hepatomas. *Exp. Cell Res.* **19**, 467—474 (1960).

[80] MAGEE, P. N., and HULTIN, T., Toxic liver injury and carcinogenesis. Methylation of proteins of rat-liver slices by dimethylnitrosamine *in vitro. Biochem. J.* **83**, 106—114 (1962).

[81] —, and FARBER, E., Toxic liver injury and carcinogenesis. Methylation of rat-liver nucleic acids by dimethylnitrosamine *in vivo. Biochem. J.* **83**, 114—124 (1962).

[82] LEE, K. Y., LIJINSKY, W., and MAGEE, P. N., Methylation of ribonucleic acids of liver and other organs in different species treated with C^{14} and H^3-dimethylnitrosamines *in vivo. J. nat. Cancer Inst.* **32**, 65—76 (1964).

[83] HEATH, D. F., and DUTTON, A., The detection of metabolic products from dimethyl-nitrosamine in rats and mice. *Biochem. J.* **70**, 619—626 (1958).

[84] MAGEE, P. N., Cellular injury and chemical carcinogenesis. In: *Cancer.* Progress vol. (R. W. Raven, ed.), p. 56—66. London: Butterworth & Co. 1963.

[85] MATSUMOTO, H., and STRONG, F. M., The occurrence of methylazoxymethanol in *Cycas circinalis* L. *Arch. Biochem.* **101**, 299—310 (1963).

[86] DRUCKREY, H., PREUSSMANN, R., SCHMÄHL D., u. BLUM, G., Carcinogene Wirkung von *N*-Methyl-*N*-nitroso-Anilin. *Naturwissenschaften* **48**, 722—723 (1961).

[87] FARBER, E., Ethionine carcinogenesis. *Advanc. Cancer Res.* **7**, 383—474 (1963).

[88] STEKOL, J. A., Biochemical basis for ethionine effects on tissues. *Advanc. Enzymol.* **25**, 369—393 (1963).

[89] WILLIAMS, R. T., *Detoxication mechanisms,* 2nd ed. New York, N. Y.: John Wiley & Sons 1959.

[90] CRAMER, J. W., MILLER, J. A., and MILLER, E. C., The hydroxylation of the carcinogen 2-acetylaminofluorene by rat liver: stimulation by pretreatment *in vivo* by 3-methylcholanthrene. *J. biol. Chem.* **235**, 250—256 (1960).

[91] MILLER, J. A., and MILLER, E. C., The carcinogenic aminoazo dyes. *Advanc. Cancer Res.* **1**, 339—396 (1953).

[92] — —, and FINGER, G., Further studies on the carcinogenicity of dyes related to 4-dimethylaminoazobenzene. The requirement for an unsubstituted 2 position. *Cancer Res.* **17**, 387—398 (1957).

[93] MUELLER, G. C., and MILLER, J. A., The metabolism of methylated aminoazo dyes. II. Oxidative demethylation by rat liver homogenates. *J. biol. Chem.* **202**, 579—587 (1953).

[94] CONNEY, A. H., MILLER, E. C., and MILLER, J. A., Substrate-induced synthesis and other properties of benzpyrene hydroxylase in rat liver. *J. biol. Chem.* **228**, 753—766 (1957).

[95] RICHARDSON, H. L., STEIR, A. R., and BORSOS-NACHTNEBEL, E., Liver tumor inhibition and adrenal histologic responses in rats to which 3'-methyl-4-

dimethylaminoazo-benzene and 20-methylcholanthrene were simultaneously administered. *Cancer Res.* **12**, 356—361 (1952).

[96] MILLER, E. C., MILLER, J. A., BROWN, R. R., and MacDONALD, J. C., On the protective effect of certain polycyclic aromatic hydrocarbons against carcinogenesis by aminoazo dyes and 2-acetylaminofluorene. *Cancer Res.* **18**, 469—477 (1958).

[97] CONNEY, A. H., MILLER, E. C., and MILLER, J. A., The metabolism of methylated aminoazo dyes. V. Evidence for induction of enzyme synthesis in the rat by 3-methyl-cholanthrene. *Cancer Res.* **16**, 450—459 (1956).

[98] WATTENBERG, L. W., LEONG, J. L., and STRAND, P. J., Benzpyrene hydroxylase activity in the gastrointestinal tract. *Cancer Res.* **22**, 1120—1125 (1962).

[99] GILMAN, A. G., and CONNEY, A. H., The induction of aminoazo dye N-demethylase in nonhepatic tissues by 3-methylcholanthrene. *Biochem. Pharmacol.* **12**, 591—593 (1963).

[100] GELBOIN, H. V., and BLACKBURN, N. R., The stimulatory effect of 3-methylcholanthrene on benzpyrene hydroxylase activity in several rat tissues: inhibition by actinomycin D and puromycin. *Cancer Res.* **24**, 356—360 (1964).

[101] CONNEY, A. H., DAVISON, C., GASTEL, R., and BURNS, J. J., Adaptive increases in drug-metabolizing enzymes induced by phenobarbital and other drugs. *J. Pharmacol. exp. Ther.* **130**, 1—8 (1960).

[102] —, and GILMAN, A. G., Puromycin inhibition of enzyme induction by 3-methylcholanthrene and phenobarbital. *J. biol. Chem.* **238**, 3682—3685 (1963).

[103] REMMER, H., and MERKER, H. J., Drug-induced changes in the liver endoplasmic reticulum: association with drug-metabolizing enzymes. *Science* **142**, 1657—1658 (1963).

[104] KAPLAN, H. S., Some implications of indirect induction mechanisms in carcinogenesis: a review. *Cancer Res.* **19**, 791—803 (1959).

[105] MILLER, J. A., and MILLER, E. C., Biochemical concepts of carcinogenesis. *Canad. Cancer Conf.* **4**, 57—79 (1961).

[106] KIT, S., Nucleic acid synthesis in the neoplastic cell and impact of nuclear changes on the biochemistry of tumor tissue: a review. *Cancer Res.* **20**, 1121—1148 (1960).

[107] BENDICH, A., Nucleic acids and the genesis of cancer. *Bull. N.Y. Acad. Med.* **37**, 661—674 (1961).

[108] DULBECCO, R., Transformation of cells *in vitro* by viruses. *Science* **142**, 932—936 (1963).

[109] HEIDELBERGER, C., *The relation of protein binding to hydrocarbon carcinogenesis.* In: CIBA Foundation Symposium on Carcinogenesis, Mechanisms of Action, p. 179—192. London: J. & A. Churchill Ltd. 1959.

[110] PITOT, H. C., and HEIDELBERGER, C., Metabolic regulatory circuits and carcinogenesis. *Cancer Res.* **23**, 1694—1700 (1963).

The Point of View of the Pharmacologist

A. C. Frazer

*Professor and Head of Department of Medical Biochemistry and Pharmacology,
University of Birmingham, Birmingham, Great Britain*

I have been asked to put before you some of the problems concerned with the carcinogenic risk that may arise from the use of drugs, especially as they may appear to a pharmacologist who is concerned with drug safety. The views expressed in this paper are my own and they do not necessarily coincide with those of any of the official bodies with which I am associated.

There are, in my opinion, certain principles which should form the basis for any attempts to control environmental hazards, especially those arising from the introduction of a new chemical substance into the human environment. The introduction of a new drug is a part of this wider problem.

1. Some Basic Principles in Safety Evaluation of Chemical Substances Introduced into the Environment

a) Any decision that aims to control the use of a new chemical substance in the environment should be based on evaluation of the balance between the benefits and the risks of using that substance.

b) The manufacturer, or perhaps in certain cases another industrial user, of a new chemical substance that is proposed for introduction into the environment should be, and should remain, responsible for his product financially, legally, scientifically and ethically.

c) No rigid plan of testing should be imposed by regulatory or other agencies on those responsible for safety evaluation; the investigator should be free to plan his own experiments in accordance with current knowledge and expertise. Of course, the studies carried out will need to be acceptable to the regulatory agencies, to whom the results must be submitted in due course.

d) Regulatory agencies will reserve the right to call for further evidence if this is considered necessary in the interests of safe use. It is important, however, that regulatory agencies should only demand further experimental work if it is likely to assist effectively in the evaluation of the human risks. It is all too easy to make demands for more experimental work. However, such demands are likely to interfere with more productive scientific work, since the available man-power and facilities in toxicology and related fields are far from adequate; demands for more experimental work should, therefore, only be made when absolutely necessary in the interests of safety.

e) The main objective of animal studies in the field of safety evaluation is to help in the assessment of the human risk. If a drug has already been extensively used in human subjects, it is probable that information relevant to human risks can be obtained more readily from a further study of any effects observed in man than from additional animal experiments. Information on safety derived from studies in man must always take precedence over observations on animals in the assessment of the human risk.

2. The Function of the Pharmacologist[1] in Development of a New Drug

The pharmacologist is concerned in obtaining as much information as possible about the effects of a new drug on biological systems. An evaluation of the cancer risk should always be included in the assessment of toxicity. The pharmacologist bases his opinion on consideration of the specifications of the drug, its chemical and physical properties, animal studies and sometimes limited investigation in human subjects. It is the pharmacologist who should decide whether it is justifiable to administer the drug to man. In coming to this decision, the balance between potential benefit and risk is assessed. Part of the risk to be considered is the carcinogenic risk.

3. Stages in the Development of a New Drug

A vast number of new substances present themselves as possible new drugs. Of these, only a small number eventually find their way into medical therapeutic use. The main steps in the emergence of a new therapeutic agent are as follows: —

a) Identification of a new substance by means of suitable specifications and study of its major pharmacodynamic effects in animals or suitable experimental preparations.

---

[1] This term is used here to cover a team of investigators commonly led by a pharmacologist, which will include chemists, biochemists, pharmacologists, toxicologists and pathologists.

b) Establishment of the pattern of absorption, distribution, metabolism and elimination, yielding an estimate of biological half-life in a number of species. Toxicological studies — acute and subacute — probably up to 90-day tests, with appropriate study of effects on the structure and function of main body cells and tissues in groups of animals receiving different levels of dosage of the new drug. In some cases, long-term toxicity studies may also be undertaken.

c) If possible, pharmacological studies in man may be carried out with the main objective of establishing similarities or differences in the metabolism, biological half-life, or distribution of the drug between the animal species already studied and man.

d) Clinical trials may be extremely limited in scope, with the simple objective of establishing whether the pharmacological effect of the drug in man is as predicted from the animal studies, and consequently, whether the drug has any therapeutic future. If it does not, the matter is likely to end here. If the drug is more promising, more extensive clinical trials will be conducted which aim to find out the most effective therapeutic use of the drug and to establish its efficacy. Toxic effects may be observed, but since only a few hundred patients are usually studied, important toxic effects occurring with an incidence of 1 in 1000 or less may well be missed.

e) Special monitoring continued for 2—3 years after marketing with an adequate system of adverse reaction reporting will help in the detection of the less common, but possibly important, toxic effects.

4. How Can the Carcinogenic Risk be Assessed?

a) By analogy. A considerable number of substances are known that induce cancerous changes. If the drug or any of its metabolites are closely related to known carcinogenic substances, the investigator will be alerted and stringent tests are likely to be demanded to assess the carcinogenic potential of the new drug. Only under exceptional circumstances, which will be discussed later, is a drug of this nature likely to be considered acceptable without detailed study of its carcinogenic potential. A drug that has no apparent relationship to known carcinogens is, of course, less suspect, but this fact alone cannot be regarded as an adequate safeguard.

b) *From consideration of chemical and biochemical properties.* The definition of drugs in such absolute terms as carcinogenic or non-carcinogenic is extremely difficult and may even be impossible. Drugs are selected because they have effects on living systems and such drugs as antibacterial agents are chosen because they have a selective cytotoxic action on invading organisms. It would hardly be surprising, however, if effects were caused by such drugs in the less susceptible cells of the host that might sometimes lead to cancerous changes. It might, therefore, be more useful to aim at classifying drugs in terms of carcinogenic potency. A powerful carcinogen that may frequently induce cancer in a short time presents quite a different problem from that associated with a substance that may give rise to an occasional tumour many years after exposure.

It has often been maintained that there is no safe-dose of a carcinogen. However, this is hardly in accord with the facts. A dose/response relationship has been established for the great majority of carcinogens. Increasing total dosage usually results in a greater incidence of tumours and a shorter induction period. It is possible to choose a sub-liminal dose of some carcinogens which does not give

rise to tumours during the normal life-span unless some co-carcinogen or promoting agent is also administered. It is indeed fortunate that an apparent safe dose does appear to exist, since most of us are exposed daily to carcinogens in the environment; it may be argued that if we lived long enough we might all eventually develop cancer. Obviously the cancer risk has to be considered in relation to all the other hazards to which we are inevitably exposed and to one or other of which we must eventually succumb. The demonstration, therefore, that a drug may cause cancer in some particular species or strain of animal at a high dosage level is not necessarily a contra-indication to its use in therapeutics. The matter must be judged in relation to the circumstances of its proposed use in man. The differentiation between potent and weak carcinogens is, of course, closely related to these dose/response relationships. Is it possible to foretell, with a reasonable chance of being right, whether a substance is likely to be, or not likely to be, a potent carcinogen?

Examination of the literature on the effects of the main known carcinogens reveals that they tend to be associated with particular effects, as indicated in Table I. This information is not exhaustive, but it is intended to illustrate this point. It looks as though it might be possible to assemble a group of measurable effects which could be studied in the course of acute and subacute toxicity tests and from which the differentiation of potent from weak carcinogens or non-carcinogens might be made. I am aware of many difficulties in this approach, but it does seem worthy of serious examination from this particular angle. The early recognition of potent carcinogens would undoubtedly be helpful, although it is obviously impossible to exclude novel mechanisms of carcinogenesis; these will

Table I

Some effects of carcinogens compiled from the literature by Miß M. G. Cutler	Delayed mitosis due to				Chromosome damage	Decreased susceptibility to toxic action due to		
	Inhibition of ATP synthesis	Inhibition of RNA and DNA synthesis	Inhibition of protein synthesis	Aster and spindle abnormalities		Enzyme deletion	Receptor deletion	Cell membrane damage
1. 2-amino-azo-fluorene	—	—	+	—	—	+	—	+
2. 2-amino-fluorene	—	—	—	—	—	+	—	+
3. Carcinogenic acenaphthenes*	—	—	—	—	—	—	—	—
4. Carcinogenic acridines	—	+	—	—	—	—	—	—
5. o-amino-azotoluene	—	—	—	+	+	+	—	+
6. 4-amino-3-hydroxydiphenyl*	—	—	—	—	—	—	—	—
7. 3,4-benzpyrene	—	+	—	—	—	+	—	—
8. Beryllium*	—	—	—	—	—	—	—	—
9. Bis (2-chloroethyl) sulphide	—	—	—	—	+	—	—	—
10. Carbon tetrachloride	+	—	+	—	—	—	—	—
11. 4-DAB	—	—	—	+	+	+	+	—
12. 1,2,5,6-DBA	—	—	—	—	+	+	—	—
13. 3,4,5,6-dibenzcarbazole*	—	—	—	—	—	—	—	—
14. Diazomethane*	—	—	—	—	—	—	—	—
15. Dimethylnitrosamine	+	—	—	+	+	+	—	—
16. 9,10-DMBA	—	+	—	+	+	—	—	+
17. Ethionine	+	+	+	+	+	—	—	—
18. Carcinogenic fluorenes	—	+	—	—	—	—	—	—
19. 2-methyl-3,4-benzphenanthrene*	—	—	—	—	—	—	—	—
20. Methyl bis (2-chloroethyl) amine HCl	—	—	—	—	+	—	—	—
21. 3-methylcholanthrene	—	—	—	+	+	+	—	+
22. 3'-methyl-DAB	—	+	—	+	+	+	+	—
23. 4'-methyl-DAB	—	—	—	+	—	—	+	—
24. Myeleran	—	—	—	+	—	—	—	—
25. Nitrosomethyl-urethan	—	—	—	+	—	—	—	—
26. 4-nitroquinoline-n-oxide	—	+	—	+	—	—	—	—
27. Phenylurethan*	—	—	—	—	—	—	—	—
28. Ionising radiations	—	—	—	—	+	—	—	—
29. Thioacetamide	+	—	—	+	+	+	—	—
30. Thiourea	—	—	—	+	+	—	—	—
31. Triethylene melamine*	—	—	—	—	—	—	—	—
32. Carcinogenic stilbenes	—	+	—	—	—	—	—	—

Pre-cancerous changes are observed only in those organs in which tumors later develop.

* Pre-cancerous changes not yet adequately studied.

need to be considered if and when they come to light.

   c) From animal studies. The only certain way of demonstrating carcinogenic action is by the induction of neoplasms in experimental animals. Various methods of administration and many different animal species and strains may be used. The methods of administration studied should include those that might be employed for the therapeutic use of the drug in man. Choice of animals is a difficult problem. Carcinogenic action with some substances may be more easily demonstrated in one species or strain of animal than another. In general, especially in the investigation of a substance of unknown carcinogenic potential, randomly outbred stocks of healthy experimental animals should be used.

A potent carcinogen is likely to give rise to tumours in significant numbers in more than one species or strain within a relatively short time. The dose/response relationship may be important.

A weak carcinogen, on the other hand, may only cause a slight change in tumour incidence in the last part of the animal's life span. Such changes need to be subjected to careful statistical analysis. Again the dose/response relationship may be of considerable interest and importance.

5. When is Full-scale Assessment of Possible Carcinogenic Action Necessary?

As already indicated, the basic concept underlying safety evaluation is the balance of benefits and risks. The continuing discovery and development of new drugs is of undoubted potential benefit to the community. While it might seem to be ideal to have every drug fully assessed for possible carcinogenic action, it should be remembered that the question asked is not whether the substance might have a carcinogenic action in some species or strain of animal when administered by any route at any dosage level, but whether the proposed use of the substance as a therapeutic agent in man is attended by any significant cancer risk? In relation to the actions and uses of drugs, these are two entirely different questions.

Unnecessary demands for full-scale carcinogenic screening tests for every new drug, not to mention the obvious need for adequate information about drugs already in use, are likely to interfere with research leading to the discovery and development of further new drugs. Apart from the high cost of such studies, they would divert a significant part of the available man-power and facilities on to basically non-productive work. It is quite impracticable to submit every potential new drug to exhaustive carcinogenic screening before it is administered to man and before its efficacy as a therapeutic agent has been reasonably established. It is necessary, therefore, to adopt a more discriminating and critical approach to this problem. The pharmacologist should always have the potential cancer risk in mind when studying the toxicology of a new drug. The scope of the studies undertaken to evaluate any carcinogenic action in detail must be judged for each case in relation to proposed use, likely benefits and actual risks.

Let us assume that it is practicable on the basis of analogy, chemical and biochemical properties, and the study of certain effects on cells and tissues, to reach some conclusion about likely carcinogenic potency. If the drug is likely to be a potent carcinogenic, it is probable that its therapeutic use will be severely restricted. In our present state of knowledge, a potent carcinogen is only likely to be used as a therapeutic agent for some condition known to be lethal within a short time. Thus, it might be used for the treatment of cancer. Detailed carcinogenic studies are not necessarily demanded at present for such substances. However, as more effective anti-cancer drugs become available, it will become necessary to evaluate in greater detail the carcinogenic and other risks involved in the use of this class of drug.

Possible weak carcinogens raise different problems. It is necessary to consider such factors as the age of the patient, the nature of the disease to be treated, the life expectancy of the patient, the route of administration and dosage levels recommended, and the extent of therapeutic control by the medical attendant. Thus, a substance that only produces occasional tumours in an animal species or strain at the end of the life span, when given at a high dosage level, may not present a significant cancer risk if used in much smaller doses for a limited period in middle-aged patients. Thus, limited use of a drug under medical care for a specific purpose, to effect the cure of a disease that is not itself without risk, may be fully justified, even though the drug has been shown to have a feeble carcinogenic action. This situation is, of course, strengthened if the life expectancy of the patient is relatively short. Discrimination and judgment in such problems calls for a study of many other factors, including the efficacy of therapeutic control, the knowledge and understanding of these problems amongst practising doctors, and the machinery needed to achieve an effective overall safeguard.

On the other hand, there are certain categories of drugs that seem to call for a full assessment of the carcinogenic potential using suitable life-span animal studies designed to detect carcinogenic action. Amongst the drugs that may require detailed study of this sort one might include drugs that may be administered in high total dosage, those that are sold over the counter and are consequently used without medical supervision, and those that may be taken daily over a substantial part of the life span, such as oral contraceptives. Drugs of this nature more closely resemble food additives than other drugs. Although the safety tests demanded by some authorities for food additives may be excessive, it is difficult to see why these investigations are demanded for food additives, which are often relatively inert substances, but not for these drugs that have well-recognised biological effects and may be taken over long periods. In due time further research may make it possible to reduce the time and effort required to achieve an adequate safeguard for both these groups.

6. Summary

i. Certain principles form the basis for control of environmental hazards; these also apply to assessment of any cancer risk involved in the use of a drug.

ii. The pharmacologist, with an appropriate scientific team, is responsible for establishing specification of a new drug and for the study of its pharmacodynamics and toxicity. The assessment of the cancer risk is a part of toxicological evaluation.

iii. The possible carcinogenic action of a drug can be evaluated by analogy, by study of effects on cells and tissues, and by appropriate animal experiments.

iv. Evaluation of the cancer risk that may arise in the therapeutic use of a drug involves such considerations as the age and life expectancy of the patient, the nature of the disease to be treated, the route of administration proposed, the dosage levels recommended and the extent of medical supervision.

v. There is no short-cut to the assessment of the balance between benefit and risk; potential cancer risk is just one facet of the overall hazards and it must be considered in proper perspective in relation to any other risks involved. Those concerned need to understand the whole problem and not just one part of it; it may be necessary to take further steps to ensure that this is so.

Discussion

Frazer (in reply to BERENBLUM): I agree that the induction of a tumour is the only sure test of carcinogenicity and that the test must be designed correctly if certain types of carcinogenicity are to be detected. However, provided we can detect potent carcinogens, is there any real necessity to identify extremely feeble carcinogens if they are only going to be used at low dosage for a short period in people whose life expectancy is unlikely to provide sufficient time for a weak carcinogen to have any effect? So far as experimental design and choice of a special animal species is concerned, this is possible when a substance analogous to some known carcinogen is being studied, but this situation may not arise in the screening of a new drug for possible carcinogenic action.

Boyland: Substances tested for carcinogenic action should be investigated without prejudice, because we know so little about the relationship between carcinogenicity and chemical structure. Oral contraceptives are a special case where it is difficult to extrapolate the results of animal experiments to the human situation.

Doll: The ability to produce morphological damage in chromosomes is a common attribute of many carcinogenic drugs and Court Brown's observations suggest that it may be possible to recognize a leukaemogenic agent by seeing whether it produces visible chromosomal damage in circulating lymphocytes in man. Are any substances known to produce cancer by a direct local effect which do not produce visible chromosomal damage in the same tissue?

Druckrey: I should like to stress the following points:

1. Drugs intended for use in pregnant women and young children should be studied especially carefully.

2. Carcinogenicity is only one of several types of irreversible and chronic toxic effect. Industry should be more aware of dangers other than carcinogenicity.

3. Professor FRAZER's insistence on the need for lifespan studies is well-founded.

4. It is reasonable to leave the decision with regard to using or not using drugs on the basis of balancing risk and benefit, to doctors in charge of individual cases. But for this purpose doctors need more knowledge of toxicology.

Frazer: When I was a medical student there were relatively few effective drugs. Today there are a great many that are extremely potent. Drugs that are potent may also be dangerous. Do practising doctors know enough about the dangers inherent in the use of potent drugs? There is a need for continuing education of the medical profession, pharmacists and the public on the proper and safe use of drugs.

Davey: I would like to congratulate Professor FRAZER on a very fair exposition of a difficult subject. A rigidity of approach in this field could seriously hamper the development of the subject, and might hold up medical advance. It is very difficult to make specific recommendations concerning what should be done to test a substance for carcinogenic action. Certainly tests should be made, but how they are done should be left to the workers concerned. I believe that we should make a distinction between substances which exert a carcinogenic effect because they interfere directly with nuclear processes and cell division, and those which produce tumours only after excessive tissue damage and excessive tissue repair.

Professor FRAZER has said that results of laboratory tests on the toxicity of drugs should be published. I agree. One of the functions of the European Society for the Study of Drug Toxicity is to provide a forum for the scientific discussion of such results, and this society actively encourages publication by sponsoring its own Journal.

Frazer: I should like to stress the importance of publication. Of course, information about an effective new drug will probably be published. However, a great many toxicity studies, and perhaps long-term investigations, are undertaken on substances that, for one reason or another, do not come on the market. This information, both negative and positive, is of considerable potential value and it would be an excellent thing if it could be made available to those concerned with drug safety.

Higginson: With regard to failure to publish, industry is not guilty alone. Many university and research laboratories also fail to publish negative results. This is important, as some compounds might be regarded as strong carcinogens on the basis of single reports, whereas several unpublished negative reports would indicate that they were weak carcinogens. With modern computer systems it should be possible to handle such negative reports. Much useful material is contained for example, in the grant reports of the National Institutes of Health.

Frazer: Thank you for a most interesting discussion. In conclusion, I should like to re-emphasise a few points. First, adequate specifications both with regard to the purity of the drug and to the limitation of impurities are essential; the problem is not an easy one, as the toxicological studies are often done on material prepared at laboratory or pilot scale; if the drug proves to be a success, a change is made to manufacturing scale and this may involve alteration of the method of synthesis; careful study of the new product in relation to the earlier specifications is necessary. Secondly, publication of experimental studies, even on unsuccessful drugs, is important. Thirdly, the safety problems of drugs already in use, combination of drugs, and even herbal mixtures, are immense. Some herbal mixtures — for example, some Jamaican bush teas — are highly toxic, or even lethal. I concentrated in my paper on the problem of new drugs for simplicity's sake. I agree that something should be done, if possible, to study some of the other problems. Fourthly, it is important to re-examine any change of use; the Safety of Drugs Committee in Britain and, I believe, the F.D.A. in the United States, regard any new use of a drug as a "new drug" for regulatory purposes.

Le Risque cancérogène des Médicaments
Réflexions d'un Clinicien

P. Chassagne

Professeur à la Faculté de Médecine, Université de Paris, Paris, France

Mes premiers mots seront pour remercier le Professeur Truhaut de m'avoir invité à prendre la parole au cours de ce symposium. J'avoue avoir hésité avant de lui donner une réponse affirmative. Devant une assemblée de savants éminents, rompus aux disciplines rigoureuses de l'expérimentation, le clinicien ne peut apporter que des impressions suggérées par un empirisme quotidien et la fréquente nécessité de prendre des décisions thérapeutiques immédiates.

Au cours du symposium de l'association européenne pour l'étude de la toxicité des drogues tenu en Janvier 1964 à Lausanne, le Professeur Truhaut a inventorié les substances cancérogènes susceptibles d'avoir un emploi thérapeutique. Cette liste, qui n'est sans doute pas close, est déjà longue et ses composants très disparates. Toutefois, il semble qu'on puisse distinguer parmi eux deux grands groupes en tenant compte uniquement du simple point de vue thérapeutique:

— ceux dont les indications sont peu fréquentes, ou le remplacement facile;

— ceux dont l'usage est quotidien, ou indispensable dans certaines circonstances.

I. Premier Groupe

a) *Les colorants* ne nous retiendront pas longtemps. Destinés à la présentation des médicaments, parfois à quelques épreuves fonctionnelles, très rarement à une application à proprement parler thérapeutique, ils peuvent facilement être choisis parmi ceux connus pour leur innocuité.

b) Le risque cancérigène du *goudron* et des *huiles* est surtout industriel. Cependant, des produits à base de goudron sont employés en dermatologie et de nombreuses préparations de ce type existent dans le commerce. Les observations publiées ayant trait à la survenue de néoplasmes cutanés à la suite de traitements de ce genre, pour exceptionnelles qu'elles soient, conduisent à écarter cette thérapeutique, dont la vogue est actuellement en diminution.

c) *L'uréthane*, ou carbamate d'éthyle, fut, un moment, utilisé comme agent leucolytique au cours de leucémies myéloïdes. Son pouvoir cancérogène est certain et parallèle aux doses ou à la durée du traitement de l'animal en expérience. Sans doute ne s'est-il pas manifesté chez l'homme. Mais ce risque, à côté d'autres accidents plus immédiats (anémie aiguë thrombopénie, aplasie médullaire, poussée leucosique), est une raison supplémentaire d'écarter l'uréthane de la thérapeutique.

d) Divers dérivés minéraux, vecteurs de rayonnements ionisants, et en particulier le *bioxyde de thorium colloïdal* ou

Thorotrast, sont doués de propriétés cancérogènes très marquées. Le thorotrast n'est pas un médicament à proprement parler, mais un moyen d'exploration dans le but d'un diagnostic. C'est ainsi qu'il a été utilisé comme produit de contraste pour des examens des sinus, des artériographies, des pyélographies rétrogrades. Il a même parfois été essayé dans un but thérapeutique, en vue de traiter des tuberculoses extra-pulmonaires, osseuses en particulier. L'accumulation de thorotrast in situ et dans différents viscères (foie, rate, ganglion, thymus) explique la fréquence des accidents survenus après un délai parfois long. On a publié l'observation d'un carcinome de la vésicule séminale 14 ans après une urétéropyélographie au thorotrast. Les observations de sarcome du foie, de la rate, des voies biliaires extra-hépatiques, des os, du rein, sont nombreuses et justifient entièrement l'exclusion totale de ce mode d'exploration, au profit d'autres de valeur égale et d'une innocuité reconnue, tout au moins du point de vue carcinogénétique.

e) Le traitement de la polyglobulie par la *chlornaphazine* a été très utilisé dans certains pays, en particulier en Scandinavie. La chlornaphazine est la dichlorodiethyl-β naphtylamine. La 2-naphtylamine est susceptible de déclencher expérimentalement l'apparition de tumeurs vésicales. Ce tropisme s'explique vraisemblablement par le métabolisme du médicament: il n'est, en effet, qu'en partie détoxiqué par le foie et ce sont les métabolites éliminés par l'urine qui sont susceptibles de développer dans l'arbre urinaire leur pouvoir cancérigène sous l'influence de β-glycuronidases toujours présentes dans l'urine. La nocivité de la β-naphtylamine est bien connue industriellement. Il était logique de prévoir que la chlornaphazine, administrée sous forme de traitement prolongé chez les polyglobuliques, entrainerait des accidents du même ordre. Une étude récente de THIELE et coll. le confirme. Elle groupe 61 malades polyglobuliques, traités par la chlornaphazine, avec des résultats hématologiques favorables dans 75% des cas. Mais, parmi 20 malades qui avaient reçu une dose totale comprise entre 100 et 175 g, on trouve 6 cas de tumeurs vésicales et, parmi 8 autres qui avaient été traités par des doses supérieures, on en dénombre 5. Sans doute, la fréquence de ces accidents est-elle en partie liée à la durée du traitement. Utilisée pour traiter la maladie de Hodgkin, où la survie ne dépasse pas quelques années, la chlornaphazine n'a pas fait apparaitre de lésions vésicales, faute de temps, sans doute. Néanmoins la cause est entendue. Un tel traitement ne peut se concevoir qu'en dernier ressort devant l'échec total des autres thérapeutiques. En fait, les résultats obtenus par les moyens actuellement à notre disposition doivent rendre ce recours inutile.

f) *Les dérivés arsenicaux* présentent la particularité d'être carcinogènes chez l'homme, alors que, chez l'animal, cette propriété n'a pas pu être mise en évidence de façon indiscutable, peut-être en raison de la toxicité du produit qui ne permet pas l'expérimentation à doses fortes. Le cancer arsenical observé en pathologie humaine, est un cancer cutané qui se développe sur les lésions d'hyperkératose, conséquence elle-même d'un traitement à doses faibles, mais de longue durée. Survenant chez des sujets relativement jeunes, sa localisation caractéristique est le scrotum (70% des cas), puis la paume des mains, la plante des pieds. Les localisations multiples ne sont pas rares. C'est, dans la majorité des cas, un épithélioma spino-cellulaire, qui, non traité, a l'évolution habituelle des autres cancers cutanés. L'existence de lésions pré-existantes peut être un point d'appel. On a décrit un carcinome arsenical développé à la périphérie d'éléments de psoriasis. La sensibilité individuelle à l'arsenic, très variable suivant les sujets, compte aussi. On connait une observation où la prise quotidienne pendant un temps assez long de 15 gouttes de liqueur de Fowler amena l'apparition d'un carcinome cutané de l'avant-bras, vérifié histologiquement. Les curieuses coutumes des arsenicophages des Alpes d'Autriche qui consomment volontairement à partir de l'adolescence et à doses progressives des produits arsenicaux, montrent que l'immunité cellulaire ne peut être acquise vis-à-vis de l'arsenic. Dans ces régions, les processus néoplasiques sont responsables de 13% de la mortalité générale et atteignent très fréquemment des sujets de moins de 30 ans.

L'arsenic a été pendant longtemps, presque une panacée, malgré les accidents généraux, parfois très graves, que ce médicament pourrait déclencher. Son règne est déclinant, pour ne pas dire terminé. Les progrès de l'art de guérir ont permis de lui substituer d'autres thérapeutiques plus efficaces et moins dangereuses.

II. Les Médicaments du deuxième Groupe

peuvent poser des problèmes plus difficiles parce que les indications de certains d'entre eux sont très fréquentes, leur action thérapeutique évidente et leur prescription indispensable dans certains cas. Nous nous limiterons à quelques uns d'entre eux et envisagerons successivement:

— les médicaments cyto-toxiques anti-cancéreux,

— les anti-thyroïdiens,

— les oestrogènes et progestatifs,

— les hydrazines, et en particulier l'isoniazide.

a) *Les médicaments cyto-toxiques,* qu'ils soient dérivés de la chloréthazine, de l'éthylène-imine, des esters disulfoniques (agents alkoylants), ou qu'ils soient des antimétabolites, sont destinés au traitement d'affections mettant en jeu, à plus ou moins brève échéance, un pronostic vital. Aussi, leurs indications, pour être limitées, n'en sont pas moins formelles. Beaucoup d'entre eux méritent la qualification de «radiomimétique», car, comme les radiations, ils sont capables à la fois d'arrêter l'évolution d'un processus tumoral et de produire des néoplasmes expérimentaux. S'agissant de malades dont on cherche seulement à assurer la survie pour quelques années, leur pouvoir carcinogénétique n'entre pas en ligne de compte.

b) *Les médicaments anti-thyroïdiens de synthèse* peuvent, dans certaines conditions expérimentales, entrainer le développement de tumeurs thyroïdiennes. Cette dégénérescence pourrait être la conséquence à la fois de l'arrêt de la sécrétion thyroïdienne et de l'hyper-sécrétion de T.S.H. qui en est la conséquence. Il semble, cependant, que la compensation du déficit thyroïdien, normalisant la sécrétion de T.S.H., n'empêche pas la survenue de tumeurs thyroïdiennes ou même l'atteinte d'autres organes, en particulier le foie. Aucune observation d'accidents de ce genre n'a été signalée en clinique humaine.

c) *Le Fer-Dextran.* Le désir d'obtenir du traitement martial une efficacité plus rapide et plus intense a conduit de nombreux auteurs à tenter de substituer à la voie orale la voie parentérale.

Les essais de traitement par voie intraveineuse ont été peu encourageants: la plupart des préparations utilisables entrainent des accidents locaux et généraux. Par ailleurs, le risque d'hémochromatose après traitement prolongé est bien connu.

Aussi, les cliniciens, et en particulier les pédiatres, ont-ils accueilli avec faveur la préparation d'un sel de fer injectable par voie intramusculaire comportant un véhicule-retard, le dextran. Certes, la tolérance locale n'est pas toujours excellente. La survenue d'une induration des plans cutanéo-musculaires, la possibilité d'une inflammation locale avec parfois réaction ganglionnaire, surtout l'apparition de pigmentation localisée plus ou moins durable, ont été observées par la plupart des auteurs. Mais ces inconvénients comptent peu en regard de la rapidité d'action et de l'efficacité durable du traitement. La brillante carrière de ce médicament a été brusquement stoppée en 1959—1960, lorsque des cancérologues anglais (RICHMOND, HADDOW et HORNING), montrèrent que des injections répétées de doses, à vrai dire élevées, à des souris entrainaient la formation in situ de sarcome dans un délai de six à huit mois chez la presque totalité des animaux. Toutefois, les mêmes expériences poursuivies chez le hamster ou le cobaye s'avérèrent négatives.

La valeur de ces expériences a été discutée: la différence de réceptivité des animaux, l'importance des doses employées (20 mg de fer par semaine chez le rat), très différentes de celles utilisées en thérapeutique, ont été les arguments avancés pour minimiser la portée des résultats expérimentaux.

Néanmoins, la vente du médicament a été suspendue dans divers pays et en particulier en France. Depuis, des enquêtes poursuivies, aussi bien chez l'enfant que chez l'adulte, ont permis de réexaminer les malades qui avaient reçu antérieurement ce traitement. Aucun incident n'a été relevé chez l'enfant. Chez l'adulte, deux observations discutables ont été signalées (métastase d'un néoplasme utérin; survenue d'une tumeur, de malignité d'ailleurs douteuse, à l'emplacement d'anciennes injections). FIELDING souligne le poids moléculaire très élevé du fer-dextran (180000) qui ne peut se mobiliser que par la voie lymphatique, rapidement bloquée. Il propose de lui substituer un fer-dextrine, ou mieux encore un fer-sorbitol, qui, expérimentalement, est incapable de provoquer des tumeurs et dont la mobilisation est plus rapide, évitant les inconvénients d'une stagnation prolongée du métal dans la zone de l'injection. Au cours des dernières années, la plupart des pays ont ré-autorisé la vente du fer-dextran. Le dernier manuel américain de posologie infantile en donne une posologie très précise. La même mesure n'a pas encore été prise en France. Pourtant, sans être irremplaçable, le fer-dextran constitue un progrès thérapeutique très appréciable. D'ailleurs, son utilisation en pratique vétérinaire (anémie des porcelets) n'a pas été interrompue et aucun accident n'a été signalé.

d) *Oestrogènes et progestatifs*. Le pouvoir cancérogène des oestrogènes est connu depuis 1932, date où fut réalisée l'expérience cruciale de LACASSAGNE, montrant que l'administration d'oestrogènes à la souris mâle peut faire apparaître un carcinome mammaire. Depuis, des expériences innombrables ont confirmé cette découverte et ont montré que cette possibilité s'étendait non seulement à la sphère génitale (corps et col utérin, testicule), mais aussi à des organes très divers (hypophyse, reins), au sang, au squelette, au revêtement cutané.

En clinique humaine, les possibilités de thérapeutiques oestrogéniques ou progestatives se sont considérablement accrues au cours des dernières années et leurs indications ont été étendues, souvent à l'excès.

Compte tenu des données expérimentales, deux ordres de questions se posent au clinicien:

1. Est-il exact que l'administration prolongée d'oestrogènes ou de progestatifs, en thérapeutique humaine, favorise l'installation d'un cancer, principalement utérin ou mammaire?

On est, dès l'abord, frappé par la rareté des observations cliniques. En ce qui concerne le cancer mammaire, on peut dire, avec Netter et Gorins, que «les épithéliomas du sein survenus au cours de l'oestrogénothérapie sont aussi rares que l'emploi des oestrogènes est universellement répandu». Cette même constatation était récemment soulignée de façon humoristique par un de nos collègues américains qui, répondant à une malade soumise à l'oestrogéno-thérapie, qui l'interrogeait sur les risques éventuels de cette thérapeutique, lui dit «Prenez des oestrogènes, vous vous sentirez mieux, mais jetez votre cigarette, qui est bien plus dangereuse». Une statistique, publiée par Wilson en 1963, porte sur 304 femmes âgées de 40 à 70 ans et soumises à un traitement oestro-génique d'une durée variable, parfois très longue (27 ans). 86 d'entre elles avaient été hysterectomisées. Les prévisions statistiques, établies sur l'ensemble de la population, faisaient escompter la découverte de 18 cancers mammaires ou utérins. Aucun n'a été mis en évidence. Une autre étude porte sur 550 femmes traitées par un progestatif de synthèse, le noréthinodrel. Deux cancers seulement ont été dépistés, ce qui peut être considéré, statistiquement, comme ne dépassant pas les limites du hasard.

Ajoutons enfin que, si l'on peut mettre en évidence les possibilités carcino-génétiques des oestrogènes chez la souris, le lapin, le hamster, il n'a pas été possible de réaliser cette expérience chez les primates.

On peut, pour conclure, dire que, dans l'espèce humaine, le déclenchement d'un cancer par oestrogénothérapie est une éventualité théoriquement possible mais, jusqu'à plus ample informé, certainement exceptionnelle.

2. Est-il exact que l'oestrogénothérapie puisse révéler un cancer latent, faire dégénérer une lésion bénigne, aggraver l'évolution d'un cancer déjà diagnostiqué?

La révélation d'un cancer latent par les oestrogènes est vraisemblable, lorsqu'elle survient après un traitement de courte durée. La coïncidence de la dégénérescence d'une maladie de Reclus et d'un traitement oestrogénique se rencontre avec une fréquence telle qu'elle ne peut être fortuite et la survenue de dégénérescence bilatérale simultanément est un argument supplémentaire. L'action favorable des oestrogènes sur un cancer mammaire pré-existant n'est pas aussi constante qu'on le dit, même s'il s'agit de la forme squirrheuse de la femme âgée. Les diverses statistiques publiées ne donnent, en moyenne, qu'un pourcentage d'amélioration compris entre 35 et 45%, si l'on veut bien fonder l'étude, non sur des impressions, mais sur des critères de valeur et n'admettre l'effet favorable que lorsqu'on constate une diminution nette, par exemple de moitié, du volume de la tumeur. Chacun connait les observations, non moins significatives, de malades atteints d'un cancer de la prostate et soumis à l'oestrogéno-thérapie, chez lesquels se développa en cours de traitement une tumeur mammaire, qu'on l'interprète comme le développement d'un cancer in situ, ou seulement la survenue d'une métastase favorisée par l'action de l'oestrogène sur la glande elle-même.

Se fondant sur l'expérience clinique, le thérapeute peut donc répondre affirmativement à la triple question posée, mais il doit aussi tempérer cette affirmation par quelques nuances, en insistant spécialement sur:

— la rareté des observations,

— la posologie élevée, continue et prolongée du médicament,

— l'importance du terrain, et en particulier du terrain hormonal. Beaucoup d'auteurs considèrent que les résultats de la thérapeutique oestrogénique sont d'autant plus favorables que l'oestrogènie physiologique est plus faible, ce qui explique les améliorations, parfois spectaculaires, observées chez les femmes âgées.

En conclusion, les résultats de l'expérimentation et les constatations de la clinique qui permettent d'affirmer le risque carcinogénétique de l'oestrogénothérapie, sans toutefois pouvoir en apprécier de façon certaine l'importance réelle, conduisent néanmoins le clinicien à une attitude générale de prudence.

Il n'est, bien entendu, nullement question de priver des malades du bénéfice d'un traitement indispensable et irremplaçable, comme c'est le cas au cours du cancer de la prostate. Mais, en dehors de ces circonstances particulières, il paraît raisonnable:

— de limiter l'oestrogénothérapie à des indications précises, sans l'étendre au traitement d'affections très diverses pour des résultats médiocres ou discutables;

— de n'administrer, sauf nécessité absolue, les oestrogènes que par doses faibles et par cures limitées et espacées;

— d'être particulièrement prudent si la malade

— est porteuse de lésions pré-existantes d'apparence bénigne (maladie de Reclus, par exemple),

— a, parmi ses ascendants ou ses collatéraux, un nombre élevé de sujets ayant été atteints de processus néoplasiques.

Enfin, les progestatifs, spécialement ceux dérivés des 19-norstéroïdes, méritent une mention spéciale. Une de leurs actions principales étant d'inhiber la fonction ovarienne, on peut s'attendre à une généralisation de plus en plus grande de leur emploi. Bien que les résultats des recherches, déjà effectuées (GRUENSTEIN et coll.) chez le rat, n'aient pas mis en valeur une action cancérogène de ces progestatifs, il semble que leur étude dans ce sens devrait être poursuivie et étendue.

e) *Hydrazine, et en particulier isoniazide.* Depuis 10 ans, les études expérimentales, poursuivies sur la souris avec l'isoniazide, ont permis de constater que l'I.N.H. pouvait avoir une action néoplasiante aboutissant au développement, non seulement d'adénomes pulmonaires, mais aussi de lésions carcinomateuses, en particulier du médiastin. Certains, même, ont constaté une atteinte hépatique et des troubles sanguins du type leucémique. Poursuivant plus loin leurs investigations, ces chercheurs ont constaté que le pouvoir cancérogène était sous la dépendance de l'hydrazine (JUHASZ, BIANCIFIORI, et RIBACCHI) qui apparait ainsi comme un des corps chimiques les plus simples doués de cette propriété. Comme nous le rappelons plus haut, certains agents anticancéreux méritent le qualificatif de «radiomimétiques», car ils peuvent à la fois déclencher le processus tumoral ou s'opposer à son développement. L'hydrazine pourrait entrer dans ce groupe, car la méthyl-hydrazine jouit de propriétés anti-cancéreuses qui sont maintenant utilisées en clinique humaine.

Parallèllement aux travaux des pharmacologues, les cliniciens, mettant à profit les remarquables propriétés antituberculeuses de l'isoniazide, l'administrèrent aux tuberculeux dans le monde entier, tant comme agent thérapeutique d'un processus en évolution que comme chimio-prophylaxie des accidents évolutifs post-primaires. L'I.N.H., s'ajoutant à la streptomycine et au P.A.S. a modifié du tout au tout la conception du traitement de la tuberculose. Le clinicien, d'abord sceptique, puis triomphant, a assisté à la guérison des tuberculoses aiguës, de la méningite tuberculeuse, à la fermeture rapide des tuberculoses excavées. Si la chimiothérapie antituberculeuse n'a pas entièrement vaincu ce fléau social, elle en a minimisé l'importance à un point tel que la mortalité tuberculeuse est devenue presque négligeable et que les spécialistes ont dû tourner de plus en plus leur attention vers l'étude des pneumopathies non tuberculeuses.

Comme chaque fois qu'apparaît un médicament très actif, on a cherché à en étendre les indications. L'amélioration de l'état général et du comportement du tuberculeux traité étant souvent manifeste et sans parallélisme avec l'évolution des lésions, on s'est demandé s'il n'y aurait pas là la possibilité d'une thérapeutique anti-dépressive, thymo-analeptique. Ainsi est né l'iproniazide, médication psychotonique, euphorisante, à action anti-tuberculeuse faible, bientôt suivi de plusieurs autres dérivés hydraziniques inhibiteurs de la mono-amine-oxydase.

Le clinicien se trouve alors dans une situation délicate: D'un côté, l'expérimentation lui montre que l'hydrazine est un facteur carcinogénétique certain. D'autre part, il a à sa disposition des médicaments hydraziniques dont l'un a fait ses preuves depuis 10 ans, et dont l'autre, d'usage plus récent, d'indications moins précises, n'en est pas pour autant moins efficace. Il n'hésitera pourtant pas longtemps sur la conduite à tenir. Il sait gré aux expérimentateurs de l'avertissement qu'ils lui donnent. Il souhaite que les recherches se poursuivent dans ce sens. Il n'ignore pas que le fait de n'avoir pas encore vu survenir d'accident chez l'homme, malgré les millions de malades traités au cours d'une décennie, n'est pas une preuve absolue d'innocuité. Néanmoins il ne lui est pas permis, en

attendant, de priver ses malades de traitements dont l'un, au moins, est une des réussites thérapeutiques les plus belles et les plus surprenantes. Il continuera donc à traiter la tuberculose par l'isoniazide et, s'il hésite parfois à prescrire un inhibiteur hydrazinique de la mono-amine-oxydase, ce ne sera pas, pour le moment, par crainte de son pouvoir carcinogénétique.

Au terme de cet exposé et comme conclusion générale, nous voudrions faire deux remarques:

A. Au Point de Vue pharmacologique

1. Sans répéter les critiques si souvent faites sur l'extrapolation des résultats expérimentaux à la pathologie humaine et fondées sur les différences de posologie, de mode d'emploi, de durée de l'expérience, nous croyons pourtant important de souligner, pour les recherches de carcinogénèse médicamenteuse comme pour certaines autres, la nécessité d'étendre les investigations aux espèces animales les plus diverses. Est-il besoin de rappeler l'extrème sensibilité du cobaye à la pénicilline, qui eût peut-être conduit à écarter cette thérapeutique, si cet animal avait été le premier ou le seul choisi par l'expérimentateur? Plus récemment, et à l'inverse, n'a t'on pas constaté qu'une ou deux espèces animales seulement pouvaient être sensibles à l'action tératogène d'un médicament hautement nocif pour l'espèce humaine? La recherche du risque carcinogénétique justifie les mêmes remarques. Comme celle des autres espèces, la sensibilité humaine est très variable suivant le médicament envisagé et pour un même médicament réputé carcinogène, suivant les individus. Le «terrain cancérogène» est une notion fort imprécise, mais l'expérience clinique en affirme l'existence, en

mettant en évidence une double sensibilité aux processus néoplasiques: sensibilité du moment liée aux conditions physiologiques ou pathologiques, sensibilité permanente constitutionnelle qu'éclaireront peut-être un jour les recherches des généticiens sur les anomalies chromosomiques des cellules cancéreuses.

2. L'étude de la toxicité d'un médicament doit, à coup sûr, comprendre des essais de carcinogénicité, mais, compte tenu de leur longueur et de leurs difficultés, il semble que l'étude des divers métabolites issus du produit considéré au cours de sa traversée dans l'organisme permettrait, d'une part, de mieux comprendre une action nocive éventuelle, d'autre part, faciliterait et écourterait les essais expérimentaux.

B. Au Point de Vue thérapeutique

En précisant les conditions d'apparition du cancer chimique expérimental: longue latence, traitement continu, influence néfaste des posologies élevées, les recherches pharmacologiques apportent des notions utiles à la thérapeutique humaine, et qui doivent orienter l'attitude du clinicien. Autant il aura peu d'hésitation à prescrire un médicament suspect pour une cure courte et en principe unique, autant il sera prudent si l'action du même médicament nécessite des traitements prolongés ou itératifs, des posologies élevées, ou s'il est destiné à des sujets en plein développement, donc particulièrement sensibles: enfant, voire foetus à travers le placenta maternel. C'est le problème, si débattu au cours des dernières années, du risque

thérapeutique. Car le risque de carcinogénèse ne doit pas être dissocié des autres accidents que le médicament peut entrainer. Il n'est pas, a priori, à considérer avec une attitude différente, d'autant que les autres risques sont, en général, plus fréquents et parfois même immédiatement graves, sans que, pour cela le médicament doive obligatoirement être abandonné. Comme le fait pertinemment remarquer dans son rapport le Pr. F. DICKENS, personne ne songe à ne plus utiliser la pénicilline parce qu'elle peut déclencher des accidents allergiques sévères, voire mortels. Le clinicien en revient donc à la règle d'or de la thérapeutique que rappelle le Pr. FRAZER dans son rapport, aux conclusions duquel nous souscrivons entièrement, et qui consiste à mettre en balance le risque du traitement et les bénéfices que le malade doit logiquement en tirer. Les progrès accomplis depuis 20 ans ont mis à la disposition des thérapeutes des produits de plus en plus actifs, mais, par là même, de plus en plus dangereux. Ils perdraient toute possibilité d'action s'il leur était interdit «d'admettre le risque individuel, implicitement et inévitablement lié à tout acte thérapeutique» (J. CHEYMOL). Ce qu'ils doivent protéger et servir, c'est l'intérêt collectif des malades. La confrontation des résultats du pharmacologue et des observations cliniques du thérapeute reste indispensable pour diminuer le plus possible le risque couru par quelques uns au profit du plus grand nombre. Aussi est-ce bien peu dire que la pharmacologie et la thérapeutique sont deux disciplines complémentaires. En réalité, elles sont inséparables.

Bibliographie

BISHOP, P. M. F., Hormones and cancer. *Clin. Obstet. Gynec.* **3**, 1109 (1960).

BONSER, G. M., L'attivita cancerogena di alcuni agenti terapeutici. *Boll. chim. farm.* **103**, 771 (1964).

FIELDING, S., Sarcoma induction by iron carbohydrate complexes. *Brit. med. J.* **1**, 1800 (1962).

GRUENSTEIN, M., SHAY, H., and SHIMKIN, M. D., Lack of effect of norethynodral (Enovid) on methyl-ethanolcholanthrene-induced mammary carcinogenesis in females rats. *Cancer. Res.* **24**, 1656 (1964).

Haddow, A., and Horning, E. S., On the carcinogeneticy of an iron-dextran complex. *J. nat. Cancer Inst.* **24**, 109 (1960).

Lacassagne, A., Apparition de cancers de la mamelle chez la souris mâle soumise à des injections de folliculine. *C. R. Acad. Sci. (Paris)* **195**, 630 (1932).

— Tumeurs malignes apparues au cours d'un traitement hormonal combiné chez des souris appartenant à des lignées réfractaires au cancer spontané. *C. R. Soc. Biol. (Paris)* **121**, 607 (1936).

— Le rôle des hormones dans la cancérisation. *Sem. Hôp. Paris* **35**, 1739 (1961).

Netter, A., Lambert, A., and Gorins, M., Cancer du corps utérin au cours de l'oestro-génothérapie. *C. R. Soc. franç. Gynéc.* **25**, 175 (1955).

Rice-Wray, E., Schulz-Contreras, M., Guer-rero, I., and Aranoa-Rosenn, A., Long term administration of norethindrol in fertility control. *J. Amer. med. Ass.* **180**, 355 (1962).

Richmond, H. G., Induction of sarcoma in the rat by iron-dextran. *Brit. med. J.* **1959** I, 947.

Thiede, J., Chevitz, E., and Christensen, B.C., Chlornaphazine as a bladder carcinogen *Acta med. scand.* **175**, 721 (1964).

Truhaut, R., Sur les risques de cancérisation pouvant résulter de l'emploi de certains agents chimiques en thérapeutique. *Proc. Europ. Soc. stud. of drug toxicity* **3**, 101 (1964).

Wilson, R. A., The roles of oestrogen and progesterone in breast and genital cancer. *J. Amer. med. Ass.* **182**, 327 (1962).

Discussion

Rudali: Professor Chassagne has justifiably commented that information with regard to toxicity and carcinogenicity should be obtained in as wide a variety of species as possible. I would like to see it made obligatory to test substances in primates. Moreover, I should like to see our contacts with veterinarians increased.

Practically the same medicines are used in veterinary medicine as are used in human medicine. I am convinced that the big veterinary schools could provide us with statistically significant data of great interest in relation to the problems we are discussing.

Schoental: I believe we are all agreed that where drugs are to be given to young people they should be tested particularly thoroughly before use. This has not been done in the case of oral contraceptives. The carcinogenic and mutagenic effects of which are not known as far as man is concerned. If it is felt that carcinogenic effects observed in rodents cannot be interpreted as indicating a cancer hazard for man then more data should be sought from experiments on primates and other species. These experiments should be carried on for more than one generation.

In the mean time the need to control population explosion should be met by the use of alternative methods of contraception.

Taylor: I feel here that it is essential that we balance risks against benefits.

Tumeurs des Cellules de Leydig du Testicule du Rat, sous l'Influence de l'o,p′-DDD*

A. Lacassagne

Professeur, Membre de l'Institut et de l'Acadèmie Nationale de Médecine, Institut du Radium, Paris, France

Je vous rappelle qu'en 1948, Neison et Woodard firent connaître l'action nécrosante qu'exerce, sur les zones fasciculée et réticulée du cortex surrénalien du Chien, un insecticide administré par voie

nous avons ajouté la même quantité d'o,p′-DDD. Effectivement, nous avons obtenu un ralentissement considérable et même l'inhibition du processus de cancérisation.

orale, le dichlorodiphényldichloroéthane (I). Dix ans plus tard, Nichols et Hennigar établirent que, dans le produit industriel, la substance active était l'isomère o,p′-DDD (II). En raison de son action élective sur l'adrénocortex, cette drogue est employée dans le traitement de certaines tumeurs de la glande surrénale.

Comme il est connu que le pouvoir cancérogène, que certains toxiques exercent sur le foie, est inhibé par l'adrénalectomie, nous avons pensé, avec ma collaboratrice Mme le Pr. Hurst, que l'administration d'o,p′-DDD pourrait n'être pas sans effet sur la production des tumeurs hépatiques chez des rats intoxiqués par le p-diméthylaminoazobenzène. Au régime d'animaux recevant quotidiennement, dans les conditions habituelles de nos expériences, du DAB au taux de 0,6 g par kilo de nourriture,

Une expérience témoin, consistant à donner, par voie orale, la même quantité d'o,p′-DDD seul, nous a permis de reconnaître à cette drogue une action oncogène dont voici les caractères.

Le traitement est bien supporté et l'état général des animaux n'est pas touché; mais il s'installe une surcharge importante du tissu graisseux souscutané et abdominal. C'est la présence d'une tumeur du testicule chez un rat traité depuis 18 mois qui attira notre attention sur cet organe. Cette action se manifeste macroscopiquement par une augmentation progressive du poids du testicule au cours des six premiers mois, qui est remplacée — entre les 10e et 12e mois — par une très forte atrophie.

---

* Résumé d'un article paru dans le Bulletin de l'Association française pour l'Etude du Cancer; 1965, **52**, 89—104.

Histologiquement, on constate que la spermatogénèse se maintient longtemps intacte. Mais, à partir du 2e mois, on remarque un épanchement albumineux intertubulaire, en même temps qu'une hyperactivité de la glande interstitielle. Vers le 9e mois, il se produit un épaississement et une transformation fibrohyaline de l'albuginée, qu'on retrouve également dans la paroi de quelques veines intratesticulaires.

A partir de ce moment, la dégénérescence de l'épithélium séminal se précise, aboutissant plus ou moins rapidement au dépeuplement total de la lignée, alors que la glande interstitielle s'hypertrophie. Il en résulte, aux environs du 12e mois, la formation de petits nodules d'aspect adénomateux, dont le volume et le nombre augmentent, et qui présentent des stades variés de tendance à la transformation carcinomateuse. En ce qui concerne le cancer constitué, voici comment nous nous sommes bornés à le décrire: «Histologiquement, il présente les traits caractéristiques, décrits par les auteurs qui ont observé de tels cancers des cellules de Leydig du Rat, qu'ils aient été considérés comme spontanés ou provoqués expérimentalement. Sa description détaillée reproduit exactement celle excellente, donnée par Roe et coll., concernant les tumeurs de la glande interstitielle du testicule obtenues au moyen du cadmium.»

Discussion

Roe: I should like to thank Professor Lacassagne for his kind remarks concerning our studies on the production of testicular tumours by cadmium. At the same time I must point out that the macroscopic and microscopic descriptions of the testicular lesions were made not by myself but by my colleague Dr. Cuthbert Dukes. Professor Lacassagne's new observations are extremely interesting.

Shabad: I should like to refer to the new and remarkable observation of Professor Lacassagne on the induction of testicular tumours by a derivative of DDT. Here is an example of a carcinogen used clinically at Bethesda by Dr. Roy Herz as a cancer chemotherapeutic agent. The stages of testicular tumour development in response to the drug in experimental animals and man are identical: first irregular hyperplasia, then nodular foci, then benign tumours, and finally malignant tumours.

I liked the more general statements of Professor Lacassagne with regard to the development of cancer. It is true that cells changed by the action of a carcinogen may be more resistant to the effects of the same carcinogen. This was seen in relation to benzpyrene-induced sarcomas by you and also by Vasiliev in our laboratories.

Finally there is the relationship between carcinogenesis and anti-tumour activity. Miss Schoental was right to say that our committee should view the evidence of carcinogenicity with pessimism. On the other hand we should not lose sight of the benefits which chemotherapeutic agents are able to offer.

Discussion générale

Réflexions de A. LACASSAGNE

Y a-t-il eu simple coïncidence, ou concordance voulue entre le choix du thème de ce colloque et la date de sa tenue ? ... je l'ignore. Toujours est-il qu'on vient de fêter au Japon le cinquantième anniversaire de la découverte de YAMAGIWA et ITCHIKAWA qui, en 1915, obtinrent expérimentalement les premiers cancers chimiques, au moyen d'un produit largement et très diversement employé, même en thérapeutique, le goudron. La date de cette réussite suivait de peu celle de MARIE, CLUNET et RAULOT-LEPOINTE, qui étaient parvenus, en 1910, à reproduire le radiocancer chez l'animal. C'est en 1932 que furent publiés les premiers cas de cancers expérimentaux, obtenus au moyen d'une hormone.

La vigtaine de rapports qui ont été présentés à ce colloque ont bien fait ressortir la grande place qu'ont prise ces trois modes de production de tumeurs, en un demi siècle. Ils ont confirmé la multiplicité et la variété de agents étiologiques des cancers; ils ont mis en évidence que beaucoup de médicaments pourraient être soit par eux-mêmes, soit par tel constituant ou par tel métabolite, des agents cancérogènes dans certaines conditions d'administration.

Tous les médicaments qui visent à freiner la croissance ou à détruire des cellules pathologiques (qu'elles soient d'origine endogène ou parasitaire) exercent presque nécessairement un certain degré d'action toxique sur des cellules saines de l'organisme. La sélectivité d'un agent déterminé, qui permet d'agir plus électivement sur les cellules pathologiques que sur les cellules normales, est affaire de dose et de son mode d'administration, que sa toxicité soit physique ou chimique.

Les radiobiologistes, à cause d'une facilité relative de contrôler l'absorption de l'énergie radiante au niveau des cellules, et de définir les lésions ainsi produites, trouvèrent assez rapidement la posologie appropriée à l'effet recherché. Les lésions produites dans le matériel chromosomique et les anomalies consécutives de la mitose avaient été bientôt reconnues, fournissant des arguments sérieux à l'hypothèse qui attribuait à des mutations somatiques l'origine de la cancérisation. En raison de la sommation des doses, on recherca les conditions de leur administration dans le temps, devant conduire soit à la stérilisation de toutes les cellules pathologiques qu'on se proposait des détruire, soit à la cancérisation expérimentale par de faibles irradiations longtemps prolongées.

Les découvertes successives de nombreuses substances oncogènes ont permis aux expérimentateurs de reconnaître de grandes analogies dans le déroulement des processus de chimio — et de radio-cancérogénèse. Dans les deux cas, des cellules-souches d'un tissu, qui survivent pendant une intoxication prolongée — tout en additionnant des changements plus ou moins irréversibles dont certains peuvent être des mutations — donnent naissance à des descendants qui, ou bien disparaissent par mort différée, ou bien se développent sous forme d'éléments tératologiques. Les stades successifs qui conduisent à la cancérisation dans le cas d'une intoxication chronique ont été particulièrement étudiés dans la peau et dans le foie.

On y assiste à une succession alternée de processus de destruction et de régénération cellulaires, cette dernière se faisant à partir d'éléments de plus en plus anormaux et de plus en plus résistants au toxique (que celui-ci soit une radiation ionisante ou une substance chimique), et aboutissant à la formation de clones de cellules cancéreuses, plus ou moins réfractaires à l'agent causal.

De tout ce qui a été dit ici, il ressort que — sans aucun doute — un risque de cancérisation peut résulter de l'emploi prolongé de certains médicaments dont les effets tardifs des faibles doses sont mal connus. Evidemment, ce risque est très faible, si on le compare à ceux provenant de l'introduction, dans l'organisme, par d'autres modes, de quantités beaucoup plus grandes soit de ces mêmes substances, soit d'autres dont le pouvoir cancérogène éventuel n'est pas mieux connu.

Le problème posé par l'évaluation du danger cancérogène des médicaments se présente de la même façon que celui résultant de l'exposition aux radiations. Pas plus que dans ce dernier cas, il semble qu'il ne faille admettre l'existence d'un seuil. Faut-il alors discuter d'une dose «*permissible*» selon la terminologie anglaise, ou «*admissible*» comme on dit de préférence en français, ce dernier qualificatif (que j'ai proposé à une commission idoine) laissant mieux entendre l'incertitude de nos connaissances et l'arbitraire de nos appréciations?

Il est certain qu'on ne peut pas empêcher les malades de réclamer toujours plus de médicaments et les médecins de les leur prescrire; de son côté, l'industrie de fabrication de nouvelles drogues en lancera toujours plus sur le marché.

Ce colloque a donc été le bienvenu; il aura certainement des résultats fructueux. Il a, une fois de plus, attiré l'attention sur l'obligation de développer les recherches sur la cancérogénèse chimique.

General Recommandations

The papers given at the Symposium cover in detail many facets of the problems relevant to carcinogenesis that may arise from the use of drugs. The recommendations that follow are of a more general nature.

1. The possibility of the occurrence of irreversible changes, which may lead to delayed effects and chronic hazards, arising from the administration of even a single dose of a drug, has not, until recently, been sufficiently recognised. Many drugs in use for many years have not been adequately tested over the long term in animals and their effects in man may have escaped notice due to inadequate record keeping. The scientific facilities available for this type of work are far from adequate and urgently need expansion. New drugs are now better tested, but efforts should be made to find out more about long term hazards associated with the use of established drugs, either natural or synthetic, from studies in man and experimental animals.

2. In evaluation of the safe use of a drug, consideration should be based on the balance of benefits and risks to the patient that may accrue from the use of that drug.

3. The following principles apply to the safety evaluation of any drug and they are relevant to the assessment of the carcinogenic risk:

a) The manufacturer should remain responsible for his product.

b) Adequate physical and chemical specifications for a new drug should be provided before biological studies are undertaken.

c) No rigid plan of testing should be imposed; the investigator should be free to plan his own experiments in accordance with current knowledge and practice.

d) Regulation agencies will reserve the right to call for further tests, but this should only be done if the tests demanded will effectively assist in assessment of the risks involved in the proposed use of the drug.

e) In view of the fact that animal tests in this field have, as their primary objective, the elucidation of the human risks, further animal studies should not be demanded if the answer is available from human experience.

4. The cancer risk should be assessed for any drug as an essential part of the general toxicological evaluation.

5. The following considerations are relevant to the assessment of the benefits arising from the use of a drug:

a) The nature and severity of the conditions to be treated.

b) The potential life span of the patient, if treated and if not treated.

c) Acceptability of the treatment proposed to the patient.

d) Efficacy of the treatment.

e) Ease of administration.

f) Reduction of unpleasant and toxic side-effects.

g) Economic advantages to the individual or the community.

h) Availability of alternative effective treatment.

6. The following considerations are relevant to the assessment of the carcinogenic risks arising from the use of a drug:

a) The age of the patient to be treated, the risk being greater in the young.

b) The physiological state of the patient, especially pregnancy and lactation.

c) The life expectancy of the patient.

d) The dosage proposed.

e) The route of administration.

f) The period of administration of the drug, the possibility of accumulation and repeated use.

g) The population at risk.

h) The extent of medical control of use.

7. Assessment of the carcinogenic risks is necessary for every drug. Particular attention should be paid to chronic toxicity studies designed to reveal possible carcinogenic action in the case of certain categories of drugs such as those that may be given to children or women during pregnancy or lactation, or those that may be administered for long periods, or drugs that may be supplied without medical control.

8. All significant information with regard to the carcinogenic hazard of any drug should be reported and made available to the medical and pharmaceutical profession. A more generally frank approach to this problem would help to dispel the undesirable aura of fear that tends to surround this field and which interferes with efficient cancer prevention.

9. Publication of all scientific work relevant to carcinogenic hazards is important and should be encouraged, even though the drug studied may have been abandoned as a possible therapeutic agent.

10. Physicians and pharmacists should appreciate the risks as well as the benefits involved in the use of drugs. The particular use to which a drug may be put is important and any change in its use may involve risks that may not have been taken into account when the original evaluation of that particular drug was made. Any intended change in the use of a drug from that recommended should be reported.

11. Physicians and pharmacists should make every effort to be informed about adverse reactions from drugs and should report such reactions as soon as possible.

12. There should be a full exploration of the possibility of further development and linkage of national medical record systems. Hospital physicians should obtain detailed histories from cancer patients regarding drugs that they may have taken in the past. Such histories might give a clue to long term adverse effects. Hospitals should not destroy case records and should make them available for retrospective studies.

13. Practising physicians and pharmacists should have a better appreciation of problems arising in the field of cancer prevention and improved opportunities for undergraduate and graduate education may be needed to achieve this.

14. Drugs obtained over the counter, including some herbal remedies, may be not free from risk and the indiscriminate or excessive consumption of such preparations should be avoided.

Recommandations générales

Les rapports présentés au Symposium étudient de façon détaillée de nombreux aspects des problèmes relatifs aux effets cancérogènes pouvant résulter de l'emploi de produits médicamenteux.

Les recommandations qui suivent sont d'un caractère plus général:

1. Jusqu'à une date récente, n'a pas été suffisamment reconnue la possibilité d'apparition, à la suite de l'administration même d'une seule dose d'un produit médicamenteux, de modifications irréversibles susceptibles de provoquer des effets retardés et des manifestations de toxicité chronique.

De nombreuses drogues en usage depuis longtemps, n'ont pas été soumises à une expérimentation adéquate à long terme chez les animaux de laboratoire et leurs effets chez l'homme peuvent être passés inaperçus du fait d'un mauvais enregistrement des observations. Les moyens scientifiques disponibles pour ce type de recherche sont loin d'être adéquats et doivent être développés d'urgence. Les drogues nouvelles sont maintenant mieux expérimentées, mais des efforts doivent être faits pour obtenir, par des études chez l'homme et les animaux d'expérience, plus d'informations sur les dangers à long terme que peut comporter l'usage de drogues connues, qu'elles soient d'origine naturelle ou synthétique.

2. Dans l'évaluation de la sécurité d'emploi d'une drogue, il s'impose de peser les bénéfices et les risques pouvant résulter pour les malades de cet emploi.

3. Les principes suivants s'appliquent à l'évaluation de la sécurité d'emploi de toute drogue et sont valables pour l'appréciation du risque cancérogène:

a) Le fabricant doit être et doit demeurer responsable de son produit.

b) Des normes physiques et chimiques adéquates doivent être fournies pour toute drogue nouvelle avant de la soumettre à des investigations biologiques.

c) Aucun protocole rigide d'expérimentation ne doit être imposé; l'expert doit être libre d'établir le protocole de ses investigations en accord avec les connaissances et la pratique courantes.

d) Les autorités chargées de l'établissement des règlementations ont le droit de demander des épreuves complémentaires, à condition que celles-ci puissent réellement contribuer à l'évaluation des risques pouvant résulter des emplois proposés pour la drogue.

e) Les investigations sur l'animal ayant comme objectif primaire, dans ce domaine, l'évaluation des risques pour l'homme, des expérimentations complémentaires ne doivent pas être demandées si la réponse cherchée peut être obtenue à partir des observations sur l'homme.

4. L'évaluation du risque cancérogène doit être effectuée pour toute drogue, en tant que partie essentielle de l'évaluation toxicologique générale.

5. Les considérations suivantes s'appliquent à l'évaluation des bénéfices pouvant résulter de l'emploi d'une drogue:

a) nature et gravité de l'état à traiter,

b) durée de vie probable du malade, s'il est traité et s'il ne l'est pas,

c) degré d'acceptabilité par le malade du traitement proposé,

d) efficacité du traitement,

e) facilité d'administration,

f) réduction des effets secondaires désagréables ou toxiques,

g) avantages économiques pour l'individu ou la collectivité,

h) existence de traitements de remplacement efficaces.

6. Sont à considérer pour l'évaluation des risques cancérogènes pouvant résulter de l'emploi d'une drogue:

a) l'âge du malade à traiter, les risques étant plus importants chez les jeunes,

b) l'état physiologique du malade, en particulier grossesse et lactation,

c) la durée de vie probable du malade,

d) la posologie envisagée,

e) la voie d'administration,

f) la durée d'administration de la drogue, les possibilités d'accumulation et de répétition des cures,

g) le nombre de sujets exposés aux risques,

h) le degré de surveillance médicale de l'emploi.

7. L'évaluation du risque cancérogène est nécessaire pour chaque drogue. Une attention particulière doit être accordée aux études de toxicité chronique conçues pour révéler d'éventuels effets cancérogènes, dans le cas de certaines catégories de drogues, telles que celles susceptibles d'être administrées à des enfants ou à des femmes en état de gravidité ou en période de lactation, celles consommées pendant de longues périodes ou celles pouvant être dispensées sans contrôle médical.

8. Toute information significative relative au risque cancérogène lié à l'usage de telle ou telle drogue doit être signalée et diffusée auprès des membres des professions médicale et pharmaceutique. Une plus franche approche de ce problème sur un plan général aiderait à dissiper l'indésirable climat de crainte qui tend à s'instaurer dans ce domaine et qui vient limiter l'efficacité de la prévention du cancer.

9. La publication de tous les travaux scientifiques relatifs aux risques cancérogènes est importante et doit être encouragée, même si l'éventuel emploi en thérapeutique de la drogue étudiée a pu être abandonnée.

10. Les médecins et les pharmaciens doivent évaluer aussi bien les risques que les bénéfices que peut comporter l'emploi des drogues. L'usage particulier en vue duquel une drogue est introduite est important à considérer et toute modification dans cet usage peut comporter des risques dont il n'a pas été tenu compte lors de l'évaluation originale de la drogue. Tout projet de modification dans les emplois de la drogue par rapport à ceux initialement recommandés doit être signalé.

11. Les médecins et les pharmaciens doivent faire le maximum d'efforts pour être informés des réactions de nocivité provoquées par les drogues et doivent signaler de telles réactions le plus rapidement possible.

12. Il s'impose d'explorer à fond les possibilités de développer davantage et de lier entre eux les systèmes nationaux d'enregistrement médical. Les médecins dans les hopitaux doivent obtenir des sujets cancéreux des informations détaillées en ce qui concerne les drogues absorbées par eux dans le passé. De telles informations pourraient constituer un fil conducteur pour la révélation d'effets nocifs à long terme. Les hopitaux ne doivent pas détruire les dossiers individuels et doivent les garder pour des enquêtes rétrospectives.

13. Les praticiens médicaux et les pharmaciens doivent être mieux infor-

més des problèmes qui se posent dans le domaine de la prévention du cancer; pour atteindre cet objectif, il peut être nécessaire d'améliorer les conditions de formation professionnelle pendant et après la scolarité.

14. Les drogues dispensées sans prescription médicale, comprenant quelques plantes médicinales, peuvent ne pas être exemptes de risques; la consommation inconsidérée ou excessive de telles préparations doit être évitée.

UICC Publications

Kaposi's Sarcoma. S. Karger AG., Basle (Switzerland) — New York (1963).

Cancer of the urinary bladder. S. Karger AG., Basle (Switzerland) — New York (1963).

Prognosis of malignant tumours of the breast. S. Karger AG., Basle (Switzerland) — New York (1963).

The lymphoreticular tumours in Africa. S. Karger AG., Basle (Switzerland) — New York (1964).

Cellular control mechanisms and cancer. Elsevier Publishing Company, Amsterdam — London — New York (1964).

Illustrated Tumor Nomenclature. Springer-Verlag, Berlin — Heidelberg — New York (1965).

Structure and control of the melanocyte. Springer-Verlag, Berlin — Heidelberg — New York (1966).

Public education about cancer; cancer education programmes in various countries. UICC, Geneva (1966).

Cancer incidence in five continents. Springer-Verlag, Berlin — Heidelberg — New York (1966).

Cancer detection. Springer-Verlag, Berlin — Heidelberg — New York (1967).

Public education about cancer; research findings and theoretical concepts. Springer-Verlag, Berlin — Heidelberg — New York (1967).

Tumour specific antigens. Munksgaard, Copenhagen (1967).

Cancer of the nasopharynx. Munksgaard, Copenhagen (1967).

Choriocarcinoma. Springer-Verlag, Berlin — Heidelberg — New York (1967).